ICSA Book Series in Statistics

The ICSA Book Series in Statistics showcases research from the International Chinese Statistical Association that has an international reach. It publishes books in statistical theory, applications, and statistical education. All books are associated with the ICSA or are authored by invited contributors. Books may be monographs, edited volumes, textbooks and proceedings.

More information about this series at http://www.springer.com/series/13402

Xinguang Chen • (Din) Ding-Geng Chen
Editors

Statistical Methods for Global Health and Epidemiology

Principles, Methods and Applications

Springer

Editors
Xinguang Chen
Department of Epidemiology
College of Public Health
and Health Professions
College of Medicine
University of Florida
Gainesville, FL, USA

Global Health Institute
Wuhan University
Wuhan, China

(Din) Ding-Geng Chen
School of Social Work
University of North Carolina
Chapel Hill, NC, USA

ISSN 2199-0980 ISSN 2199-0999 (electronic)
ICSA Book Series in Statistics
ISBN 978-3-030-35259-2 ISBN 978-3-030-35260-8 (eBook)
https://doi.org/10.1007/978-3-030-35260-8

This Springer imprint is published by the registered company Springer Nature Switzerland AG.
The registered company address is: Gewerbestrasse 11, 6330 Cham, Switzerland

Preface

Global health is a newly established scientific discipline. It has been emerged along with globalization to deal with challenging medical and health issues that either have a global impact or cannot be solved without collaborative and collective efforts across countries, regions, and even the whole globe. Typical global health questions include health care systems and inequality, HIV epidemic and control, influenza, tobacco control, drug and substance use prevention, mental health issues, and environmental pollution.

As a new discipline in public health and medicine, there is a growing demand for statistical methods to advance the global health. Advancement of global health and global health research also needs the participation of epidemiologists. In a more general sense, global health can be considered as an application of epidemiology in global health. Guided by these thoughts, in this book, we have collected a series of statistical methods for global health and epidemiology in three broad parts.

Part I consists of six chapters with focus on data and sampling for global health and epidemiology. Chapter 1 (by Xinguang Chen and Bin Yu) focuses on introduction to existing sources of data that have great potential and been conventionally used in global health and epidemiology research. Chapter 2 (by Hao Chen and Keerati Ponpetch) introduces sources of satellite imagery data that has emerged as a new source of data particularly important for global epidemiological research. Chapter 3 (by Xinguang Chen and Hui Hu) devotes to the GIS/GPS-assisted probability sample—a newly systematized and highly cost-effective method to draw probability samples in both resource-limited and developed countries. Chapter 4 (by Yan Wang and Xinguang Chen) covers a new method for survey studies to collect data on sensitive questions with a construal-level theory supported method. Chapter 5 (by Andrea Hussong, Veronica Cole, Patrick Curran, Daniel Bauer, and Nisha Gottfredson) describes the techniques for harmonization of data collected by different studies. Lastly, Chap. 6 (by Guanhong Miao, Hanzhi Gao, Yan Wang, and Samuel Wu) introduces a series of methods for privacy-preservation data sharing.

Part II of the book consists of another six chapters with focus on the most essential statistical and epidemiological methods. This part starts with Chap. 7 (by

Bin Yu) that describes the methods and techniques for global mapping, which is fundamental for global health research to describe geographic patterns of morbidity and mortality. Chapter 8 (by Xinguang Chen and Ding-Geng Chen) introduces a newly established 4-dimensional approach for descriptive analysis, including count, population-based rate, geographic area-based rate, and both population and geographic area-based rate. Chapter 9 (by Xinguang Chen) describes an innovative application of the classic epidemiological method of age-period-cohort (APC) model to investigate historical trend in population health with more recent data. Chapter 10 (by Ding-Geng Chen, Xinguang Chen, and Huanzhen Qin) covers a new approach to solve the APC model based on the Moor-Penrose generalized inverse matrix theory. Chapter 11 (by Xinguang Chen) describes the use of mixed effects model in analyzing data from cross-cultural studies to study health behaviors among adolescents in Hong Kong, Macao, Taipei, Wuhan, and Zhuhai. Chapter 12 (by Yang Yang) illustrates the geographically weighted regression in global epidemiology and global health research.

Lastly, Part III of the book consists of four chapters covering advanced and highly innovative methods for global health and epidemiology. This part starts with Chap. 13 (by Ropo Ogunsakin and Ding-Geng Chen) on Bayesian spatiotemporal modeling of infectious diseases with application to Malaria in Nigeria. Chapter 14 (by Kai Yang and Peihua Qiu) introduces an advanced disease surveillance model considering geographic correlation. Chapter 15 (by Xinguang Chen, Kai Wang, and Ding-Geng Chen) introduces a new cutting-edge analytical method for quantum change–cusp catastrophe modeling of continuous data with application in analyzing the testosterone in bifurcating the age-related changes in prostate-specific antigen (PSA) as a commonly used biomarker for prostate cancer screening and diagnosis. The last chapter of this book, Chap. 16 (by Ding-Geng Chen and Xinguang Chen), introduces the same cutting-edge cusp catastrophe modeling method for analyzing binary data and discusses the methodology development.

Selection of the statistical methods for this book is guided by a global and epidemiological perspective, considering the unique needs for global health research that is often cross-cultural, cross-country, cross-geographic areas, and global. Such large-scope research often involves resource-limited regions, countries, and places. The methods included in this book are specifically designed to meet these needs.

It is our hope that the publication of this book will facilitate researchers and graduate students in the fields of epidemiology and global health to advance their research agenda, promoting advancement of global health. We also expect feedback from those who use the methods in their research to further improve the methods covered in the book and to collect and develop additional methods for global health and global epidemiology.

We are deeply grateful to those who have supported in the process of creating this book. We thank all the contributing authors to this book for their enthusiastic involvements and their kindness in sharing their professional knowledge and expertise. Our sincere gratitude goes to all the chapter reviewers for their expert reviews of the book chapters, which lead to a substantial improvement in the quality of this book. We thank all the reviewers for providing thoughtful and in-depth evaluations of the papers contained in this book. We gratefully acknowledge the professional support of Ms. Laura Aileen Briskman from Springer who made the publication of this book a reality. We would also thank the support and encouragement from the editors of ICSA Book Series in Statistics, Professors Jiahua Chen and Ding-Geng Chen.

We welcome readers' comments, including notes on typos or other errors, and look forward to receiving suggestions for improvements to future editions. Please send comments and suggestions to any of the editors.

Gainesville, FL, USA Xinguang Chen
Chapel Hill, NC, USA (Din) Ding-Geng Chen
July 2019

Contents

List of Contributors

Daniel J. Bauer, PhD Department of Psychology and Neuroscience, University of North Carolina at Chapel Hill, Chapel Hill, NC, USA

(Din) Ding-Geng Chen School of Social Work, University of North Carolina, Chapel Hill, NC, USA

Hao Chen Department of Environmental and Global Health, University of Florida, Gainesville, FL, USA

Xinguang Chen Department of Epidemiology, College of Public Health and Health Professions, College of Medicine, University of Florida, Gainesville, FL, USA
Global Health Institute, Wuhan University, Wuhan, China

Veronica T. Cole, PhD Wake Forest University, Winston-Salem, NC, USA

Patrick J. Curran, PhD Department of Psychology and Neuroscience, University of North Carolina at Chapel Hill, Chapel Hill, NC, USA

Hanzhi Gao Department of Biostatistics, University of Florida, Gainesville, FL, USA

Nisha C. Gottfredson, PhD Gillings School of Public Health, University of North Carolina at Chapel Hill, Chapel Hill, NC, USA

Hui Hu Department of Epidemiology, University of Florida, Gainesville, FL, USA

Andrea M. Hussong Department of Psychology and Neuroscience, University of North Carolina at Chapel Hill, Chapel Hill, NC, USA

Guanhong Miao Department of Biostatistics, University of Florida, Gainesville, FL, USA

Ropo Ebenezer Ogunsakin University of Pretoria, Pretoria, South Africa

Keerati Ponpetch Department of Environmental and Global Health, University of Florida, Gainesville, FL, USA

Huaizhen Qin Department of Epidemiology, University of Florida, Gainesville, FL, USA

Peihua Qiu Department of Biostatistics, University of Florida, Gainesville, FL, USA

Kai Wang Harvard University, Cambridge, MA, USA

Yan Wang Department of Epidemiology, University of Florida, Gainesville, FL, USA

Samuel S. Wu Department of Biostatistics, University of Florida, Gainesville, FL, USA

Kai Yang Department of Biostatistics, University of Florida, Gainesville, FL, USA

Yang Yang Department of Biostatistics, School of Public Health and Health Professions & Emerging Pathogens Institute, University of Florida, Gainesville, FL, USA

Bin Yu Department of Epidemiology, University of Florida, Gainesville, FL, USA

List of Reviewers

David Ansong University of Carolina at Chapel Hill, Chapel Hill, NC, USA

Kanisha C. Brevard University of Carolina at Chapel Hill, Chapel Hill, NC, USA

(Din) Ding-Geng Chen School of Social Work, University of North Carolina, Chapel Hill, NC, USA

Xinguang Chen Department of Epidemiology, College of Public Health and Health Professions, College of Medicine, University of Florida, Gainesville, FL, USA
Global Health Institute, Wuhan University, Wuhan, China

Liang Mao University of Florida, Gainesville, FL, USA

Shamiel D. Nelson University of Florida, Gainesville, FL, USA

Shannon Rich University of Florida, Gainesville, FL, USA

Jenny Shapio University of Florida, Gainesville, FL, USA

Anni Yang Colorado State University, Fort Collins, CO, USA

About the Editors

Xinguang Chen, MD, PhD, is an elected fellow of the American College of Epidemiology and currently a tenured professor of epidemiology at the University of Florida. He is also a chair professor at Wuhan University Global Health Institute, editor-in-chief for Global Health Research and Policy, associate editor for *Global Health Journal*, and an advisory board member of the WHO-China Information Collaboration Center at People's Publication House of China. Professor Chen is well known for his international and intercultural research on challenging medical and health issues, including HIV/AIDS, substance use, physical activity, cardiovascular disease, and cancer. In 2014, Professor Chen published a paper with the *Yale Journal of Biology and Medicine* on global health for medical and health education. His research is guided by cross-cultural, transdisciplinary, and global perspectives, and it is characterized by advanced statistical and epidemiological methods and models particularly suitable for resource-limited settings. He has received continuous NIH funding for his methods and epidemiological research since the 1990s, and his research extends from the United States to China, Southeast Asia, and Latin America. He has published more than 280 manuscripts in peer-reviewed journals, four authored books, and several book chapters and encyclopedia entries.

(Din) Ding-Geng Chen, PhD, is an elected fellow of the American Statistical Association, the Wallace Kuralt Distinguished Professor at the School of Social Work, and a professor of biostatistics at the Gillings School of Global Public Health, University of North Carolina at Chapel Hill, USA. He is also an extraordinary professor at the Department of Statistics, University of Pretoria, South Africa. He was a professor in biostatistics at the University of Rochester and the Karl E. Peace Endowed Eminent Scholar Chair in Biostatistics at Georgia Southern University, USA. He is also a senior statistics consultant for biopharmaceuticals and government agencies with extensive expertise in Monte Carlo simulations, clinical trial biostatistics, and public health statistics. Professor Chen has more than 200 referred professional publications, and he has co-authored/co-edited 28 books on clinical trial methodology, meta-analysis, and public health applications. He has been invited nationally and internationally to give speeches on his research.

Part I
Data Acquisition and Management

Chapter 1
Existent Sources of Data for Global Health and Epidemiology

Xinguang Chen and Bin Yu

Abstract Many research questions in global health and epidemiology can be addressed using data from existing sources over the world. In the first chapter of this book, we provide a summary of data sources most commonly accessed for global health and epidemiological research. We focus on sources that provide relevant data by country on geographic area, population size and age composition, population mobility, socioeconomic status, cultural and legal characteristics, and morbidity and mortality. Specific examples from the World Bank, the World Health Organization, other global organizations, and well-known large-scale cross-country survey studies are emphasized.

Keywords Data science · Source of data · Global health · Statistics · Epidemiology

1.1 Introduction

Global health and epidemiology research uses data to quantitatively investigate medical and health issues at national, international, regional and global levels. Collecting such data is challenging even for conducting a project limited to a local community, a county, a state, a country, not to mention for a research project with a global focus. Fortunately, through decades of efforts, a number of national, international and global agencies, such as the United States, the United Nations,

X. Chen (✉)
Department of Epidemiology, College of Public Health and Health Professions, College of Medicine, University of Florida, Gainesville, FL, USA

Global Health Institute, Wuhan University, Wuhan, China
e-mail: jimax.chen@ufl.edu

B. Yu
Department of Epidemiology, University of Florida, Gainesville, FL, USA
e-mail: byu@ufl.edu

X. Chen, (Din) D.-G. Chen (eds.), *Statistical Methods for Global Health and Epidemiology*, ICSA Book Series in Statistics,
https://doi.org/10.1007/978-3-030-35260-8_1

the World Bank, and the World Health Organization, have collected and compiled large amounts of important data by country. The data compiled by these agencies are highly valuable for global health and epidemiological research, such as data on geographic area, population, socioeconomic status, press freedom index, birth rates, death rates, leading causes of death, tobacco use, numbers of doctors, hospital beds, and healthcare expenditures, to name a few. Data from most of these sources are available for use free of charge. To facilitate global health and epidemiological research, in the first chapter of this book, we describe existing data from a number of important sources commonly accessed in research.

1.2 Country Codes, Population and Geographic Area Data

Population size and geographic area are essential data elements used for global health and epidemiological research. Such data are often used by researchers to gain a mastery of the basic conditions across all countries and to identify countries of interest against the global picture.

1.2.1 Standard Country Codes

When using country-level data, it is important to consider numerous ways in which countries are named or abbreviated, as this has implications for database construction and navigation. For example, the following four names, the USA, the U.S., the United States, and the United States of America all represent one country. When we read or hear about any of these names, we know it is referred to the United States. However, when you input these four different names into a search algorithm to construct a dataset, the algorithm may consider each as a different country for statistical analysis.

To facilitate analysis using data by country, The International Organization for Standardization (ISO) has created and maintains the ISO 3166 Standard—Codes for the Representation of Names of Countries and their Subdivisions (ISO, 2018). The ISO 3166 standard codes consist of three parts: ISO 3166-1, ISO 3166-2 and ISO 3166-3. ISO 3166-1 is widely used representing the names of countries and their subdivisions. ISO 3166-1contains three parts: (a) two-letter country codes (also known as alpha 2), representing individual countries using two English letters. For example, AF: Afghanistan, CN: China, and US: United States. These two-letter codes are also used to define three-letter country codes and internet country codes. (b) three-letter country codes (also known as alpha 3), representing individual countries using three English letters. With this three-letter country code system, AFG = Afghanistan, CHN = China, USA = the United States. (c) Numeric codes, using three digits to representing individual countries. With this code system, 004 = Afghanistan, 156 = China and 840 = the United States.

The Table below is a screen shot from the Wikipedia showing the codes for 248 countries and territories in the world (Table 1.1).

Table 1.1 A snap shot from Wikipedia's list of the 248 countries and territories in the world

ISA 3166 [1]			ISO 3166-1 [2]		
Country name [9]	Official state name [5]	Sovereignty [5, 6, 7]	Alpha-2 code [9]	Alpha-3 code [9]	Numeric code [9]
Afghanistan	The Islamic Republic of Afghanistan	UN member state	AF	AFG	004
Akrotiri and Dhekelia—See United Kingdom, The					
Aland Island	Åland	Finland	AX	ALA	248
Albania	The Republic of Albania	UN member state	AL	ALB	008
Algeria	The People's Democratic Republic of Algeria	UN member state	DZ	DZA	012
American Samoa	The Territory of American Samoa	United States	AS	ASM	016
Andorra	The Principality of Andorra	UN member state	AD	AND	020
Angola	The Republic of Angola	UN member state	AO	AGO	024
Anguilla	Anguilla	United Kingdom	AI	AIA	660
Antarctica [a]	All land and ice shelves south of the 60th parallel south	Antarctic Treaty	AQ	ATA	010
Antigua and Barbuda	Antigua and Barbuda	UN member state	AG	ATG	028

Country name codes are created for 249 countries in the world, of which 193 countries are sovereign states and member countries of the United Nations. The country name codes can be assessed at the website: https://en.wikipedia.org/wiki/List_of_ISO_3166_country_codes.

1.2.2 Population Data by Country

Population data are particularly important for global health and epidemiology. Population size is the basis to compute many epidemiological and health indices, such as prevalence and mortality rates; the number of persons at risk and the number of persons who need specific healthcare services.

Most countries with national censuses publish population data regularly or irregularly. One source which publishes population data for individual countries is the database by the World Bank (2018). The database is available at: https://data.worldbank.org/indicator/SP.POP.TOTL.

This database provides data on population size by country for all member countries of the World Bank (189 of total 195 countries). Detailed data are also available on population breakdown by sex and 5-year age group. These population data were collected through the following sources: The United Nations Population Division, the World Population Prospects (2017 Revision); the Census reports and other statistical publications from national statistical offices; the Eurostat: Demographic Statistics; the United Nations Statistical Division; the Population and Vital Statistics Report in different years; the U.S. Census Bureau (International Database); and the Secretariat of the Pacific Community (Statistics and Demography Program) (World Bank, 2018). These sources can be accessed to help researchers gain a better understanding of the data collection process.

Data are easily downloadable in excel file format. As an illustration, data presented in Table 1.2 provide an example of a part of the data we manually obtained from the website for 10 selected countries.

Table 1.2 Population data of 10 selected countries in the world, data source: world bank

Country name	Alpha 3-code	Total population (1000)	Male (1000)	Female (1000)
Afghanistan	AFG	35,530.08	18,309.89	17,220.19
Argentina	ARG	44,271.04	21,667.87	22,603.17
Australia	AUS	24,598.93	12,254.51	12,344.43
Brazil	BRA	209,288.28	102,855.02	106,433.26
Canada	CAN	36,708.08	18,213.75	18,494.33
China	CHN	1,386,395.00	714,405.30	671,989.70
Egypt	EGY	97,553.15	49,324.99	48,228.16
France	FRA	67,118.65	33,000.44	34,118.21
India	IND	1,339,180.13	693,958.76	645,221.37
Japan	JPN	126,785.80	61,915.09	64,870.71

1.2.3 Geographic Area Data by Country

Like population, geographic area is another key piece of data important to researchers, as well as policy-makers, planners, and public workers alike to understand, comprehend, and advance global health and epidemiology. Relative to population size and composition that change rapidly over time, geographic area of a country is much more stable. Sources of geographic data are available from the following websites:

1. Internet World Stats (https://www.internetworldstats.com/stats.htm),
2. Wikipedia (https://en.wikipedia.org/wiki/List_of_countries_and_dependencies_by_area)
3. The World Bank (https://data.worldbank.org/indicator/ag.lnd.totl.k2).

1.2.4 Data from the Internet World Stats

In this web-based data source, you can access to the compiled data by simply using the URL address: https://www.internetworldstats.com/list1.htm#AF. Detailed data on area size of individual country are organized in different way. After gaining access the web address, simply click the hyperlink: Click here for Countries by Alphabetic Order (ISO 3166), you will see a table listing all the information contained there. Very importantly, in this website, individual countries are identified using the ISO 2-letter code, an obvious plus for data processing in global health and epidemiologic research (Internet World Stats, 2019).

In addition to the geographic area, this website contains information on total population, the number of internet users, internet penetration rate, and the date the data were acquired. Data on internet usage from this website are highly valuable for global health and epidemiology to address many challenge issues in contemporary society. As an example, Table 1.3 is a snapshot of the data from the Internet World Stats.

1.2.5 Data from Wikipedia

Wikipedia also publishes data on area size by country (Wikipedia, 2019a). Furthermore, it provides more detailed data on the area of land and water for individual countries, which are very useful for global health and epidemiology. For information purpose, Table 1.4 presents a screen shot of the first page of the website. The figure shows that data from this source include world total and country-specific data on the total area size, land area, water area, and % water. A note is also added to each entry describing additional information for the data.

Table 1.3 A snapshot of the data from the Internet World Stats

Country or region name	Symbol	Size (sq. km.)	Population (2018 est.)	Internet users	Internet penetration (%)	Data date
Afghanistan	AF	645,807	36,373,176	5,700,905	15.7	Dec/2017
Africa	–	**30,221,535**	**1,287,914,329**	**453,329,534**	**35.2**	**Dec/2017**
Aland Island	AX	1580	28,666	n/a	n/a	Dec/2017
Albania	AL	28,748	2,911,428	1,916,233	65.8	Mar/2017
Algeria	DZ	2,381,741	42,008,054	18,580,000	44.2	Mar/2017
American Samoa	AS	197	55,653	22,000	39.5	Mar/2017
Andorra	AD	464	68,728	83,728	100.0	Mar/2017
Angola	AO	1,246,700	20,655,513	5,951,453	22.3	Mar/2017
Anguilla	AI	96	14,906	12,557	84.2	Mar/2017
Antarctica	AQ	13,209,000	2700	4400	100.0	Mar/2017
Antigua & Barbuda	AG	442	93,659	60,306	64.4	Mar/2017
Argentina	AR	2,777,409	44,272,125	24,758,206	78.6	Mar/2017
Armenia	AM	29,743	2,934,152	2,126,716	72.5	Dec/2017
Aruba	AW	193	104,588	91,532	87.5	Mar/2017
Asia	–	**39,365,000**	**4,207,588,157**	**2,023,630,194**	**48.1**	**Dec/2017**
Australia	AU	7,682,557	24,641,662	21,176,595	85.9	Mar/2017
Austria	AT	83,858	8,592,400	7,273,168	84.6	Mar/2017
Azerbaijan	AZ	86,530	9,923,914	7,999,431	80.6	Dec/2017
Bahamas, The	BS	13,962	397,164	333,143	83.9	Mar/2017
Bahrain	BH	694	1,418,895	1,278,752	90.1	Mar/2017
Bangladesh	BD	142,615	166,368,149	80,483,000	48.4	Dec/2017
Barbados	BB	431	289,680	217,260	75.0	Dec/2013
Belarus	BY	207,600	9,608,058	5,204,685	54.2	Dec/2013
Belgium	BE	30,518	10,449,361	8,586,240	82.2	Dec/2013
Belize	BZ	22,966	340,844	108,048	31.7	Dec/2013
Benin	BJ	112,622	10,741,458	1,232,940	11.5	Jun/2016

Table 1.4 Geographic information from Wikipedia

Rank	Sovereign state/dependency	Total in km^2 (mi^2)	Land in km^2 (mi^2)	Water in km^2 (mi^2)	% water	Notes
–	World	510,072,000 (196,940,000)	148,940,000 (57,510,000)	361,132,000 (139,434,000)	70.8	
1	Russia	17,098,246 (6,601,670)	16,377,742 (6,323,482)	720,500 (278,200)	4.21	Largest country in the world (10.995% of the world's land mass); its Asian portion makes it the largest country in Asia, and its European portion of roughly 3,960,000 km^2 (1,530,000 sq. mi) makes it the largest country in Europe.[Note 2]
–	Antarctica	14,000,000 (5,400,000)	14,000,000 (5,400,000)	0 (0)	0	13,720,000 km^2 (5,300,000 sq. mi) (98%) of land area is covered by ice. Though not itself a country, areas are claimed by a number of countries [Note 3]
2	Canada	9,984,670 (3,855,100)	9,093,507 (3,511,023)	891,163 (344,080)	8.93	Largest English-speaking and French-speaking country and the largest country in the Western Hemisphere by total area (second largest by land area, after United States), with the largest surface area of water. Total area and water area figure include area covered by freshwater only, and do not include internal water (non-freshwater) of about 1,600,000 km^2, or territorial water of 200,000 km^2.[4,5]
3	China	9,595,961 (3,705,407)	9,326,410 (3,600,950)	270,550 (104,460)	2.82	Second largest country in Asia (thought the largest located wholly within the continent), and second largest country in the world by land area Excludes Taiwan, disputed territories with India, and disputed island in the South China Sea. Figure for total area

An obvious issue for data from this source is that it does not use the ISO 2-alpha or 3-alpha code as the name to identify individual countries. When processing such data, you have to manually code the variable for country name yourself. Territories not identified by the ISO names are also included in this data source if they are adequately large. You can exclude these territories if they are not the focus of your research.

Lastly, Wikipedia highlights at the top of the web page that there are disputes regarding the neutrality and accuracy. Attention should be paid to this issue when data from this source are used for publication.

1.3 Data for Socioeconomic Status and Vital Statistics

After having data on population and geographic area, we naturally want to obtain data on social economic status and vital statistics for individual countries. Such data can be obtained from official publications of individual countries (e.g., statistical yearbooks, or annual national reports or something alike). However, a better approach would be to access data that have been compiled for research. Although there are often 1 or 2-year delay than the data published by individual countries, compiled data are often adjusted for between-country differences, and thus can be directly used in research. You can find such compiled data from two important sources: Data from the World Health Organization (WHO), particularly data reported in the Country Profile published by WHO and the Database from the World Bank.

1.3.1 Data from the World Health Organization

World Health Organization produces *World Health Statistics*, an annual snapshot of the health status of all the member countries across the globe (WHO, 2019e). The report can be accessed at the web address: https://www.who.int/gho/publications/world_health_statistics/en/. In addition to a summary of global health status, the report provided detailed data on a long list of medical and health issues ranging from infectious diseases, non-communicable diseases, mental health, maternal child health, immunization, sanitation and environmental health, alcohol and tobacco use, road safety, violence. Annual pdf report since 2005 can be downloaded for data extraction.

After gain access into the website described above, you can see the detailed statistics by clicking on the button "By section" from two options. This link will bring you to a page where you will see the following six selections: (1) Global health observatory data, (2) Data repository, (3) Reports, (4) Country statistics, (5) Map gallery, and (6) Standards.

Each of these links leads you do a different type of data. For example, when clicking on Country statistics, you will see all countries being listed alphabetically. By clicking the name of a country, you can find the detailed vital statistics by category for the country, including (a) country summary of statistics, (b) country life tables, and (c) disease and injury country estimates.

It is worth noting that data from this source of WHO are for member countries only. No data can be found for non-member countries. In addition, data availability by country also varies from year to year. As expected, data are available for more member countries in more recent years than in early years.

1.3.2 *Data from the World Bank*

The World Bank collects, compiles and updates their data on total and per capita GDP (gross domestic productivity, in US dollars) and annual GDP growth (World Bank, 2019). GDP is the single most widely used indicator for economic level and growth of a country. In addition to GDP, other data important for global health and epidemiology include percentage of primary school enrollment, percentage of population under poverty, per capita CO_2 emission (metric tons), and life expectancy at birth (years). You can access these data using the following URL address: https://data.worldbank.org/country.

After access to the web site, you may also find information for several important large-scale national and international surveys, which may contain the data you need but not listed in the compiled data. You may also gain access to data for individual participants who took part in the survey for in-depth modeling analysis. Two typical examples are the World Bank Group Country Survey and the Demographic and Health Survey for different countries conducted in different years.

The World Bank Group Country Survey is an opinion survey that is designated to measuring and tracking Bank's clients, partners, and other stakeholders' perception of World Bank. Country Surveys explore perceptions of the World Bank's work (speed, effectiveness, relevance, etc.), knowledge, and engagement on the ground for work improvement. Typical survey respondents are national and local governments, multilateral/bilateral agencies, media, academia, the private sector and civil society. The earliest survey was conducted in 2011, and such data provide some information about socioeconomic status of the member countries.

1.4 Data on Important Social, Legal and Religious Factors by Country

1.4.1 *Data for Measuring Press Freedom*

When studying social influence on health, freedom of speech is an important factor (Chen, Elliott, & Wang, 2018). One important global organization, the Reporters Without Borders collected data and created a Press Freedom Index (PFI) by country

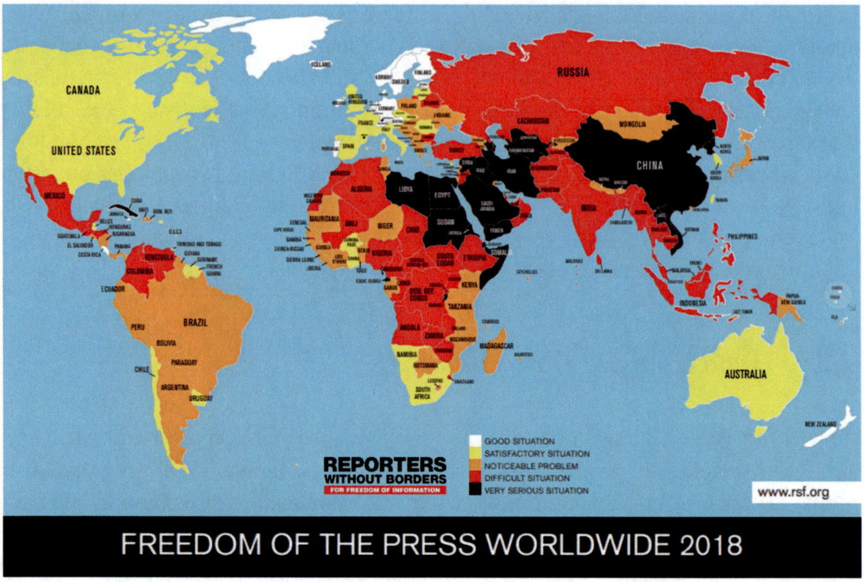

Fig. 1.1 Global pattern of PFI, 2018. Note: The figure was derived from the Reporters Without Borders website (https://rsf.org/en/ranking)

annually (Reporters Without Borders, 2018). Data for the compiled PFI since 2002 can be accessed through the website: https://rsf.org/en/ranking. This PFI index is a composite score which measures six aspects of press freedom, including (1) pluralism, (2) media independence, (3) media environment and self-censorship, (4) legislative framework, (5) transparency, and (6) the quality of the infrastructure that supports the production of news and information. An online questionnaire is developed with 87 items to obtain data for measuring these six aspects. Respondents of the questionnaire are primarily media professionals, lawyers and sociologists. Data regarding the abuses and acts of violence against journalists are also collected. The index scores are calculated by combining questionnaire data and the data regarding abuses and violence against journalists. Figure 1.1 shows the global pattern of PFI with light color indicating more press freedom and dark color indicating less press freedom in 2018 (Reporters Without Borders, 2018).

1.4.2 World Index of Moral Freedom

Likewise, data from the World Index of Moral Freedom (WIMF) can also be used in global health and epidemiology research. This index consists of five domains: (1) religious freedom, (2) bioethical freedom, (3) drugs freedom, (4) sexual freedom, and (5) family and gender freedom (Foundation for the Advancement of Liberty, 2016).

1. The domain of religious freedom measures the level of free practice of any religion or levels of religious-control in a country.
2. The domain of bioethical freedom measures the level of freedom in individual's decision-making on matters posing bioethical questions, such as legal control of abortion, euthanasia and other practices (e.g., surrogacy or stem cell research) pertaining to bioethics.
3. The domain of sexual freedom measures the freedom of sexual intercourse, pornography and sex service among consenting adults.
4. The domain of family and gender freedom assesses the level of freedom among women, LGBT individuals and unmarried couples living together (Kohl, 2016).

The highest score for each domain is 20 points with a total score of 100 points for the composite WIMF. With the WIMF core, the following criteria is used to rank a country:

1. Countries with the highest moral freedom: WIMF score: 90–100 points
2. Countries with very high moral freedom: WIMF score: 80–90 points
3. Countries with high moral freedom: WIMF score: 60–80 points
4. Countries with acceptable moral freedom: WIMF score: 50–60 points
5. Countries with insufficient moral freedom: WIMF score: 40–50 points
6. Countries with low moral freedom: WIMF score: 20–40 points
7. Countries with very low moral freedom: WIMF score: 10–20 points
8. Countries with the lowest moral freedom: WIMF score: 0–10 points

A total of 160 countries are ranked using this index. The first edition of WIMF report was published in 2016 (http://www.fundalib.org/wp-content/uploads/2016/04/World-Index-of-Moral-Freedom-web.pdf). Results from the report indicate that the Netherlands was scored the highest among all countries in the world (WIMF = 91.70), with 10 countries having WIMF scores higher than 75 points.

1.4.3 Country Profile of Religions

Religion is another important factor for global health and epidemiological research. Religion may exert effect on people's physical, mental and social well-being. People with different religions present different patterns of health problems and risk behaviors, such as mental health problems and suicide (Koenig, 2009; Stack & Kposowa, 2011). However, it is challenging to measure religion. Wikipedia is one source that provides information on specific religions by country (Wikipedia, 2019b). In one Wikipedia entry entitled "Religions by country", data regarding religions for individual countries are provided using tables and maps. In the table, you can obtain data on population breakdown by religion, country and continent.

Religions listed in the table on the website include Christian, Islam, Hindu, Buddhist, Folk religion, Jewish, and Other religion. For example, the religion profile for the United States consists of Christian (73.83%), Islam (0.9%), Hindu (0.6%), Buddhist (1.2%), Jewish (1.8), irreligion (16.40%). An emerging area of global health and epidemiology research seeks to understand how religion impacts health.

1.5 Data on Disease Statistics

1.5.1 Data for Global Cancer Statistics

Data for cancer statistics by country are available from existing sources, including the World Cancer Research Fund & American Institute for Cancer Research and the WHO Cancer Country Profile.

World Cancer Research Fund & American Institute for Cancer Research (https://www.wcrf.org/) is a leading authority on cancer prevention research with focus on diet, nutrition and physical exercise, and their influence on cancer (World Cancer Research Fund International, 2019). Data on specific cancer by country are available through their website (https://www.wcrf.org/dietandcancer/cancer-trends), such as lung cancer, breast cancer, prostate cancer, colorectal cancer, and other important cancers. Data are also available regarding risk factors for different types of cancers and recommendations for cancer prevention.

Data from WHO Cancer Country Profile can be accessed through the website (https://www.who.int/cancer/country-profiles/en/). Data included in the profile were obtained either from original studies or estimated by WHO (2014a). This source contains information by country regarding levels and time trends of morbidity and mortality overall and by cancer types, risk factors, availability of national cancer plans, monitoring and surveillance, primary prevention policies, screening, treatment and palliative care.

1.5.2 Data for Global Cardiovascular Disease Statistics

Data regarding cardiovascular disease (CVD) by country and gender, can also be accessed through the WHO website (https://www.who.int/cardiovascular_diseases/en/). Data by four global regions (Americas, Europe, Eastern Mediterranean, and Pacific region) are also available in addition to data for individual member countries (WHO, 2019a). Mortality attributable to CVD, cancer, diabetes or chronic respiratory disease, by region and by country can also be accessed through the website (http://apps.who.int/gho/data/view.sdg.3-4-data-reg?lang=en). Data in CVD mortality, overall and by gender in most countries are available since 2000.

1.5.3 Data for Global Infectious Disease Statistics

Infectious disease data can be accessed through the WHO website (https://www.who.int/csr/resources/databases/en/). Outbreak case counts are compiled by country and year (WHO, 2019b). The covered infectious diseases include, but are not limited to, Ebola, Yellow fever, Hantavirus, Chikungunya, Cholera, Dengue, Viral Hepatitis, Influenza, Malaria, Measles, and Zika virus (https://www.who.int/csr/don/archive/disease/en/).

Additional data on select infectious diseases are available through the Global Burden of Disease (http://apps.who.int/gho/data/node.home), including HIV/AIDS, Tuberculosis, Malaria, Cholera, Influenza, and Meningitis.

1.5.4 Data for Causes of Death in the United States

Mortality data by causes of death are of great significance in global health to determine the future prevention and treatment strategies and policies. The availability of such data varies fom countries to countries. One well-established source of mortality data is the Wide-Ranging Online Data for Epidemiologic Research (WONDER) managed and provided by the Centers for Disease Control and Prevention (CDC) in the United States. All the data can be publically accessed through the designated website (https://wonder.cdc.gov/). CDC WONDER manages a large number of collections of data for public use to address various research topics, including births, deaths, cancer diagnoses, tuberculosis cases, vaccinations, environmental exposures and population estimates and many other related topics.

Researchers can gain access to the data by log into the CDC WONDER website first; take time to explore the topic areas of your interest, and download the data. Using suicide mortality data as an example. (1) Go to the website https://wonder.cdc.gov/. (2) Click on the "Topics" tab to explore and find the topic area of your interest. The suicide should be within the "Leading Causes of Death" category under "Death". (3) Go back to request data by clicking on "WONDER Systems" tab, select the "Detailed Mortality". In this page, carefully review and signed the consent to abide by the terms of data use restriction. After review, click on "I Agree" at the bottom of the page to proceed. (4) In the tab named "Request Form", specify the data you need and how they are tabulated, including locations to cover, demographic factors, time duration, and days of a week. (5) Specify the cause of death using one of five methods: (a) ICD-10 Codes, (b) ICD-10 130 Cause List (Infants), (c) Drug/Alcohol Induced Causes, (d) ICD-10 113 Cause List, and (e) Injury Intent and Mechanism. Codes for suicide deaths can be selected from (d) the ICD-10 113 Cause list by finding the title: #Intentional self-harm (suicide) ($_{*}$U03,X60-X84,Y870) and choose two entries under this title; or from (e) the Injury Intent Mechanism by choosing "Suicide" from for data acquisition. After all selections are completed, click the "Send" tab at the bottom of the page, the data you request will come in another page. The data can be saved for further use.

1.6 Data on Global Tobacco and Substance Use

Data for substance use/abuse are very important for global health and epidemiology. Among various substances, tobacco and alcohol have been studied the most comprehensively. As such, sources of data for these two substances are highlighted in this chapter. However, data for other substances, such as marijuana, opioids and other prescription and illicit drugs can be obtained following the same approach.

1.6.1 Tobacco Use and Prevention

Tobacco use is highly prevalent around the world, and global tobacco prevention and control programs have been established and implemented since the 1950s when Dr. Doll and Hill demonstrated the association of tobacco smoking and lung cancer in the United Kingdom (Doll & Hill, 1956). Data on tobacco use, prevention and control can be accessed through WHO website (http://apps.who.int/gho/data/node.main.TOBCONTROL?lang=en). In the "Monitor" section, you can obtain data on age-standardized prevalence of tobacco use for adults and youth by country and by gender.

In addition to data from WHO, another important sources for data on tobacco use is the World Health Statistics (https://www.who.int/gho/publications/world_health_statistics/en/). The World Health Statistics provides an overview of a number of tobacco-related health problems. Data on the prevalence rate of tobacco smoking by region and by year are also available from the World Health Statistics.

A third source for data on tobacco use and control is the Global Tobacco Surveillance System (GTSS) (https://www.cdc.gov/tobacco/global/gtss/index.htm). The GTSS aims to enhance country capacity to design, implement and evaluate tobacco control interventions, and monitor key articles of the World Health Organization's (WHO) Framework Convention on Tobacco Control and components of the WHO MPOWER technical package (CDC, 2018). The GTSS consists four surveys, including Global Youth Tobacco survey (https://www.who.int/tobacco/surveillance/gyts/en/), Global School Personnel Survey (https://www.paho.org/hq/index.php?option=com_content&view=article&id=1749:2009-global-school-personnel-survey-gsps&Itemid=1185&lang=en), Global Health Professions Student Survey (https://www.who.int/tobacco/surveillance/ghps/en/), and Global Adult Tobacco Survey (https://www.who.int/tobacco/surveillance/survey/gats/ind/en/).

1.6.2 Alcohol Use

Alcohol use and abuse is a risk factor for many health-related problems, including cardiovascular diseases, cancer, suicide and other diseases (Harris, 2013). One important data source of alcohol use and abuse is the Global Information System on Alcohol and Health (GISAH) (WHO, 2019c), available at (http://apps.who.int/gho/data/node.main.GISAH?lang=en). Various topics are covered in the data, including levels and patterns of alcohol consumption, consequence of alcohol, alcohol control policies, alcohol use disorders and alcohol dependence, presented by country and year.

Another available data source for alcohol use and abuse is the World Health Statistics (WHO, 2019e). Data from this source can be accessed through the website (http://apps.who.int/gho/data/node.sdg.tp-1?lang=en). Data on prevalence of use and amount of alcohol consumption per capita are available by region and year. For example, the global average alcohol consumption was 6.4 L of pure alcohol per person aged 15 or older. The highest alcohol consumption was observed in Europe (9.8), followed by Americas (8.0), Western Pacific (7.3), Africa (6.3), Southeast Asia (4.5) and Mediterranean (0.6).

1.7 Data for Measuring Suicide by Countries in the World

Suicide is a significant global health problem with a long history, and it occurs throughout the lifespan. The rate of suicide provides a reliable measure of the happiness among people in a country (Bray & Gunnell, 2006). Data estimated by the World Health Organization indicate that nearly 800,000 people die due to suicide every year, which is equivalent to one person dying from suicide every 40 s (WHO, 2014b).

To monitor suicide by country over time, WHO has compiled data on rates of suicide by country, including crude rates and age-standardized rates, overall and by gender. These data can be accessed at the website (https://www.who.int/mental_health/prevention/suicide/suicideprevent/en/). As an example, Fig. 1.2 shows the global pattern of suicide mortality in 2016 based on the data from this source.

1.8 Data on Physicians, Nurses and Hospital Beds

Statistics on physicians, nurses, and hospital beds are important for evaluating health resources and healthcare systems. World Bank compiled such data and made it available at their website: https://data.worldbank.org/indicator/SH.MED.PHYS.ZS. Typical data include the numbers of physicians, hospital beds and nurses and midwives per 1000 population. According to the most recently available global

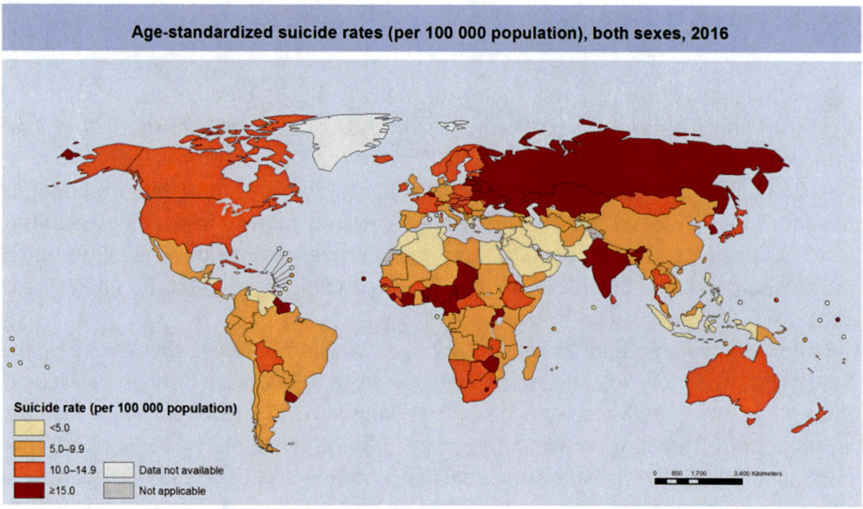

Fig. 1.2 Global pattern of suicide mortality in 2016. Note: The map was derived from the WHO website (https://www.who.int/mental_health/prevention/suicide/suicideprevent/en/)

data, in 2011–2013, worldwide on average among 1000 population, there were 1.5 physicians, 3.1 nurses/midwifes and 2.7 hospital beds (World Bank, 2016).

1.9 Important Surveys with International and Global Coverages

The data sources described in Sects. 1.1–1.8 contained only aggregate data, and no individual-level data can be obtained from these sources. In this section, we will introduce several large-scale international and global surveys that offer data at the individual level.

1.9.1 The Demographic and Health Surveys

The Demographic and Health Survey (DHS) (DHS, 2019) is listed under the World Bank website. Although not conducted by World Bank, you can access to DHS using the following web address: https://www.dhsprogram.com/Who-We-Are/About-Us.cfm. The DHS Program is funded by the U.S. Agency for International Development (USAID). The DHS also receives contributions from other donors and participating countries. The goal of DHS is to collect data and provide evidence to advance global understanding of health and population trends in developing countries.

Initiated in 1984, through a partnership with Johns Hopkins Bloomberg School of Public Health/Center for Communication Programs and other agencies, and currently implemented by ICF, a well-known scientific consulting agency, DHS collects and disseminates national representative national data on fertility, family planning, maternal and child health, gender, HIV/AIDS, malaria and nutrition for over 90 developing countries.

1.9.2 Global School-Based Student Health Survey

The Global School-Based Student Health Survey (GSHS) is a collaborative surveillance project designed to help countries measure and assess the behavioral risk and protective factors in ten key areas among students in the age range of 13–17 years (WHO, 2019d). Survey topics in GSHS include alcohol and drug use, dietary behaviors, hygiene, mental health, physical activity, sexual behaviors, tobacco use and violence and unintentional injury. A total of 103 countries have participated in the project. The data and other related information can be accessed at the following website (https://www.who.int/ncds/surveillance/gshs/en/).

1.9.3 Health Behavior in School-Aged Children

Health Behavior in School-Aged Children (HBSC) (http://www.hbsc.org/) aims to collect data on health and well-being, social environments and health behavior among school-aged children (HBSC, 2019). HBSC started in 1984 with five participating countries. After its interception, HBSC has become a major cross-sectional survey with a total of 49 member countries across Europe and North America. HBSC is conducted every fourth year among students aged 11, 13 and 15 years. The topics covered by HBSC include body image, bullying and fighting, eating behaviors, health complaints, injuries, life satisfaction, obesity, oral health, physical activity and sedentary behavior, relationship with family and peers, school environment, self-rated health, sexual behavior, socioeconomic environment, substance use (alcohol, tobacco and cannabis), and weight reduction behavior. Data collected by HBSC can be accessed through inquiry at the website https://www.uib.no/en/hbscdata.

1.9.4 International Social Survey Program

The International Social Survey Program (ISSP) (http://www.issp.org/menu-top/home/) is the largest cross-nation research effort in social science (ISSP, 2019). It was initiated in 1984 by the United States, Australia, Great Britain and Germany.

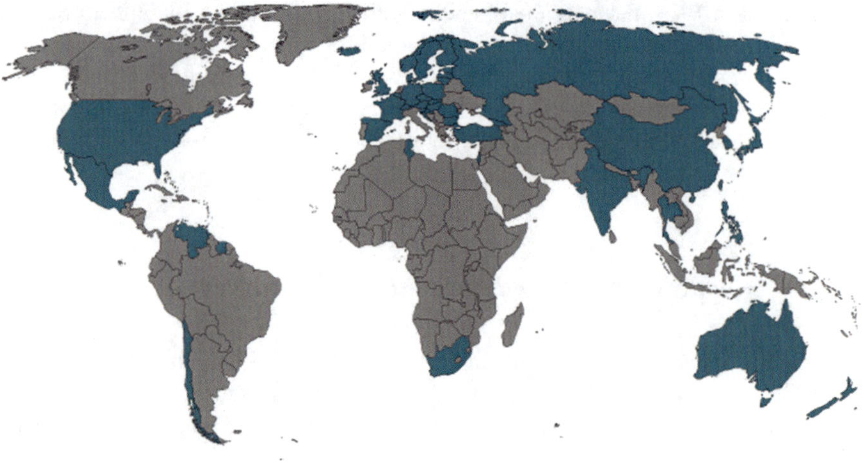

Fig. 1.3 Member countries in the ISSP. Note: The map was derived from ISSP website (http://w.issp.org/members/member-states/)

Now the ISSP collaboration has 61 participating countries. The topics covered by the ISSP include role of government, social network, social inequality, family and changing gender roles, work orientations, religion, environment, national identity, citizenship, leisure time and sports, health and health care. ISSP data by year and by topic area can be accessed through the designated website (http://www.issp.org/data-download/by-topic/). Figure 1.3 presents the participating countries of the ISSP all over the world for references.

1.9.5 Multiple Indicator Cluster Survey

Multiple Indicator Cluster Survey (MICS) (https://www.unicef.org/statistics/index_24302.html) was established to collect data at the household level. The MICS was originally developed in response to the World Summit for Children to measure progress of an internationally set of mid-decade goals (UNICEF, 2014). To date, more than 300 surveys have been conducted by MICS in more than 100 countries, filling the gap of data on well-being of children and women. Data collected through MICS are used to help shape policies for the improvement of the lives of women and children.

To date, six rounds of surveys by MICS have been conducted, including the first round (1995–1996), second round (2000), third round (2006), fourth round (2009–2013), fifth round (2012), and sixth round (2016). The seventh round for 2019 is in the design stage and new data are anticipated by 2020 or 2021. The MICS uses five main questionnaires for data collection as described below:

1. Household questionnaire, covering contents on household characteristics, energy use, insecticide treated nets, water and sanitation, handwashing, salt iodization and water quality;
2. Individual questionnaire for women, covering contents on background, mass media, fertility and birth history, maternal and newborn health, post-natal health, contraception, genital mutilation, attitudes towards domestic violence, victimization, marriage, sexual behaviors, HIV/AIDS, tobacco and alcohol use, and life satisfaction, etc.;
3. Questionnaire for children under five, covering contents on birth registration, early childhood development, child discipline and functioning, breastfeeding and dietary intake, immunization, and anthropometry, etc.;
4. Questionnaire for children age 5–17, covering contents on labor, discipline, functioning, parental involvement and foundational learning skills; and
5. Questionnaire for men, covering contents on mass media, fertility, attitudes towards domestic violence, marriage/union, sexual behaviors, HIV/AIDS, circumcision, tobacco and alcohol use, and life satisfaction.

The survey design, data and reports by MICS reports by country and year are available through the website (http://mics.unicef.org/surveys).

1.9.6 World Health Survey

The World Health Survey (https://www.who.int/healthinfo/survey/en/) was implemented by WHO in 2002–2004 in 70 member countries. The goal is to collect information about health of adult populations and healthcare system (WHO, 2019f). The total sample size of the survey was over 300,000 people. Figure 1.4 presents the participating countries of the World Health Survey. Data by country collected through this important effort can be accessed through the website: (http://apps.who.int/healthinfo/systems/surveydata/index.php/catalog/whs).

1.9.7 The World Mental Health Survey Initiative

The World Mental Health Survey Initiative (WMH) is a project of the Assessment, Classification, and Epidemiology (ACE) Group at the WHO which coordinates the implementation and analysis of general population epidemiologic surveys covering mental, substance use, and behavioral disorders in countries of all WHO Regions (https://www.hcp.med.harvard.edu/wmh/) (WMH, 2005). A total of 28 countries participated in the WMH with a total sample size in excess of 155,000. The aim of WMH is to obtain accurate estimates about the prevalence rates and correlates of mental, substance and behavioral disorders. Disorders considered in WMH

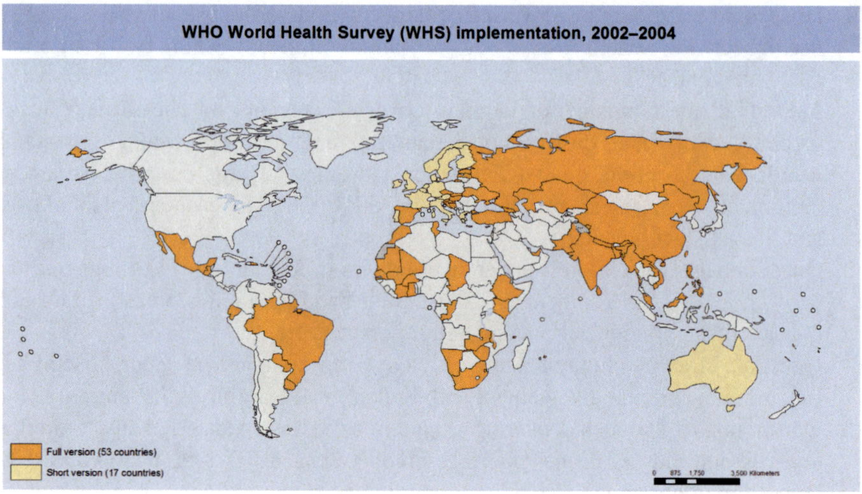

Fig. 1.4 Countries enrolled in World Health Survey. Note: The map was derived from World Health Survey website (https://www.who.int/healthinfo/survey/whs_001.png?ua=1)

include anxiety disorders, mood disorder, disorders that share a feature of problems with impulse control and substance disorders (e.g. alcohol abuse and dependence, drug abuse and dependence, nicotine). All disorders are assessed based on the definitions and criteria of the Diagnostic and Statistical Manual of Mental Disorders, Fourth Edition (DSM-IV) and the ICD-10 Classification of Mental and Behavioral Disorders.

1.9.8 World Value Survey

The World Values Survey (WVS) (www.worldvaluessurvey.org) is conducted through a global network of social scientists who study the changing values and their impact on social and political life (WVS, 2018). The WVS started in 1981, and the survey participants were from approximately 100 countries. The WVS seeks to help scientists and policy-makers understand the changes in beliefs, values and motivations of people throughout the world. Since 1981, a total of six waves of WVS have been completed with the most recent survey completed in 2014. WVS data are available free of charge at the following website (http://www.worldvaluessurvey.org/WVSContents.jsp).

1.10 Summary

Research in global health and epidemiology requires data collected in a standardized and systematic fashion by multiple countries to address important medical and health problems with worldwide significance (Chen, 2014; Harris, 2013; Nock, 2012; Webber, 2005). There is a growing trend in data collection through international and global collaborations. Data collected through such collaborative efforts are free and widely available for use. As the first chapter of this book, we introduced several sources of data readily accessible online and routinely used in research and practice. However, this is not an exhaustive list, and more resources are available. The information covered in this chapter provides a mode for researchers who are interested in using existing data to advance their horizon in global health and epidemiological research.

References

Bray, I., & Gunnell, D. (2006). Suicide rates, life satisfaction and happiness as markers for population mental health. *Social Psychiatry and Psychiatric Epidemiology, 41*(5), 333–337. https://doi.org/10.1007/s00127-006-0049-z

CDC. (2018). *GTSS*. Retrieved March 8, 2019, from https://www.cdc.gov/tobacco/global/gtss/index.htm

Chen, X. (2014). Understanding the development and perception of global health for more effective student education. *The Yale Journal of Biology and Medicine, 87*(3), 231–240.

Chen, X., Elliott, A. L., & Wang, S. (2018). Cross-country Association of Press Freedom and LGBT freedom with prevalence of persons living with HIV: Implication for global strategy against HIV/AIDS. *Global Health Research and Policy, 3*(1), 6. https://doi.org/10.1186/s41256-018-0061-3

DHS Program. (2019). *The DHS program*. Retrieved March 21, 2019, from https://dhsprogram.com/Who-We-Are/About-Us.cfm

Doll, R., & Hill, A. B. (1956). Lung cancer and other causes of death in relation to smoking; a second report on the mortality of British doctors. *British Medical Journal, 2*(5001), 1071–1081.

Foundation for the Advancement of Liberty. (2016). *Moral freedom in the world*. Retrieved March 8, 2019, from http://www.fundalib.org/en/468-2/

Harris, R. E. (Ed.). (2013). *Epidemiology of Chronic Disease: Global Perspectives*. Burlington, MA: Jones & Bartlett Learning.

HBSC. (2019). *HBSC*. Retrieved March 21, 2019, from http://www.hbsc.org/

Internet World Stats. (2019). *Country list by geographical regions*. Retrieved March 20, 2019, from https://www.internetworldstats.com/list1.htm#AF

ISO. (2018). *ISO 3166 country codes*. Retrieved January 10, 2019, from https://www.iso.org/iso-3166-country-codes.html

ISSP. (2019). *International social survey program*. Retrieved March 21, 2019, from http://www.issp.org/menu-top/home/

Koenig, H. G. (2009). Research on religion, spirituality, and mental health: A review. *Canadian Journal of Psychiatry, 54*(5), 283–291. https://doi.org/10.1177/070674370905400502

Kohl, A. (2016). *World index of moral freedom 2016: How free is your country from state-imposed moral constraints?* Retrieved March 7, 2019, from http://www.fundalib.org/wp-content/uploads/2016/04/World-Index-of-Moral-Freedom-web.pdf

Nock, M. K. (2012). *Suicide: Global perspectives from the WHO world mental health surveys*. Cambridge: Cambridge University Press.

Reporters Without Borders. (2018). *2018 world press freedom index*. Retrieved March 21, 2019, from https://rsf.org/en/ranking

Stack, S., & Kposowa, A. J. (2011). Religion and suicide acceptability: A cross-national analysis. *Journal for the Scientific Study of Religion, 50*(2), 289–306. https://doi.org/10.1111/j.1468-5906.2011.01568.x

UNICEF. (2014). *Multiple indicator cluster survey (MICS)*. Retrieved March 21, 2019, from https://www.unicef.org/statistics/index_24302.html

Webber, R. (2005). *Communicable disease epidemiology and control: A global perspective*. Wallingford: CABI. https://doi.org/10.1079/9780851999029.0000

WHO. (2014a). *Cancer country profiles 2014*. Retrieved March 21, 2019, from https://www.who.int/cancer/country-profiles/en/

WHO. (2014b). *Preventing suicide: A global imperative*. In: World Health Organization (Ed.) (p. 89). Geneva: World Health Organization.

WHO. (2019a). *Cardiovascular diseases (CVDs)*. Retrieved March 21, 2019, from https://www.who.int/cardiovascular_diseases/en/

WHO. (2019b). *Databases and information systems*. Retrieved March 21, 2019, from https://www.who.int/csr/resources/databases/en/

WHO. (2019c). *Global information system on alcohol and health*. Retrieved March 21, 2019, from https://www.who.int/gho/alcohol/en/

WHO. (2019d). *Global school-based student health survey (GSHS)*. Retrieved March 21, 2019, from https://www.who.int/ncds/surveillance/gshs/en/

WHO. (2019e). *World health statistics*. Retrieved March 21, 2019, from https://www.who.int/gho/publications/world_health_statistics/en/

WHO. (2019f). *World health survey*. Retrieved March 21, 2019, from https://www.who.int/healthinfo/survey/en/

Wikipedia. (2019a). *List of countries and dependencies by area*. Retrieved March 21, 2019, from https://en.wikipedia.org/wiki/List_of_countries_and_dependencies_by_area

Wikipedia. (2019b). *Religions by country*. Retrieved March 21, 2019, from https://en.wikipedia.org/wiki/Religions_by_country

WMH. (2005). *The world mental health survey initiative*. Retrieved March 21, 2019, from https://www.hcp.med.harvard.edu/wmh/

World Bank. (2016). *Physicians (per 1,000 people)*. Retrieved March 8, 2019, from https://data.worldbank.org/indicator/sh.med.phys.zs

World Bank. (2018). *Population, total*. Retrieved December 25, 2018, from https://data.worldbank.org/indicator/SP.POP.TOTL

World Bank. (2019). *Countries*. Retrieved March 21, 2019, from https://data.worldbank.org/country

World Cancer Research Fund International. (2019). *World cancer research fund international*. Retrieved March 21, 2019, from https://www.wcrf.org/

WVS. (2018). *WVS database*. Retrieved March 21, 2019, from http://www.worldvaluessurvey.org/wvs.jsp

Chapter 2
Satellite Imagery Data for Global Health and Epidemiology

Hao Chen and Keerati Ponpetch

Abstract In this chapter, we describe commonly accessible sources of satellite imagery data free of charge for research. Exemplary data include lightening for development level, $PM_{2.5}$ for pollution, temperature, recitation deforestation. We cover the sources of such data, methods to access, and utilization of them as a measure of the macro-environment in research, overall and zoom in down to specific country, district and community/neighborhood levels. Examples are used to illustrate the process, including R codes, screen shots, and tables.

Keywords Global health · Satellite imagery data · Epidemiology · Environment health

2.1 Introduction

Environmental changes can be natural or anthropogenic and examples of such changes include air pressure, wind, rain, fog, air pollution, and deforestation, to name a few. Of these changes, the anthropogenic factors are commonly investigated in research related to population health and targeted for interventional methods to improve public health. For example, many studies discovered that exposure to ambient air pollution is associated with increased morbidity and mortality and heightened social and economic burden (Dockery et al., 1993; Lelieveld, Evans, Fnais, Giannadaki, & Pozzer, 2015). World Health Organization estimates that ambient air pollution in both urban and rural areas has caused an excess of 4.2 million premature deaths worldwide in 2016 (WHO, 2018). There is a great research need to establish the association between the environmental factors and many adverse health outcomes at the national, international and global levels. Traditional methods such as air quality index (AQI) collected through specific monitoring

H. Chen (✉) · K. Ponpetch
Department of Environmental and Global Health, University of Florida, Gainesville, FL, USA

X. Chen, (Din) D.-G. Chen (eds.), *Statistical Methods for Global Health and Epidemiology*, ICSA Book Series in Statistics,
https://doi.org/10.1007/978-3-030-35260-8_2

techniques, have been widely used in research; however, such data are often limited for addressing larger scale health problems, including air pollution and population health for all countries across the globe.

To better understand the association between the environmental factors and adverse health outcomes at the macro level, satellite remote sensing (RS) has generated an important source of data with unique perspectives and functions for research in global health and epidemiology. Digitizable information from this source of data can be used to measure many environmental parameters, such as particulate matter (PM) from air pollution, temperature, and vegetation coverage. These quantitative measures can then be used to examine the association between these environmental factors and health outcomes at the macro level. Another feature of RS data is that consistent observational records can be generated with the data to describe key environmental factors at different scales, from local to countrywide, continental, and further to global (Sorek-Hamer, Just, & Kloog, 2016).

Utilization of satellite observations in the environmental health studies in the United States started in 2009. In those early studies, one type of RS data—the Aerosol Optical Depth (AOD) were used to expand the $PM_{2.5}$ exposure matrix to obtain spatially complete PM surface, which provided a better measure of $PM_{2.5}$ concentrations for research to examine environmental pollution and coronary heart diseases (Hu, 2009; Hu & Rao, 2009; Sorek-Hamer et al., 2016). In addition to the etiology of diseases, RS data are highly valuable for exposure assessment over time and future prediction of incidence of diseases. This feature is very important to inform decision-making and planning in development and implementing prevention strategies and to evaluate interventional results. For example, temperature and precipitation data can be used to predict the prevalence of mosquito-associate disease such as dengue and malaria (Thomson et al., 2017).

Many governmental, academic, and industrial organizations have devoted much effort to collect and compile RS data with a number of satellites lunched for environmental monitoring. To promote the utilization, remote sensing data from a range of sources become widely accessible to the public free of charge. The question is where to find and how to acquire such data to address specific research questions in global health and epidemiology. To facilitate the use of RS data, in this chapter, we will introduce the commonly used sources of data that are readily available and free of charge (see Table 2.1). For each data sources, examples are used to demonstrate how to acquire the datasets needed. In addition, advantages and limitations of the data are discussed.

2.2 USGS Data

USGS stands for the US Geological Survey, and USGS is the first source of data we introduce in this chapter. USGS data consist of some most typical satellite imagery data commonly used in research. Researchers can access to the very informative USGS data through the Earth Explorer.

Table 2.1 Examples of RS data source

Satellite source	Date of operation	Developer	Resolution	Data hosting sites
Landsat 1–3	1972–1983	NASA	80 m	Earth explorer, Earthdata
Landsat 4	1982–1992	NASA	80 m	Earth explorer, Earthdata
Landsat 5	1982–	NASA	29/30 m	Earth explorer, Earthdata, INPE
Landsat 7	1999–2020	NASA	15/30 m	Earth explorer, GloVis, INPE
Landsat 8	2013–	NASA	15/30 m	Earth explorer, GloVis, INPE
GOES-R	2016–	NOAA	0.5–2.0 km	Earthdata, CLASS
Sentinel-1	2014 (A)/2016 (B)	ESA	5 m- 4 km	Sentinel satellite data
Sentinel-2	2015 (A)/2017 (B)	ESA	10, 20, 60 m	Sentinel satellite data
Sentinel-3	2016 (A)/2018 (B)	ESA	500 m	Sentinel satellite data
ALOS	2006–	JAXA	2.5 m	Global ALOS 3D world
ERS	1991 (1)/1995 (2) 2000 (1)/2001 (2)	ESA	25 m	Earth observation link (EOLi), sentinel satellite data
Himawari-8/9	2014–	JMA	0.5, 1.0 km	Himawari monitor
Terra and Aqua	1999 (Terra)/2002(aqua)	NASA	250 m	Earth explorer, Earthdata

2.2.1 *Introduction of Earth Explorer (EE)*

Earth Explorer (EE) provides a useful tool to access the satellite and aerial image data that can be used to measure biology and ecosystem, climate and land use change, energy, environmental health, geology, water, and natural hazards. EE also features free downloading data over chronological timelines. Specific data can be accessed using a wide range of search criteria including address/place, path/row, coordinates, google map options, dates range, result options, mass media search, and etc. It also provides access to Landsat data products such as MODIS and AVHRR land surface and Hyperion's hyperspectral data from NASA, which have covered the landscape images with consistent spectral bands since 1972. It is worth noting that changes in land coverage is especially important when studying the ecological systems and their relationship with human health (USGS, 2013).

The interface of EE is user-friendly, and the website is easy to navigate through. An application, named as Bulk Download is provided for researchers to obtain more than one type of data to address complex research questions.

2.2.2 Steps to Access USGS Data Using EE

To demonstrate steps to access the USGS data using EE, we used Landsat source as an example. As expected, the Landsat data are available free of charge. What you need to do before accessing is to register as a data user.

Step 1. Access to USGS data using EE interface with the URL: https://earthexplorer.usgs.gov/. After gaining access to the website, you will see the following on our computer screen—the EE interface for data accessing (Fig. 2.1).

Step 2. Set your search criteria.

This step can be completed by clicking on the "Search Criteria" tab. In this part, you define the region of interest, timeline for the aerial and satellite imagery data. For example, search criteria as shown in Fig. 2.2:

1. Click on the "Predefined Area" tab and then the "Add Shape".
2. Open the box under "State", and select a state, here we use "Florida" as an example state; open the box "Area Type" and the select "State"; and then click "Add".

Step 3. Enter the time range for the data you plan to download.

This step is easy, and it can be completed by clicking the "Date Range" tab and then fill in the time period for data and then hit data sets (Fig. 2.3).

Step 4. Select data to download.

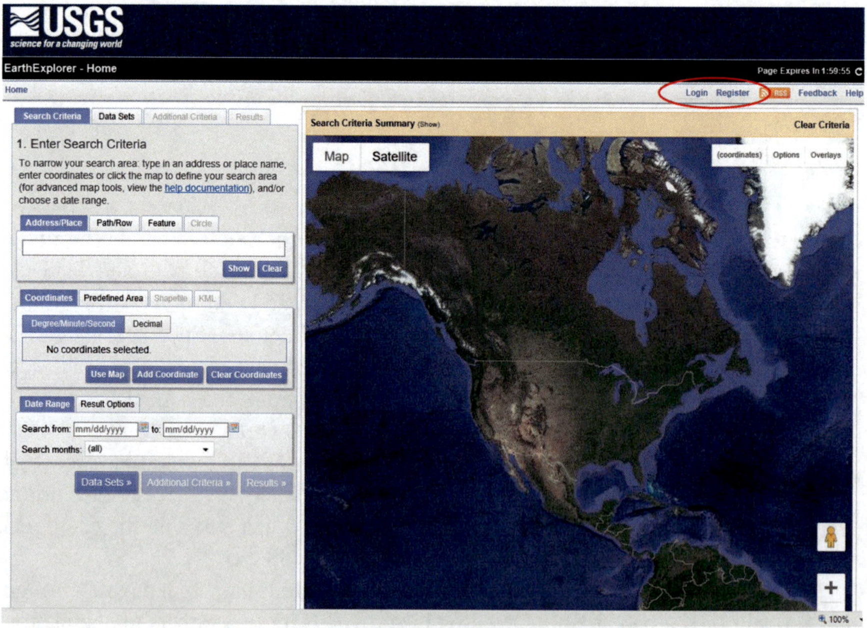

Fig. 2.1 Homepage of USGS Earth Explorer. Red circle shows the tabs for "Register" and "Login"

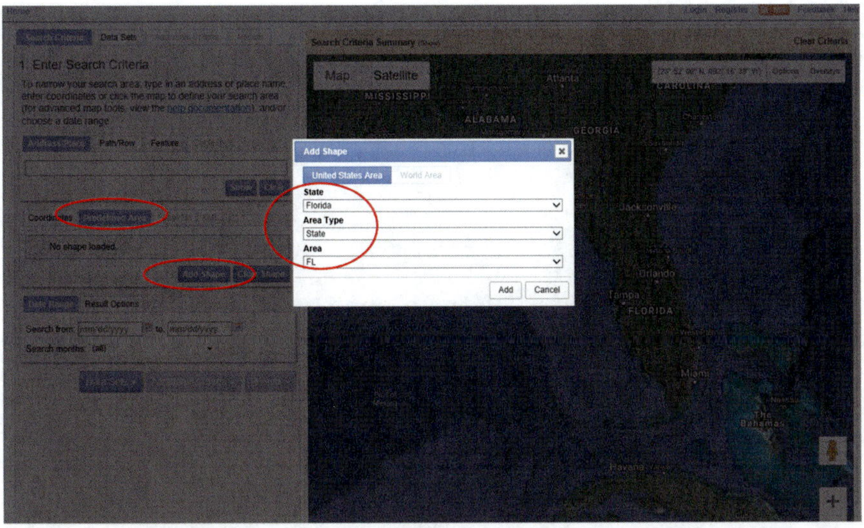

Fig. 2.2 Example of accessing data source using predefined area function. Red circles showed the tabs described in step 2

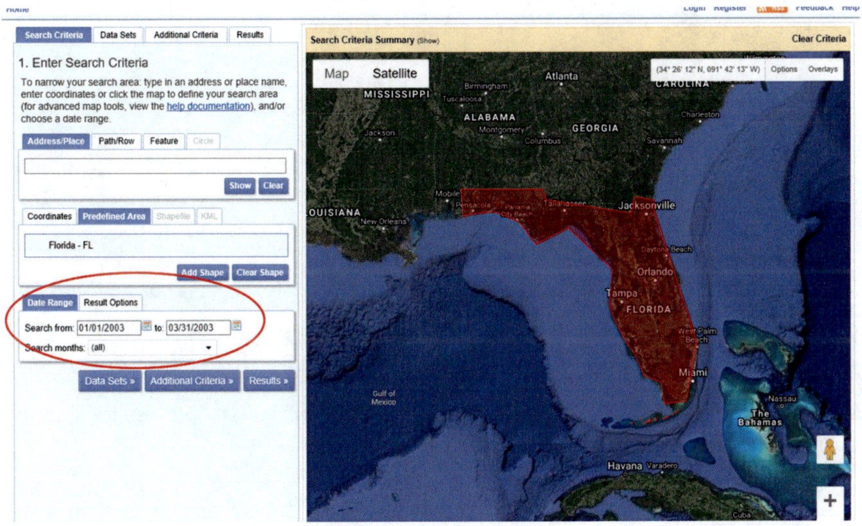

Fig. 2.3 Enter date range. Red circle shows the tabs to enter dates

Click the "Data sets" tap, you will see a long list of many options to download the remote sensing data, including the aerial imagery, Landsat, LiDAR, MODIS, etc. The data were also categorized into different levels for quality purposes. Here we chose eMODIS NDVI as the example dataset by: first select "Vegetation Monitoring" from the list and then select eMODIS NDVI (Fig. 2.4).

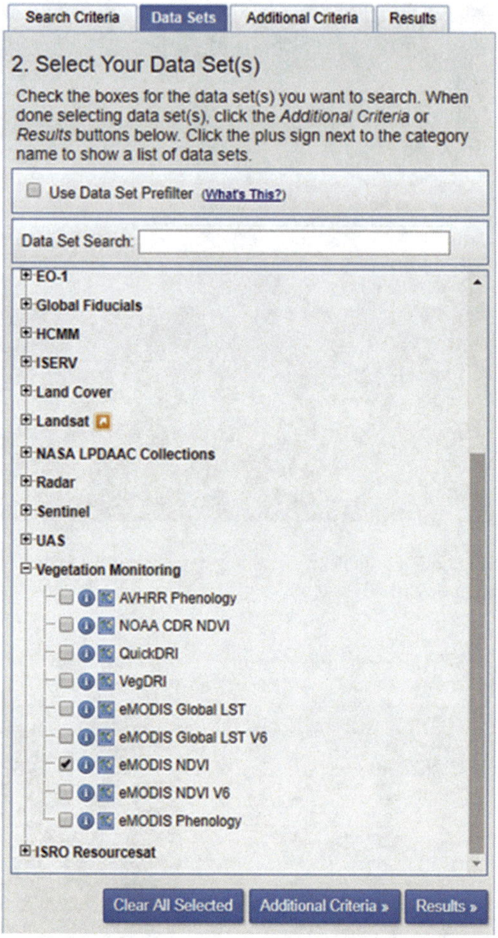

Fig. 2.4 Select data sets

Step 5. Application of filters to remove noise (optional).

Click the "Additional Criteria" tab, choose the image of interest to filter out scenes with too much cloud.

Step 6. Download data.

This step is completed by clicking on the "Results" tab as shown below. The screen provides options for you to browse, preview and download the data as shown below (Fig. 2.5).

Step 7. Loading dataset to R.

For researchers who are familiar with R program, the follow codes can be used to complete the previous steps. These codes can be modified to any other types of data (Fig. 2.6).

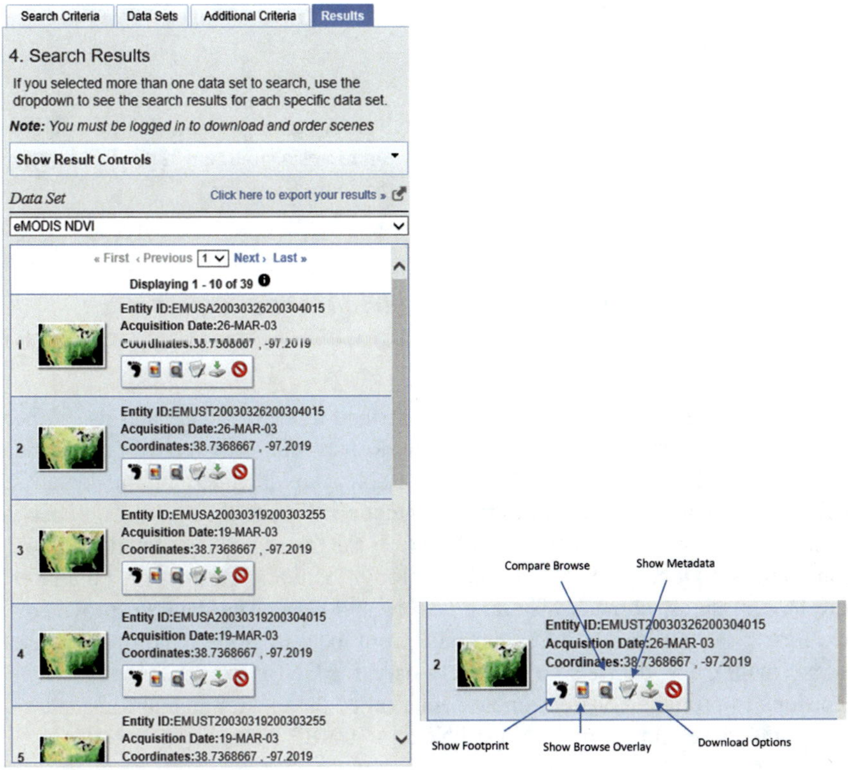

Fig. 2.5 Download data sets

```
library(tiff)
library(raster)

#import FL administrative bundary--RASTER---
FL<-'U:/RS_EH/Data/FL boundary/FL_raster/FL_Ras.tif'
FLR = raster(FL)
plot(FLR, col='gray')

#import raster 'NDVI1KM' downloaded from EE
ND<- raster("U:/RS_EH/Data/NDVI1KM/NDVI.tif")
ND
plot(ND)

#Crop NDVI1KM with FL boundary
c<-crop(ND,FLR)
plot(c)

mask<-mask(x=c, mask=FLR)
plot(mask)
```

Fig. 2.6 R codes to load the same dataset from USGS

2.3 UNEP Data of United Nations Environmental Program (UNEP)

UNEP stands for the United Nations Environmental Program (UNEP). UNEP provides another important source of satellite and aerial imagery data. Researchers can access UNEP data using the Environmental Data Explorer.

2.3.1 Introduction of the Environmental Data Explorer of UNEP

The Environmental Data Explorer is an interface used by UNEP and its partners to prepare the Global Environment Outlook Report and other related environment assessments. Data for more than 500 variables are included in this database, including air pollutant emissions, water, vegetation, climate change, disaster, health, and among many others. These variables cover the themes, many of which are very important for global health and epidemiology, including freshwater, population, forests, emissions, climate, disasters, health, and GDP. The data are provided in two forms: (a) statistics at different scale (from local to global) and (b) geospatial forms (maps). The datasets are routinely used for UNEP to make evidence-based decisions to promote coherent implementation of the environmental dimension of sustainable development in the United Nations (UNEP, 2018).

2.3.2 Steps to Access UNEP Data

Step 1: Go to the website.

Data access can be completed after getting to the website: http://geodata.grid.unep.ch/. After getting into the website, you will see the following page (Fig. 2.7), which assist you navigate the UNEP data with the Environmental Data Explorer.

As shown in Fig. 2.7, you can see that Environmental Data Explorer contains two options (methods) to access the data: (a) Keyword search by filling in the first box "Enter words to search"; and (b) Search using the existed category by opening the second box and selecting the categories of your interest. After clicking the "Search" bottom, additional criteria are available for users to further refine the data selection and download.

As an illustration, we will introduce the first approach in detail. When you are familiar with the first approach, the second approach would be easy to follow. The approach of keyword search can be completed in the following steps:

Step 2. Start data search by entering a keyword(s).

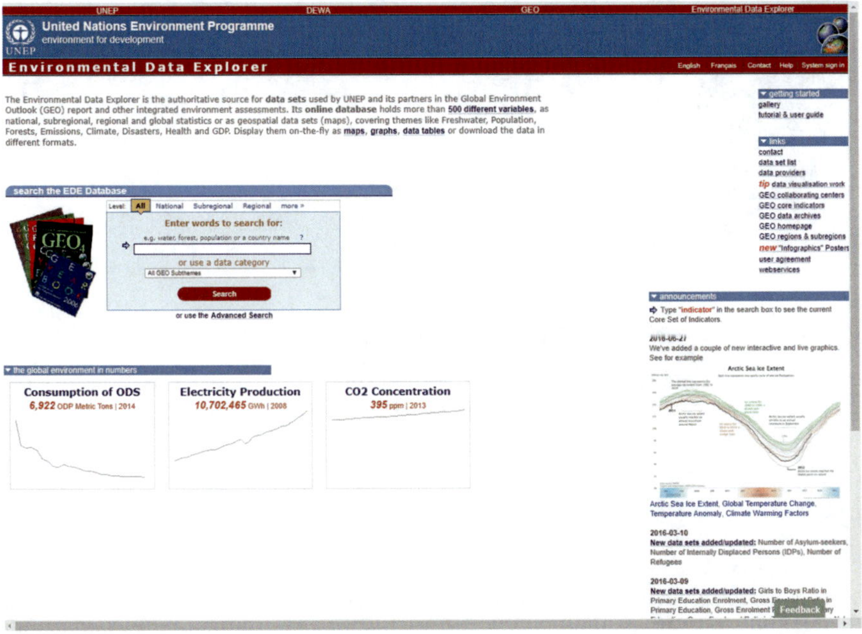

Fig. 2.7 Home page of the Environmental Data Explorer of UNEP

Use annual temperature as an example. Type the words "annual temperature" in the box "Enter words to search for", then "Search", you will see a screen as in Fig. 2.8.

Step 3. Choose the dataset of interest.

For example, select "Average Monthly Maximum Temperature-January", click the "Continue" tab at the bottom of the screen (Fig. 2.9).

Step 4. Display and download the datasets.

There are three data options as shown in the screen in Fig. 2.10, including "Draw Map", "Show Metadata" and "Download Data". By selecting each of them, you can get a map and save it for use. You can also review and download the data.

Step 5. Applying datasets to R.

R codes can be used in statistical program to achieve the steps in the sample described above.

1. Import data into R using the following code:

```
#Download Tmax.tif into R
Tmax<- raster("U:/RS_EH/Data/tmax_1_tif/tmax_1.tif")
Tmax
plot(Tmax) #Display as a map
```

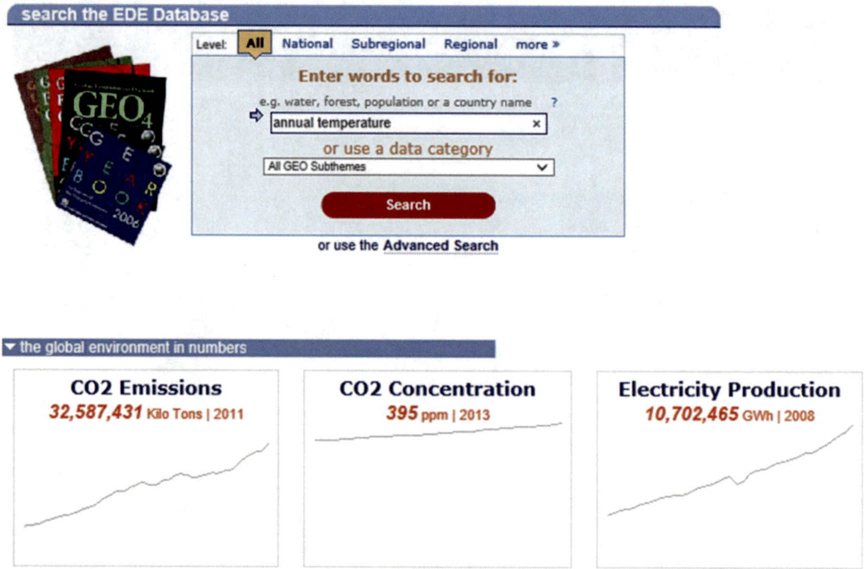

Fig. 2.8 Search keyword "annual temperature" in the Environmental Data Explorer

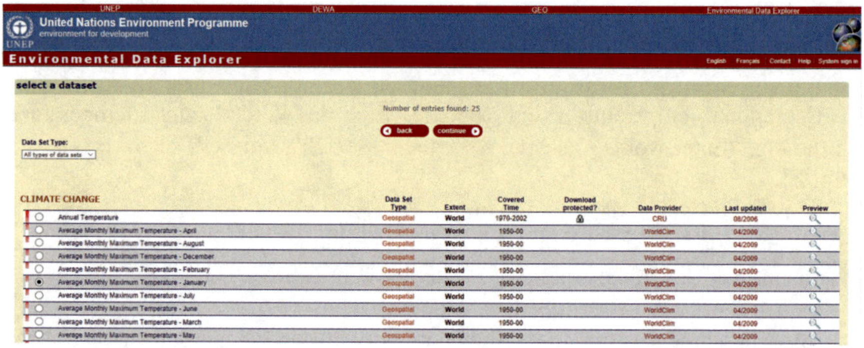

Fig. 2.9 Examples of data sets in the Environmental Data Explorer

2. Crop Tmax data to Florida boundary in R

```
#Download Tmax.tif into R
Tmax<- raster("U:/RS_EH/Data/tmax_1_tif/tmax_1.tif")
Tmax
plot(Tmax) #Display as a map

#Crop Tmax to Florida boundary
Temp<- crop(Tmax, FLR)
plot(Temp)
```

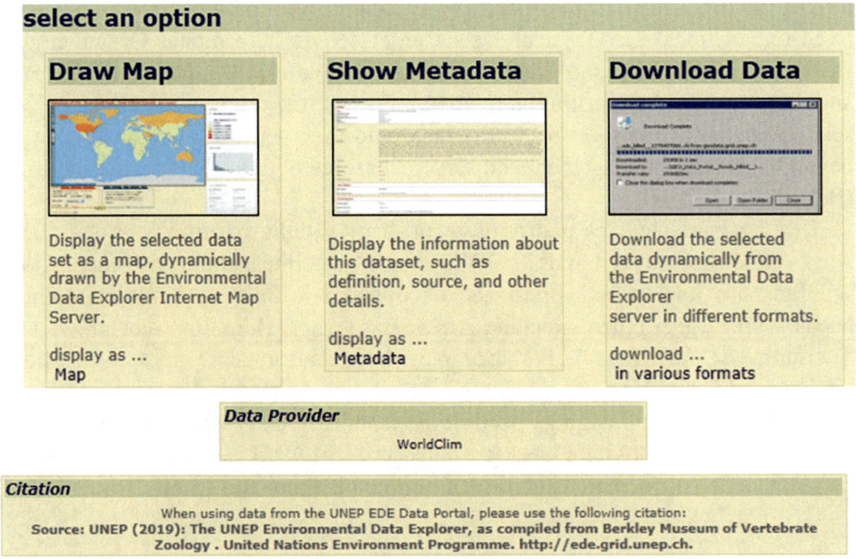

Fig. 2.10 Data access options in the Environmental Data Explorer

2.4 NASA Earth Science Data

NASA Earth Science Data consist of another important and very comprehensive source of data. Data from this source are often used in many types of research, including medical and health related studies.

2.4.1 Introduction of the Earth Science Data

NASA Earth Science Data (also called EARTHDATA) are compiled by and powered by EOSDIS (the Earth Observing System Data and Information System). EOSDIS covers a wide spectrum of data on earth sciences including ocean surface, field campaigns, polar processes, land cover change, cryosphere, digital elevation, atmosphere dynamics and composition, and interdisciplinary research, and among others (Behnke, Mitchell, & Ramapriyan, 2018). EOSDIS also features a set of 12 discipline-based Distributed Active Archive Centers (DAACs) across the United States. These centers include: EROS Data Center (EDC) Land Processes, Goddard Space Flight Center (GSFC), Jet Propulsion Laboratory (JPL) Physical Oceanography DAAC (PO-DAAC), Langley Research Center (LaRC), National Snow and Ice Data Center (NSIDC), Oak Ridge National Laboratory (ORNL), Socioeconomic Data and Applications Center (SEDAC) at the Consortium for International Earth Science Information Network (CIESIN), Global Hydrology Resource

Center (GHRC) at Marshall Space Flight Center, National Climatic Data Center (NCDC), National Geophysical Data Center (NGDC), National Oceanographic Data Center (NODC), and Satellite Active Archive (SAA) of National Oceanic and Atmospheric Administration (NOAA). Each of the center was collocated with scientific expertise in their respective field and they perform many tasks that are beyond basic data management and serve over three million users across the world (Behnke et al., 2018).

The database includes platforms from many satellites including Aqua, Terra, Aura, TRMM, Calipso, Landsat, GOES, NOAA satellites, and many others. These satellites use numerous instruments to collect data to meet different scientific needs. Typical instruments include AIRS, Barometer, Humidity Sensor, MODIS, Thermometer, VIIRS, etc. For example, the data for AOD or aerosol optical thickness (ADT) which describes the air pollution levels can be measured by the Moderate Resolution Imaging Spectroradiometer (MODIS) using the satellite Aqua and Terra over most of the globe on a daily basis. MODIS can measure the spectral radiance in 36 channels in resolution of between 250 nm and 1 km.

2.4.2 Steps to Access Earth Science Data

The tool available for use to access NASA Earth Science Data is the EARTHDATA Search. Launched in 2018, this online search tool contains many methods to search the data you need and download them for use. NASA's data policy ensures that all NASA data are fully available, open and without restrictions. In the following, we use the vegetation coverage data as an example to demonstrate how to use the search engine to get data from the Moderate Resolution Imaging Spectroradiometer (MODIS). We demonstrate the process in several steps.

Step 1: Registration and login.

Visit the website https://urs.earthdata.nasa.gov/ for registration. EARTHDATA requires registration and login for data access (Fig. 2.11).

Step 2. Visit the Homepage.

After login, visit the homepage by clicking the EARTHDATA logo on the top left corner in Fig. 2.11. Then click "FIND DATA" on the bottom right corner in Fig. 2.12.

Step 3: Search data using a keyword(s).

Type a keyword of interest for searching, for example "vegetation". The EARTHDATA allows you to define your search based on keywords, platforms, instruments, etc. on the left side of the webpage. We defined our search with keyword "Land Surface", platform "Aqua", and instrument "MODIS". After search, we obtained 28 matching collections as shown in Fig. 2.13.

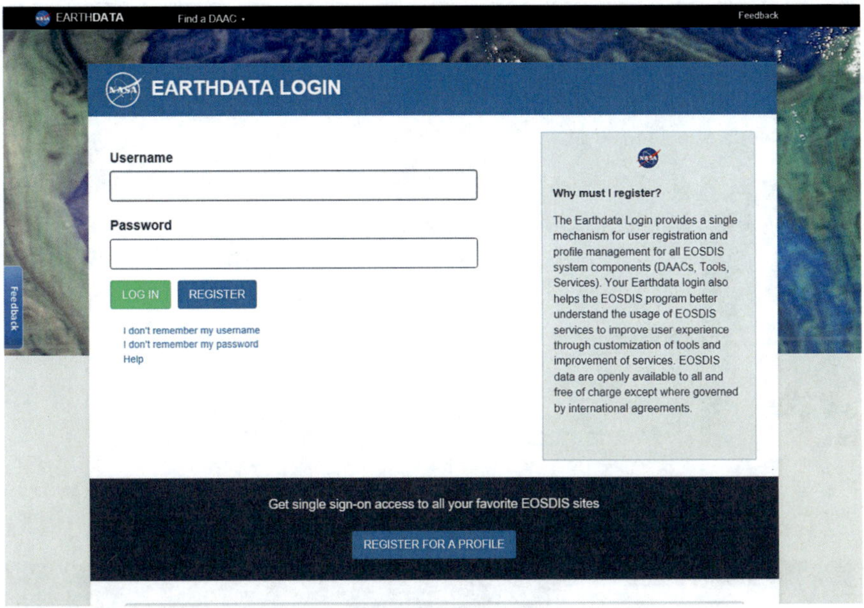

Fig. 2.11 Login and registration webpage for EARTHDATA

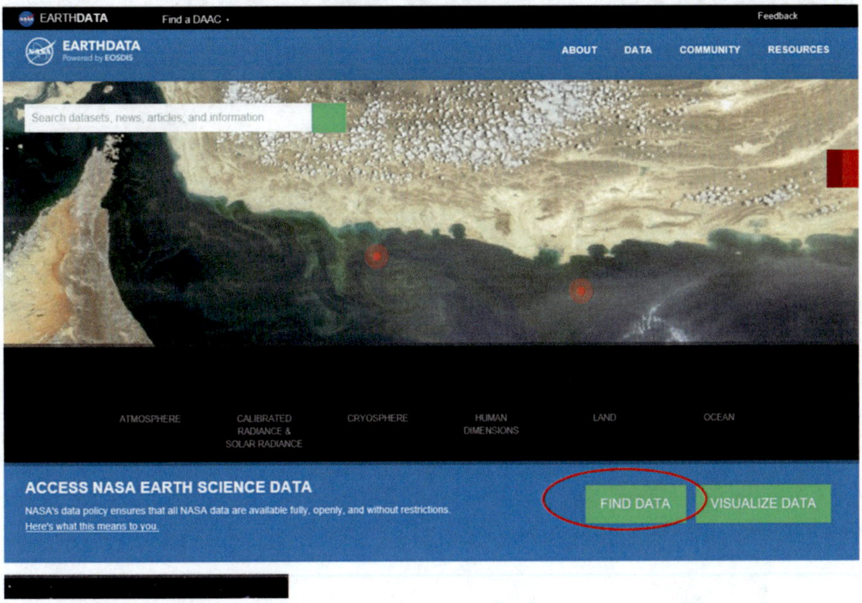

Fig. 2.12 Homepage for EARTHDATA. Red circle shows the "FIND DATA" tab

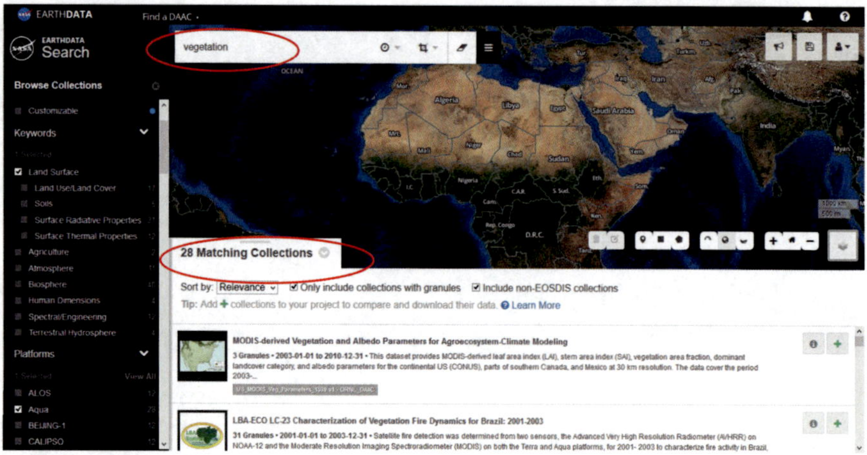

Fig. 2.13 Search data on EARTHDATA. Red circles show the “keyword box” and the number of searching results

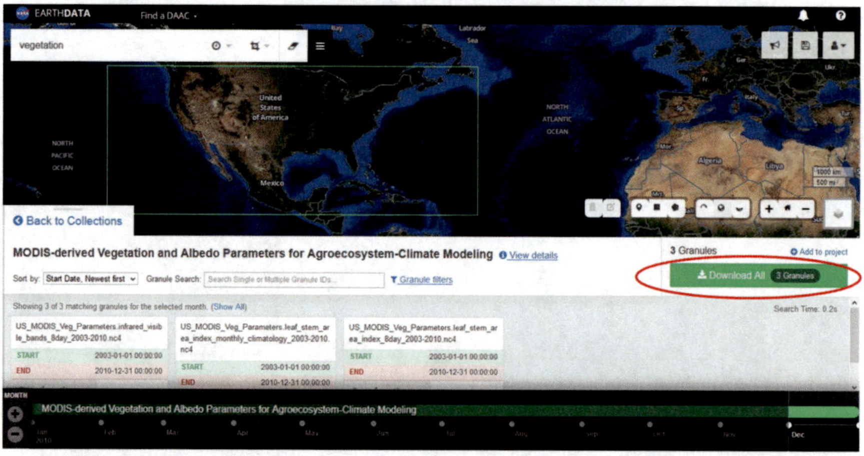

Fig. 2.14 Choose and download datasets on EARTHDATA. Red circle shows the “Download” tab

Step 3. Download the data of interest.

In this example, we select, from all the 28 options, the MODI-derived Vegetation and Albedo Parameters for Agroecosystem-Climate Modeling datasets for downloading (Fig. 2.14).

2.5 Sentinel Satellite Data

Sentinel Satellite data are compiled by the European Space Agency (ESA). Data from this source also covers many topics commonly investigated in global health.

2.5.1 Introduction of the Sentinel Satellite Data

Data from this source provide the highest resolution remote sensing data covering the whole globe generated using sentinel satellites. Five satellites will be contributing to the datasets including (ESA, 2014):

1. Sentinel-1: weather, day and night images used for land and ocean observation;
2. Sentinel-2: high resolution images for land which can reach as low as 10 m and there are as many as 12 spectral bands including red, green, blue and the near-infrared;
3. Sentinel-3: datasets for land and ocean observation;
4. Sentinel-4 and -5: datasets for atmospheric composition monitoring from geostationary and polar orbits respectively.

The Copernicus Open Access Hub (formerly known as Sentinels Scientific Data Hub) is a user-friendly interface that provided users to search and acquire RS data of interest. This interface is jointly operated by the European Commission, ESA, and the European Environment Agency. All data from this source are available for users free of charge.

2.5.2 Steps to Access the Sentinel Satellite Data

To show the process of data acquisition using the interface Copernicus Open Access Hub, we will provide an example using the AOD data. It takes several steps to acquire data using the ESA's interface:

Step 1: Visit the homepage and register.

The interface of the Copernicus Open Access Hub can be accessed through the website: https://scihub.copernicus.eu/dhus/#/home. Download the data from the Hub requires registration/sign up and login as shown in Fig. 2.15. After registration, you will receive an email to validate your registration. After validation, you will be able to login.

Step 2. Set search criteria.

Once the search tap is clicked, it will provide information for all the available sentinel data from different satellites. Further refinement can be made to select more specific datasets by the "advance search" function.

As mentioned, we will use AOD as the example parameter. The example data were collected using the Multi-Spectral Instrument, carried by SENTINEL-2 satellite to measure AOD. We choose Frankfurt am Maine, Germany as the target area and type "platformname: Sentinel-2" in the search box. A total of 50 products were returned and shown in Fig. 2.16.

Step 3. Choose datasets and download.

After data search is completed and the data of interest are located, take a review of the data, and make further changes when needed. Finalize the

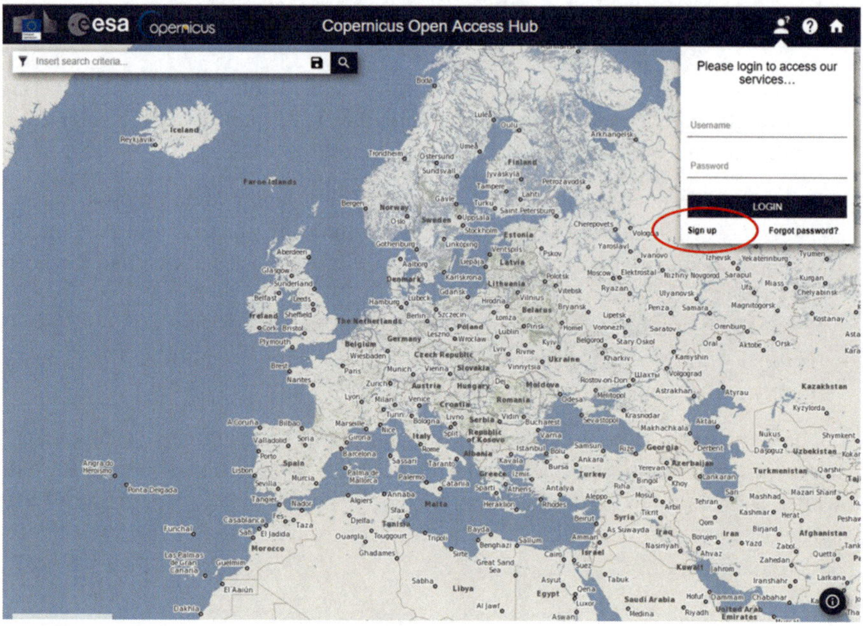

Fig. 2.15 Registration and login for the Copernicus Open Access Hub. Red circle shows the "sign up" tab for registration

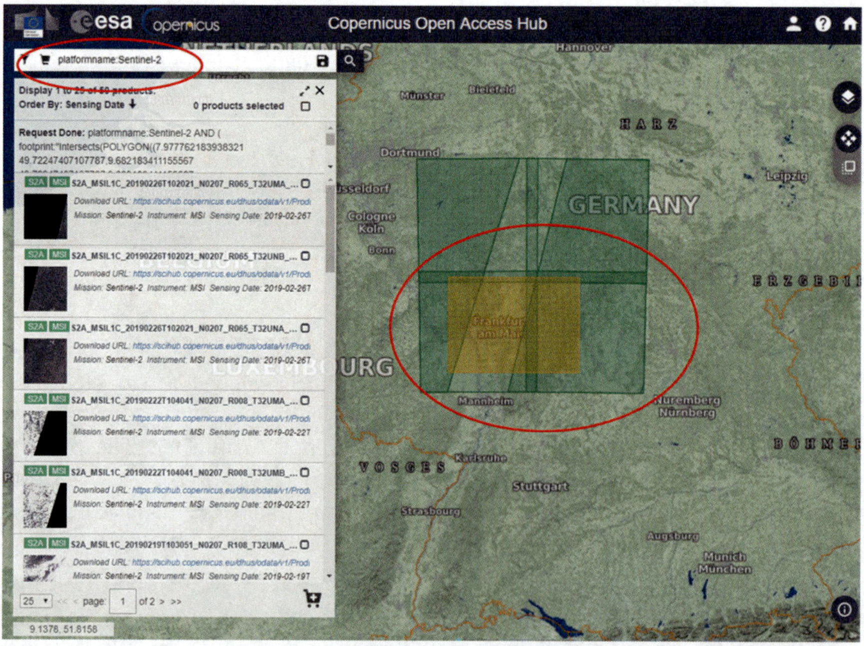

Fig. 2.16 Search function of the Copernicus Open Access Hub. Red circles show the search box and area of interest in the map

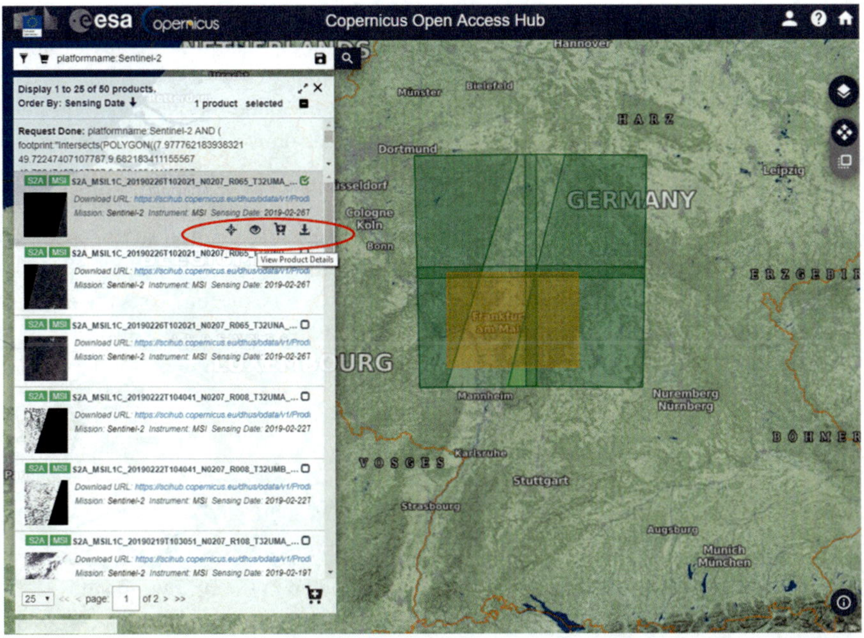

Fig. 2.17 Choose and download data from the Copernicus Open Access Hub. Red circle shows the viewing and downloading options

selection and download the data following the online instructions from the website. It is sometimes time-consuming in downloading data from this source, particularly when the dataset is big. As an example, we choose "S2A_MSIL1C_20190226T102021_N0207_R065_T32UMA_20190226T135911" dataset to show. There are also viewing and downloading options available (Fig. 2.17).

2.6 Global ALOS 3D World Data

Global ALOS 3D world of the Japanese Aerospace Exploration Agency (JAXA) provides satellite sensing data with high resolution. The data have been widely used in the health science studies.

2.6.1 Introduction of the Global ALOS 3D World

The ALOS (Advanced Land Observing Satellite) 3D World of JAXA (Japanese Aerospace Exploration Agency) release datasets from the global digital surface model (DSM) with a horizontal resolution of approximately 30 m. The data are available free of charge since May 2015. Data from this source are considered the most precise global-scale elevation data that were compiled with images acquired by the ALOS satellite "DAICHI". The dataset is highly expected to be applied in scientific research and education where endeavors are made to investigate the map development, water resource investigation, as well as damage prediction of natural disasters. However, the application of the data is hampered for practice use by the significant extent of data gaps and questionable use of fill data. It is recommended to use the datasets through significant process and in combination with other data sources. Overall download volume for the global data is more than 250 GB. The large file is due to the reason that the data contains two sets; one employs the mean of the higher resolution data points while the other one represents the average. Subtle differences of images generated by the two are noticeable (Takaku & Tadono, 2017; Takaku, Tadono, Tsutsui, & Ichikawa, 2016).

2.6.2 Steps to Access the ALOS 3D World Data

Data from this source can be accessed and downloaded in the following steps:

Step 1. Visit the homepage and registration.

The search engine to access ALOS 3D World of JAXA data can be found through: https://www.eorc.jaxa.jp/ALOS/en/aw3d30/. Go to the homepage using the link (Fig. 2.18).

Scroll down the homepage and find the following link to enter registration page (https://www.eorc.jaxa.jp/ALOS/en/aw3d30/registration.htm). An email will be sent to the registered email for confirmation and password after completing registration (Fig. 2.19).

Find the dataset link on the homepage as shown here and click to enter the data page (http://www.eorc.jaxa.jp/ALOS/en/aw3d30/data/index.htm). Enter the username (the registered email address) and password to access the data map as shown in Fig. 2.20.

Step 2. Search data.

Click the area of interest. Here we choose Florida for example (Fig. 2.21). You can choose even smaller square for more detailed data.

Step 3. Download data.

Following the online instructions to download the selected data as shown in the red circle in Fig. 2.21.

2.7 Earth Online Data

Earth Online (EO) is another product based on ESA's Earth Catalogue Service and provides many sources of remote satellite sensing data that can be applied in the health science.

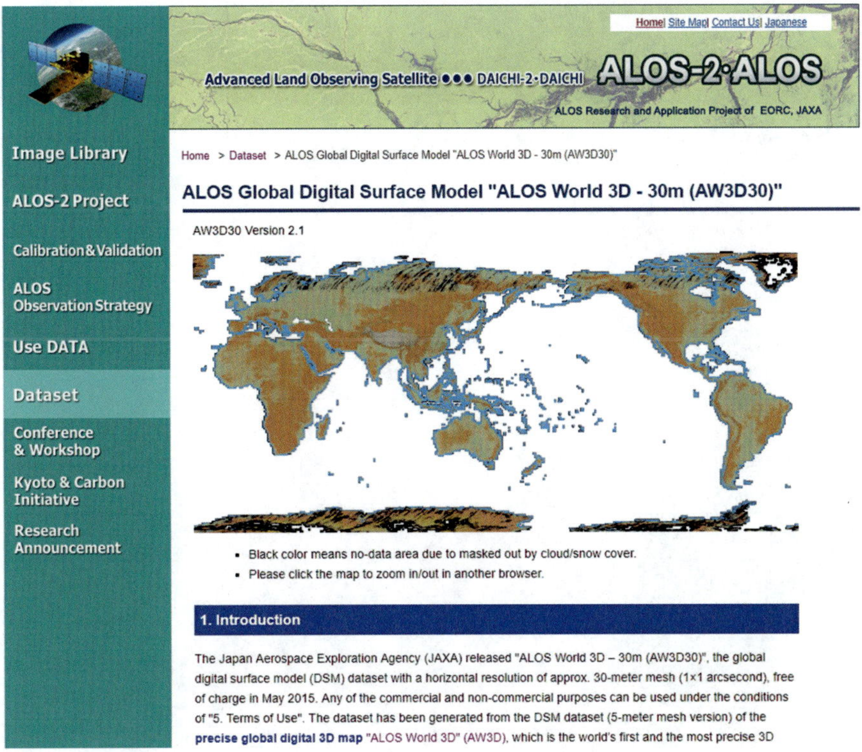
Home| Site Map| Contact Us| Japanese
Advanced Land Observing Satellite ●●● DAICHI-2·DAICHI
ALOS-2·ALOS
ALOS Research and Application Project of EORC, JAXA
Image Library
ALOS-2 Project
Calibration&Validation
ALOS Observation Strategy
Use DATA
Dataset
Conference & Workshop
Kyoto & Carbon Initiative
Research Announcement
Home > Dataset > ALOS Global Digital Surface Model "ALOS World 3D - 30m (AW3D30)"
ALOS Global Digital Surface Model "ALOS World 3D - 30m (AW3D30)"
AW3D30 Version 2.1
Black color means no-data area due to masked out by cloud/snow cover.
Please click the map to zoom in/out in another browser.
1. Introduction
The Japan Aerospace Exploration Agency (JAXA) released "ALOS World 3D – 30m (AW3D30)", the global digital surface model (DSM) dataset with a horizontal resolution of approx. 30-meter mesh (1×1 arcsecond), free of charge in May 2015. Any of the commercial and non-commercial purposes can be used under the conditions of "5. Terms of Use". The dataset has been generated from the DSM dataset (5-meter mesh version) of the precise global digital 3D map "ALOS World 3D" (AW3D), which is the world's first and the most precise 3D

Fig. 2.18 Homepage of the Global ALOS 3D World

2.7.1 Introduction to the EO Data

EO is formerly known as Earth Observation Link (EOLi). As of Jan. 4th, 2019, EOLi catalogue and ordering services has been upgraded and presented as the ESA simple online catalogue that was hosted by EO. The mission of EO, is to supply scientists and decision makers objective and continuous data and images of planet earth by satellite remote sensing technology, so that informed decisions will be made to understand and protect our environment. EO provides interface to browse the metadata and preview of images of Earth Observation data acquired by the satellites ERS and Envisat. The service also provides downloadable products of various processing levels. The data from EO comprise of topics in agriculture, atmosphere, earth surface, water, land, ocean and coasts, snow and ice, and natural disasters. EOis a JAVA application which is supported on all major computing platforms including Windows, Linux, MaxOS X and other Unix systems.

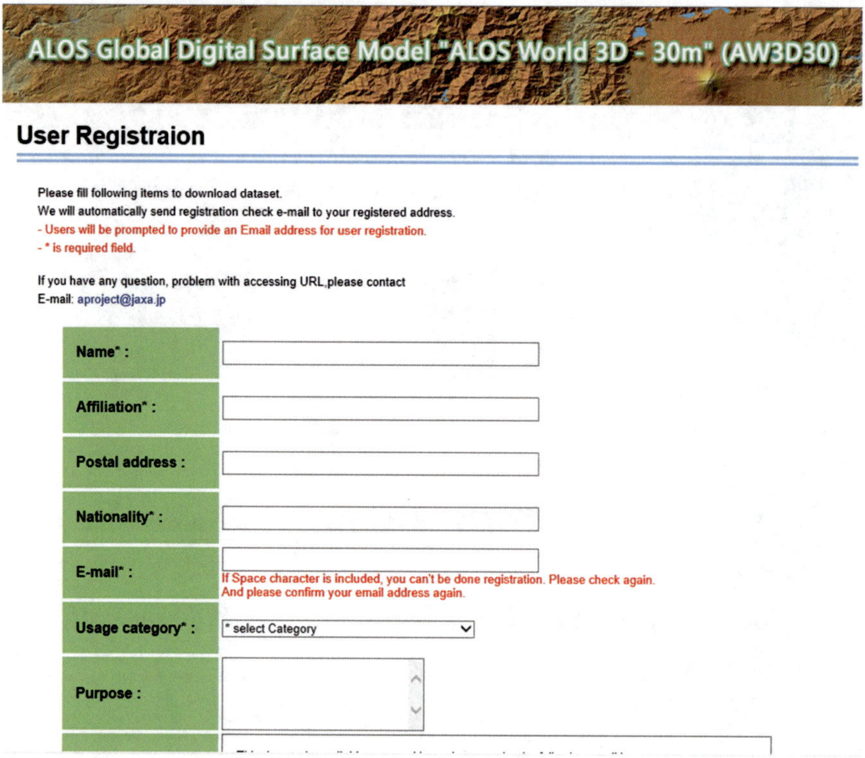
ALOS Global Digital Surface Model "ALOS World 3D - 30m" (AW3D30)
User Registraion
Please fill following items to download dataset.
We will automatically send registration check e-mail to your registered address.
- Users will be prompted to provide an Email address for user registration.
- * is required field.
If you have any question, problem with accessing URL,please contact
E-mail: aproject@jaxa.jp
Name* :
Affiliation* :
Postal address :
Nationality* :
E-mail* :
If Space character is included, you can't be done registration. Please check again.
And please confirm your email address again.
Usage category* :
* select Category
Purpose :

Fig. 2.19 Registration page on the Global ALOS 3D World

2.7.2 *The Steps of Access Earth Online Data*

The method described in Sect. 2.4 for Sentinel satellite data access can be used here to access the EO data. As an example, we use the atmosphere data to show the steps for data acquisition.

Step 1. Registration.

Go to the Earth Online application site: https://earth.esa.int/web/guest/home, and complete the registration online as shown in Fig. 2.22. A confirmation email will be sent to the registered email for validation.

Step 3. Choose data of interest.

Once login, click the "Data Access" tab and choose subtab "Browse Data Products". Then select "Atmosphere" as shown in Fig. 2.23.

Step 3. Data selection.

After clicking the "Atmosphere", a list of atmospheric data appears. As an example, you can select "GOMOS Level 2 - Atmospheric constituents' profiles - User Friendly Product (NetCDF.GOMOS_UFP)" Fig. 2.24.

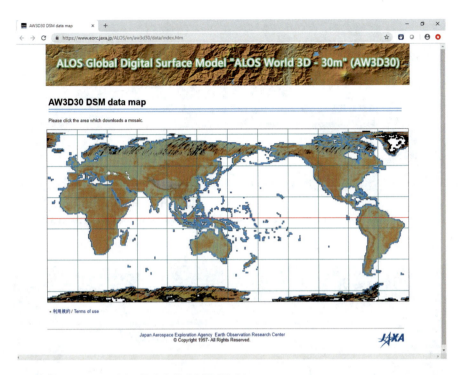

Fig. 2.20 Data map of the Global ALOS 3D World

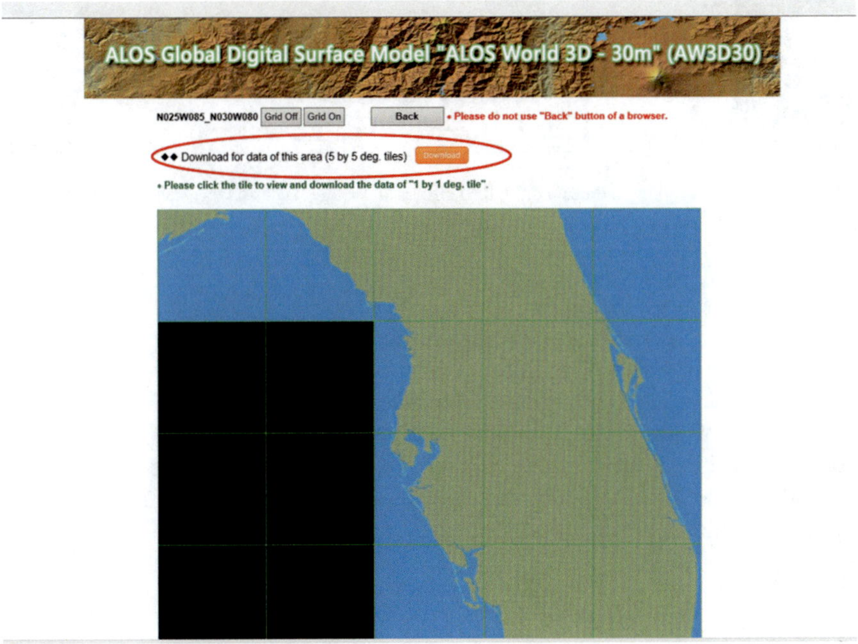

Fig. 2.21 Data map of Florida in the Global ALOS 3D World

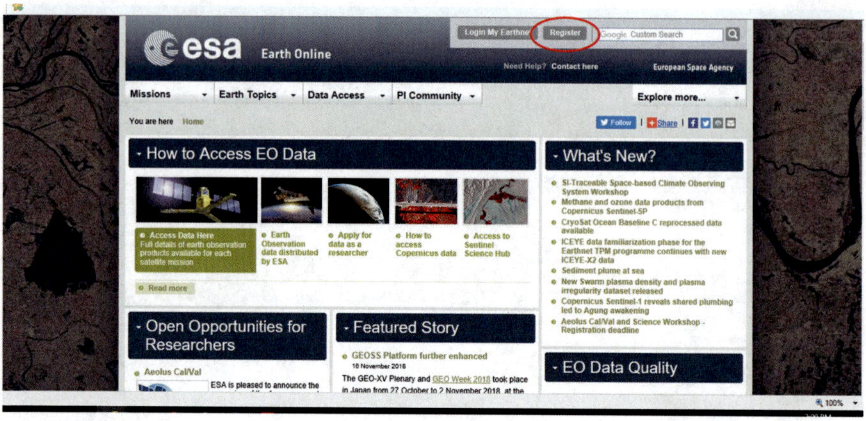

Fig. 2.22 Homepage and registration tap of EO data. Red circle shows the "Register" tab

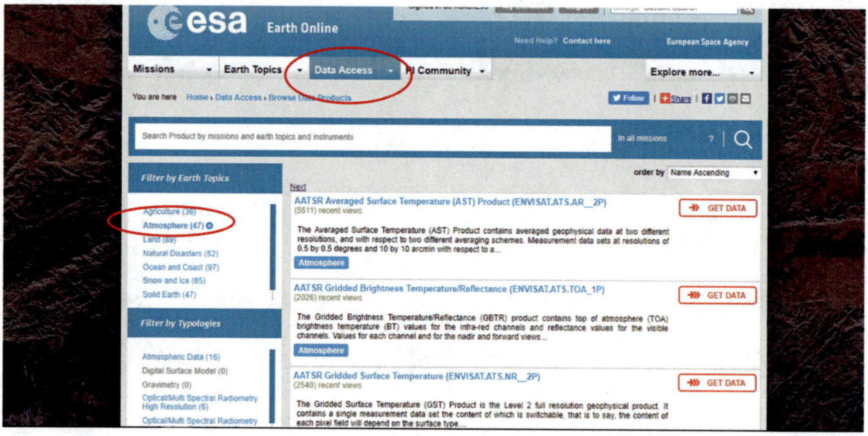

Fig. 2.23 Data search from the EO data. Red circles show the "Data Access" tab and result number for "Atmosphere" category

Step 4. Download the datasets.

The dataset you selected will become available to download after your request is granted by the data host (Fig. 2.25).

To file an access request, click on the "My Earthnet" on the top of the webpage. Information of study area, primary application domain, and a brief executive summary will be needed for the request (Fig. 2.26). The length of waiting time depends on the data categories (e.g. fast registration with immediate access, fast registration with approval, or procedures requiring evaluation).

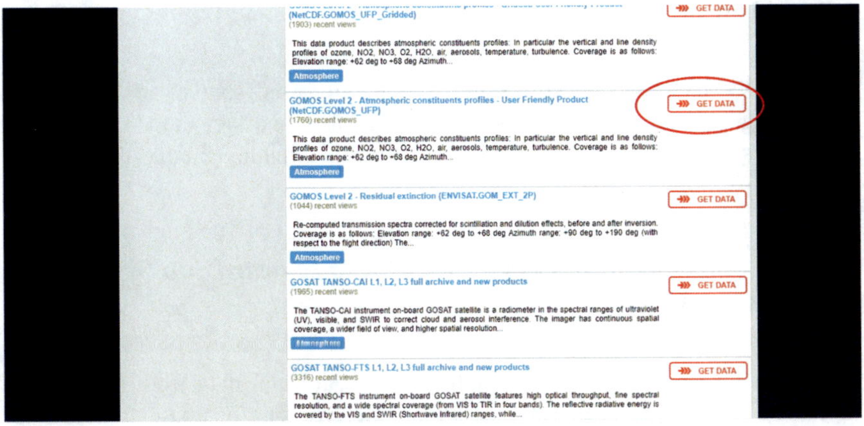

Fig. 2.24 Data selection from the EO data. Red circle shows the "GET DATA" tab

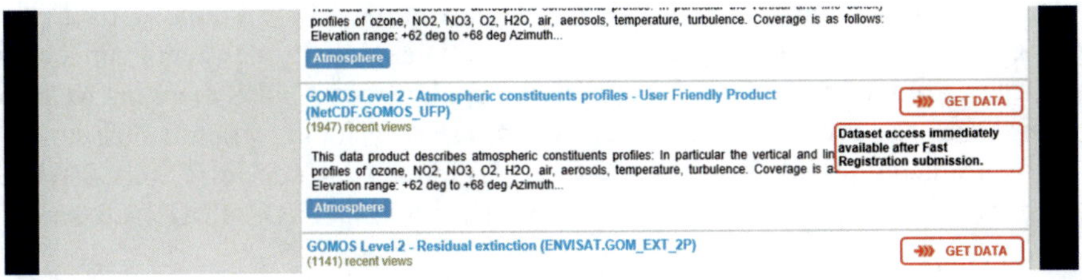

Fig. 2.25 Data access requires Registration submission

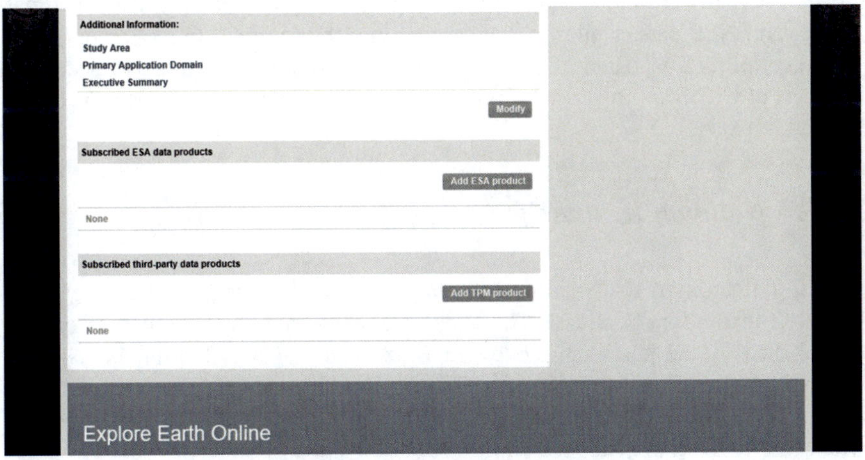

Fig. 2.26 Fast registration to gain data access in EO data

2.8 Additional Sources of Data

Till now, we have introduced six most commonly used sources of satellite and aerial imagery data. Additional sources are available, and they could be useful for researchers to address specific global health and epidemiological questions.

2.8.1 Comprehensive Large Array-Data Stewardship System (CLASS)

CLASS is an electronic library that hosts environmental data from the National Oceanic and Atmospheric Administration (NOAA). The database from CLASS encompasses NOAA and US Department of Defense (DOD) Polar-orbiting Operational Environmental Satellite (POES) data, NOAA's Geostationary Operational Environmental Satellite (GOES) data, and derived data. POES collects data on a variety of land, ocean, and atmospheric conditions globally daily and supports a wide spectrum of environmental monitoring applications. GOES monitors weather events such as storms, tornados and natural disasters including wildfire, dust storms, and volcanic eruption. Other notable CLASS products include Joint Solar Satellite System (JPSS), Sea Surface Temperature data (SST), RADARSAT, and among others.

Though there is a lot of data in CLASS, but it's less user-friendly compared with EE of USGS and the Sentinel Science Data Hub of ESA. But CLASS has developed hardware and software evolution plans for near-term upgrades for climate model and NPP data, while looking further into the future with its Target System Architecture (TSA) (Rank, 2011). The free registration is required to access the datasets of CLASS. (https://www.bou.class.noaa.gov/saa/products/welcome).

2.8.2 National Institute for Space Research (INPE)

INPE, the acronym for National Institute for Space Research in Portuguese, is a research institution in Brazil. The agency hosts a remotely-sensed data catalog, established by the partnership between Brazil and China called the China-Brazil Earth Resources Satellite Program (CBERS). The satellite imagery data are mainly from China-Brazil Earth Resources Satellites 2, 2b and it also includes satellites from USA, UK, India, etc.

The most important feature for INPE database is that the satellite data only covers South America and Africa. The image recorded by the camera are 27 km by width and have 2.7-m spatial resolution. To access the dataset, registration with email address is required as the datasets will be sent to the email address provided. This is the link to access the catalog: http://www.dgi.inpe.br/CDSR/.

2.8.3 Himawari Monitor Data of Japanese Meteorological Agency (JMA)

Himawari-8 is main satellite of JMA to carry out the mission for advanced Himawari Imager (AHI) for improved numerical weather prediction accuracy and enhanced environmental monitoring (Yang et al., 2018). The satellite was launched in October 2014. AHI of JMA provides high spatial—temporal resolution data on PM levels using a vertical-humidity correction method. AHI also shares similar spectral and spatial features as the Advanced Baseline Imager (ABI) that is planned for use in the American GOES-R satellites (Yang et al., 2018).

User registrations is also required to access the data catalog. The dataset can be freely accessible through the website: https://www.eorc.jaxa.jp/ptree/index.html.

2.8.4 The AErosol RObotic NETwork (AERONET)

NASA and PHOTONS (PHOtometrie pour le Traitement Operationnel de Normalisation Satellitaire) established a ground-based remote sensing aerosol network called AERONET (Holben et al., 1998). AERONET provides spectral AOD data around the globe and its data quality can be achieved through AERONET: level 1.0 (unscreened), level 1.5 (cloud screened), and level 2.0 (cloud screened and quality assured). Free data are available through following link: https://aeronet.gsfc.nasa.gov/new_web/data.html.

2.8.5 Bhuvan India Geo-Platform of ISRO

Bhuvan is a platform that integrating remote sensing data from satellites that were launched by India including satellites Hyperspectral, Cartosat, Oceansat and Resourcesat. The mapping service allows users to develop both 2D and 3D representation of earth surface, but most tailored to view India. The imagery datasets include satellite images for more than 300 cities in the country and partly North Indian Ocean, and the resolution of the images can be as small as 1 m.

Registration and log-in is required to access and download the datasets. Outside of India, only a few products are available including Normalized Difference Vegetation Index (NDVI) Global Coverage, CartoDem Version-3R1 for SAARC countries, and Climate products for North Indian Ocean. Here is the website link to access the datasets: https://bhuvan.nrsc.gov.in/bhuvan_links.php.

2.9 Conclusion Remark

Data from all the sources described in this chapter will facilitate research to address pressing medical and health issues by incorporating global and remote sensing data. Such data are particularly valuable to assess environmental factors where there is insufficient monitoring; and they have already been introduced in environmental health research over a decade. In addition to filling in the spatial gap, data from these sources will add time series data to extend the temporal data gap. These remote sensing data provide large scale of monitoring of environment changes over time, such as the observation of vegetation levels in a country over decades. Such long period of observation will provide valuable information of how vegetation coverage change affects human health. Lastly, we have to admit that satellite remote sensing data is still in progress. More research efforts are required to ensure data quality. As many sources of satellite data are publicly available free of charge, more research is possible to test the data quality and its result can be used for improvement. We are confident that the utilization of the RS data will promote the research in global epidemiology and global health.

References

Behnke, J, Mitchell, A, & Ramapriyan, H. (2018). *NASA's earth observing data and information system - Near-term challenges*. In: 9th PV2018 Conference, United Kingdom: Harwell.

Dockery, D. W., Pope, C. A., 3rd, Xu, X., Spengler, J. D., Ware, J. H., Fay, M. E., ... Speizer, F. E. (1993). An association between air pollution and mortality in six U.S. cities. *The New England Journal of Medicine, 329*, 1753–1759.

European Space Agency (ESA). (2014). *Overview: Copernicus monitoring system*. Retrieved from March 4 http://www.esa.int/Our_Activities/Observing_the_Earth/Copernicus/Overview3

Holben, B. N., Eck, T. F., Slutsker, I., Tanre, D., Buis, J. P., Setzer, A., ... Smirnov, A. (1998). AERONET - a federated instrument network and data archive for aerosol characterization. *Remote Sensing of Environment, 66*, 1–16.

Hu, Z. (2009). Spatial analysis of MODIS aerosol optical depth, PM2.5, and chronic coronary heart disease. *International Journal of Health Geographics, 8*, 27.

Hu, Z., & Rao, K. R. (2009). Particulate air pollution and chronic ischemic heart disease in the eastern United States: A county level ecological study using satellite aerosol data. *Environmental Health, 8*, 26.

Lelieveld, J., Evans, J. S., Fnais, M., Giannadaki, D., & Pozzer, A. (2015). The contribution of outdoor air pollution sources to premature mortality on a global scale. *Nature, 525*, 367–371.

Rank, R. (2011). *Comprehensive large array-data stewardship system: Infrastructure and architecture improvements for NPP and GOES-R*. In Seventh Annual Symposium on Future Operational Environmental Satellite Systems, Washington State Convention Center.

Sorek-Hamer, M., Just, A. C., & Kloog, I. (2016). Satellite remote sensing in epidemiological studies. *Current Opinion in Pediatrics, 28*, 228–234.

Takaku, J., & Tadono, T. (2017). *Quality updates of 'Aw3d' global Dsm generated from Alos prism*. In 2017 IEEE International Geoscience and Remote Sensing Symposium (Igarss) (pp. 5666–5669).

Takaku, J., Tadono, T., Tsutsui, K., & Ichikawa, M. (2016). *Validation of 'Aw3d' global Dsm generated from alos prism*. In Xxiii Isprs Congress, Commission Iv. (Vol. 3, pp. 25–31).

Thomson, M. C., Ukawuba, I., Hershey, C. L., Bennett, A., Ceccato, P., Lyon, B., & Dinku, T. (2017). Using rainfall and temperature data in the evaluation of National Malaria Control Programs in Africa. *The American Journal of Tropical Medicine and Hygiene, 97*, 32–45.

United Nations Environment Programme (UNEP). (2018). *Why does UN Environment matter?* Retrieved from https://www.unenvironment.org/about-un-environment/why-does-un-environment-matter

USGS. (2013). *Earth explorer help document*. In USGS (Ed.).

World Health Organization (WHO). (2018). *Ambient (outdoor) air quality and health.* Retrieved from October 1 http://www.who.int/news-room/fact-sheets/detail/ambient-(outdoor)-air-quality-and-health

Yang, F. K., Wang, Y., Tao, J. H., Wang, Z. F., Fan, M., de Leeuw, G., & Chen, L. F. (2018). Preliminary investigation of a new AHI aerosol optical depth (AOD) retrieval algorithm and evaluation with multiple source AOD measurements in China. *Remote Sensing, 10*, 748.

Chapter 3
GIS/GPS-Assisted Probability Sampling in Resource-Limited Settings

Xinguang Chen and Hui Hu

Abstract It is rather challenge to draw probability samples for epidemiology and global health research that involves specific geographic area and resource-limited countries and regions. Based on authors' published work, in this chapter we introduce an innovative probability sampling method using the GIS technology for probability spatial sampling, the GIS and GPS technologies to connect the sampled geographic area with residential houses and residents, and the random digits method to select individual participants. With this method, data requirement and cost are minimized while implementation can be achieve in a short period. Most part of the method has been tested and used in a developing country to sample rural residents, rural-to-urban migrants and urban residents.

Keywords Probability sampling · GIS/GPS technologies · Survey studies · Statistics

3.1 Study Population and Samples

A significant contribution made by statistics to the modern scientific research is the establishment of the concepts of *study population* and *sample*. It is with these two concepts researchers can work with only a small number of participants as a sample selected from the study population, collect data from the sample, and

X. Chen (✉)
Department of Epidemiology, College of Public Health and Health Professions, College of Medicine, University of Florida, Gainesville, FL, USA

Global Health Institute, Wuhan University, Wuhan, China
e-mail: jimax.chen@ufl.edu

H. Hu
Department of Epidemiology, University of Florida, Gainesville, FL, USA
e-mail: huihu@ufl.edu

X. Chen, (Din) D.-G. Chen (eds.), *Statistical Methods for Global Health and Epidemiology*, ICSA Book Series in Statistics,
https://doi.org/10.1007/978-3-030-35260-8_3

derived information from the collected data using statistical methods, and then use the derived information to inference the characteristics of the study population.

When seeing the word "population", most researchers naturally visualize the total number of people living in a country as in demography. In statistics, study population, also known as *target population is* the group of people from which researchers select samples, collect data and conduct analysis to draw scientific conclusions about a specific research question(s). For example, if one wants to study the mortality rate for the United States, all people living in the United States consist of the target population. If one wants to study cigarette smoking among rural-to-urban migrants in China, all Chinese who migrate from rural areas to urban area in China will be the study population. If one want to study the prevalence of HIV infection among men who have sex with men (MSM) in an African country, all MSM in that country will be the target population. If one wants to study the impact of internet use on mental health, all persons who use internet would be the study population.

From the description above, we can see different types of study population. Some study population is *permanent*, such as all the residents in a country that are used to study morbidity, mortality, and access to healthcare; some other populations are *transient*, such as seasonal migrant populations and refuge populations; while some other populations are *conceptual, hidden or virtual*, such MSM, sex works, the internet users, drug dealers. In our society today, we have to pay more attention to medical and health problems among transient, conceptual and hidden populations than the permanent populations because of the increased diversity along with globalization and increased power and freedom for all individuals in every societies (Pieterse, 2015).

3.2 Non-probability Sampling

Sampling is the process by which a pre-determined number of individuals is selected from the target population. Establishment of many sampling methods makes it possible for scientists to collect data from a very small number of individuals selected from a large population, and use the data to understand a research question for the whole population. For example, by collecting data from a sample of approximately 2000 adult residents that are eligible to vote in the United States, a researcher can predict the likelihood of a candidate running for the President Position of the country with high accuracy, usually plus minus 5% of error.

Before establishment of the probability sampling method (detailed in the next section), two methods were used to draw study samples, one being named as *purposeful sampling* and another *convenience sampling*. These methods have been used in research up to now because of their high efficiency and low cost. However, we must be aware that data collected from such samples are not valid to help derive the statistics for the study population.

3.2.1 Purposeful Sampling

Purpose sampling is also known as judgmental sampling. Today, this sampling method is often used in small scale and exploratory studies, such as pilot study to establish a theory or generate a set of hypotheses for a large-scale project. For example, if a researcher wants to examine stress associated with migration for immigrants from another country in the United States, he/she may purposefully selected a number of migrants in different ages and gender with different length of migration in the United States, and assess the levels of stress. Such data will be useful for a researcher to establish study hypothesis, plan for data collection and statistical analysis.

In addition to hypothesis generation, purposeful sampling method is used in selecting participants to conduct *formative studies*, test and evaluate the *feasibility of a large project*; or conduct *pilot, focus-group* studies to establish protocols for data collection and develop measurement instruments and survey questionnaire. For example, if a researcher want to develop a questionnaire to assess HIV risk behaviors among MSM, he/she can select and recruit a small number (2–3) of MSM with different racial/ethnic backgrounds (white, black, Hispanic), educational levels (high school or less, college or more), living in different neighborhoods (urban core, suburb, rural area). He/she will then collect data from these participants through individual or group interview on topics related to HIV, sex, drugs, etc. With information from such focus-group study, researchers may be able to develop a survey questionnaire for a full-scale research.

Advantages for the purposeful sampling method is that it is highly feasible, can be completed in a short period to generate needed data. One big limitation is that data derived from purposeful samples cannot be generalized to the whole study population.

3.2.2 Convenience Sampling

A method more complex than the purposeful sampling is convenience sampling. This method is also known as *accidental* sampling or *natural* sampling. With this method, researchers select participants as sample by considering primarily the feasibility. Such samples are often selected in a convenient location/time where/when eligible participants often pass by. For example, in many psychological studies, researchers set up a booth at the cafeteria, and recruit students who come to there for meals. Market researchers also recruit shoppers at the front gates of a shopping mall to examine people's purchasing behaviors. Medical researchers can recruit patient participants in the waiting area of an outpatient clinic for health service access and utilization research. HIV researchers can sample truck drivers on selected rest areas by a free ways where most drivers take break.

3.3 Probability Sampling

Probability sampling consists of a group of methods that can be used to select a pre-determined number of individuals from the target study population, including simple random sampling, systematic sampling, stratified random sampling, and multilevel/multistage random sampling. These methods have been described in great details in almost all books in statistics, demography and epidemiology, and two of my best reference books are (1) *Survey Methodology* by Groves et al. (2009) and Sampling Techniques by Cochran (1977). Essentially, when using a probability sampling method to select participants from a study population, it will help us achieve the following goals to strengthen a research study:

3.3.1 Know the Probability for Sampling

First of all, probability sampling method will allow researchers to know the probability or chance by which an individual from the study population can be selected. Using simple random sampling method will ensure an equal probability to select any individual from the target population while using other methods will result in varying but still known probabilities for individual participants to be sampled.

3.3.2 Independent Identical Sample Distribution

Second, by using a probability sampling method, selected individual participants in a sample are mutually independent from each other. The selected participants thus follow the sampling distribution. If a sample is selected using the simple random method with the same probability for all individuals, all participants in the sample will follow the independent and identical distribution, often abbreviated as *i.i.d, iid or IID*. Therefore, data collected from a probability sample can be analyzed using most statistical methods that are based on random samples.

3.3.3 Generalizability to the Study Population

Last, results derived from a probability sample can be generalized to the whole study population with quantified confidence—which is the ultimate goal for researchers to investigate medical and health issues with a global impact. In another word, probability sample is a prerequisite to ensure *external validity* of a research study.

3.4 Challenges to the Classic Probability Sampling Methods and Alternatives

Although the advantages for a probability sample are well known, a careful investigation of the published research studies, particularly journals with original articles that are primarily based on survey data, including the very prestigious peer-reviewed journals, such as *Journal of Acquired Immune Deficiency Syndrome* and *AIDS and Behavior*, less than 10% of them used a probability sampling method for participant selection (Chen et al., 2018). There are a number of factors that may have prevented researchers from using probability sampling method to select participants in their research studies. In this chapter, we described three major barriers, including (1) the lack of new methods to overcome difficulties associated with technological development, (2) difficulties in defining a study population, and (3) timing—obtain the results in short period.

3.4.1 Methodology Barriers

Lack of appropriate methods appears to be the first barrier that prevent scientists to use probability sampling methods (Chen et al., 2015; Landry & Shen, 2005). For example, many probability sampling methods based on landline telephone using digital dialing have been well-established and widely used in research to select sample (Cochran, 1977; Kish, 1965). Despite the high feasibility and efficiency, this category of methods has several limitations. Using telephone number for sampling will miss the households that do not have a landline telephone. In the United States, approximately 3–5% of the households without a landline phone will be missed. People in these households are more likely to be low in socioeconomic status and/or racial/ethnic minorities with more medical and health problems, such as overweigh and obese, cardiovascular diseases, violence, and drug use (Groves et al., 2009).

More challenging than the incomplete coverage to the telephone number-based digital dialing method is the replacement of landline telephone with numerous new communication technologies, including smart phone, internet and mass media. Few people now still use a landline telephone for communication, totally ruling out of the possibility to randomly select phone numbers and contact the individuals by calling them one by one. Although telephone numbers are still used to date, the telephone is moving with people, not fixing in one physical location. Also, persons with more than one phone are common, preventing researchers from directly using such phone numbers to build the sampling frame (Chen et al., 2018).

3.4.2 Hard-to-Reach or Hidden Populations

A prerequisite for probability sampling is that the study population can be defined operationally for enumeration to construct the sampling frame. However, in modern survey studies, a number of study populations can be described conceptually but cannot be defined operationally. Typical examples include, but are not limited to: Illegal immigrants, mobile populations such as seasonal workers in the United States from Mexico, rural migrants working in urban cities in China, male and female sex works, lesbian, gay, bisexual and transgender populations, drug dealers, substance users, and persons living with HIV.

In survey studies, we consider this type of population as hard-to-reach or hidden populations. Although these populations can be defined conceptually, no sampling frame can be established for probability sampling because we simply do not know the total number of these population and exactly where they are. Even if we know the total number of this population and can identify each of them to construct a sampling frame, we do not know if we can reach the sampled individuals since it is very hard if not impossible to know where they live.

3.4.3 Urgency to Know Study Results

As we all know that it will take time to complete a study if participants are selected using a probability sampling method, but addressing many urgent medical and health issues requires timely data (Heeringa & O'Muircheartaigh, 2010). The most well-known examples that need quick data include epidemiological studies of outbreaks and vaccination of infectious diseases, such as Zika (Boeuf, Drummer, Richards, Scoullar, & Beeson, 2016), severe acute respiratory syndrome (SARS) (Tong, 2005), Ebola (Weyer, Grobbelaar, & Blumberg, 2015), and HIV/AIDS. New approaches have been attempted for quick sampling without using a validated sampling frame. Methods often used in reported studies include the capture-recapture method derived from agriculture and wild life studies (Tilling, 2001); the venue-day-time sampling, where participants are selected from locations within a time range when participants are often present (Mansergh et al., 2006); and respondent-driving sampling (RDS), in which study participants are selected by starting with a few seed participants to nominate and recruit others within their network connections (Heckathorn, 1997, 2002).

Although these methods allow for timely sampling of study participants, data collected from these types of samples cannot be analyzed using the conventional statistical methods due to a number of limitations inherited with the methods. For example, in both venue-day-time method and RDS, selected participants are nested with each other, violating the requirement of identical and independent distribution (IID) for statistical analysis; while data from the capture-recapture must be analyzed using method specifically devised for the sampling methods, mostly for closed population. In addition, despite rigorous efforts to improve these alternative methods, the validity of these methods in ensuring probability and representative samples remains unclear.

3.4.4 Application of GIS/GPS Technologies in Probability Sampling

Advancement in geographic information systems (GIS) and global positioning systems (GPS) have encouraged researchers to develop new probabilistic sampling methods with adequate geographic and population coverage and minimal data requirements and can be complete in a short period (Chen et al., 2015; Galway et al., 2012; Landry & Shen, 2005; Shannon, Hutson, Kolbe, Stringer, & Haines, 2012). A number of GIS/GPS-assisted methods have been developed for probability sampling to deal with specific settings, such as sampling mobile or migrant populations (Chen et al., 2015; Landry & Shen, 2005), selecting participants in remote and rural areas (Escamilla et al., 2014; Haenssgen, 2015; Kondo, Bream, Barg, & Branas, 2014; Wampler, Rediske, & Molla, 2013) and other special conditions (Galway et al., 2012; Murray, O'Green, & McDaniel, 2003).

A thorough review of the published sampling method studies reveals that GIS/GPS-assisted sampling methods can be characterized as the *geographically stratified multi-stage sampling*. Using this approach in sampling, a seven-step procedure must be followed:

1. Define the targeted population and geographic area you want to study,
2. Using GIS data to construct the primary sampling frame (PSF) and define residential area to determine the primary sampling units (PSUs),
3. Randomly select PSU on computer with a pre-determined probabilistic scheme (e.g., simple random, proportion to or stratified by population density),
4. Randomly select households from each sampled PSU through random routes, random section, or other methods; and construct the secondary sampling frame (SSF) by enumerating the selected households,
5. Select a pre-determined number of participants randomly from each sampled SSF,
6. Estimate sample weights using information from the previous steps across all sampling stages,
7. Compute descriptive statistics, such as mean, standard deviation, proportion, rate and ratios for the study population, considering the sample design used in participant selection and finalized sampling weights.

3.5 Challenges to the Existing GIS/GPS-Assisted Probability Sampling Methods

Sampling methods building upon the GIS/GPS technologies bring new hope for scientists to apply probability sampling method in modern global health and epidemiology. However, a careful review of the reported methods for probability sampling assisted by GIS/GPS technologies have several limitations that have to be addressed, such as pre-determination of sample size, which caused a study project to be terminated earlier than planned (Landry & Shen, 2005); determination of residential area from non-residential housing; method for stratification, and estimation of geographic sampling weights.

3.5.1 Challenges to Determine Sample Size Before Sampling

Determination of sample size is critical for planning a research project. However, with the reported GIS/GPS-assisted sampling method, researchers cannot determine the sample size until the sampling procedure is completed. This is because a GIS/GPS-assisted sampling method often consists of two interrelated steps: Sampling geographic area first and then sampling households and individual participants in the sampled geographic areas. Sample size would be easy to determine for a study that draws geographic samples only. However, it is not possible to pre-determine exactly how many persons in the study population in a randomly selected geographic area before the area is selected and fully enumerated.

One method attempted by researchers is to enumerate all of them in a randomly selected geographic area to construct the SSF, assuming an average number of participants per geographic units. This method has been proven infeasible for a study involves high and large variation in population density, complex residential arrangement, and the presence of high-rise multi-function buildings in selected geographic areas (Landry & Shen, 2005). For example, the chance to select a geographic area with high-rise building with several hundreds of residents would not be small in a modern city. However, it will be very costly and time-consuming to enumerate a randomly selected geographic area with high-rise residential building with a large number of residents.

3.5.2 Challenges to Distinguishing Residential from Non-residential Housing

To correctly estimate sampling weights, researchers must be able to distinguish between residential housing and non-residential housing. Only the geographic area with residential housing is needed to estimate sampling weights. Methods attempted for distinguishing the two have proven to be time-consuming. For example, in a previous study, we printed out the satellite imagery maps for all sampled geographic areas, worked together with local people to mark out the areas with residential housing in the sampled geographic area, and re-computed the residential areas and used in estimating sample weights. This method is not only time-consuming but also error prone, underscoring the need for better approaches (Chen et al., 2015).

Recent development in new methods provides tools to recognize visually or digitally the residential area/housing with widely available aerial imagery data (Chang et al., 2009; Escamilla et al., 2014; Haenssgen, 2015; Pearson, Rzotkiewicz, & Zwickle, 2015; Wampler et al., 2013). These methods are often computerized, thus fast and inexpensive, and can be used in diverse settings. With this approach, researchers can involve resource-limited countries for large scale international and global project for epidemiological research. For example, in study to separate the residential houses from other types of house using aerial images, Pearson et al. (2015) corrected identified 93.3% of 175 households that are residential. Although the error rate of 6.7% is low, this study was conducted in pastoral area with a semi-nomadic residential patterns, a setting relatively easy for random sampling than in the more complex residential arrangements in urban settings. Methods are needed to draw probability samples in more complex settings.

3.5.3 Challenges Due to Heterogeneity in Population Density

A third challenges for GIS/GPS-assisted sampling is that we need to deal with the large heterogeneity in population density in addition to the complex residential arrangement. The classic stratification could be a method to deal with this issue. In GIS/GPS-assisted sample, a grid network system is used to divide the geographic areas of the target population into mutually exclusive cells, named as *geounits*. If population data for individual jurisdictions are available, a stratified method can be used to randomly sample geounits as we used in our previous research (Chen et al., 2015). However, population data by jurisdiction may not always be available in resource-limited and low- and middle-income countries. Therefore, it would be challenge to draw random samples with the available GIS/GPS-assisted sampling methods.

Recently, people start to use night-time satellite images as a measure of population density but this approach appears to not useful for rural areas and resources-limited countries/places, and countries/areas that do not depend on electricity for daily activities (Schneider, Friedl, & Potere, 2009). In order to use GIS/GPS-assisted sampling method to conduct global health research, additional improvements have to be made over the current methods to suitable for many different conditions.

3.5.4 Challenges to Determine the Geographic Sample Weights

A last but not least challenge is to determine the geographic sample weights. This sound ridiculous at the beginning since the geographic sample weight would be an inverse of the geographic sampling ratio. The challenge stemmed from the fact that although conceptually there is a clear difference between residential areas and non-residential areas; but in fact it is very hard if not impossible to determine them for sampling. This is because there is not clear and scientifically accepted boundaries between residential and non-residential areas and a lack of information on the number of residents living in a sampled geographic area at a specific date and time (Kondo et al., 2014; Landry & Shen, 2005; Shannon et al., 2012).

To illustrate the challenge, Fig. 3.1 shows a sampled geographic area marked by the red box with four households A, B, C and D. In this case, how can we separate the residential areas from non-residential areas? The biggest challenge is how to divide the large blank space between the school (a non-residential house) and the four residential houses.

In this chapter, we will introduce an integrative GIS/GPS-assisted sampling methods with techniques to overcome almost all of the key challenges described above and with potential to incorporate new development in technology in the future. This method is based our previous research, including GIS/GPS-assisted sampling in different articles (Chen et al., 2015, 2018; Chen & Hu, 2018; Heeringa, 2018).

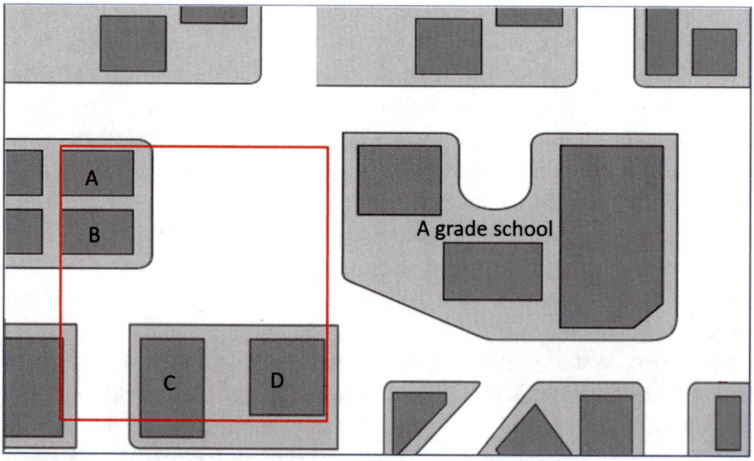

Fig. 3.1 Difficulties in determination of the residential geographic areas. Red square: A sampled geographic area with households A, B, C, D and a school nearby in a street block

3.6 GIS/GPS Assisted Multi-stage Probability Sampling

We developed the Integrative Multi-Stage GIS/GPS-Assisted Probability Sampling Method based on our previous studies and others as summarized in Sect. 3.5. The purpose is to provide a cost-effective sampling method with high feasibility in both developed and resource-limited settings for global health research. We will introduce the method in several steps after an overall summary.

3.6.1 *Introduction to the Method*

The Integrative GIS/GPS-assisted multi-stage probability sampling method is summarized in Fig. 3.2. Using this method to draw probability samples must go through four technically different stages after preparation. Before sampling, researchers will make preparations, including computer and GIS software (e.g., ArcGIS or any other software that contain geographic data and can process geographic information), collecting data from local sources that are available and useful for sampling, including aerial imagery data, updated local maps, and total population data. Effort should also be used to identify one or two residents in the study area who are familiar with all the streets and households and have time and be willing to assist.

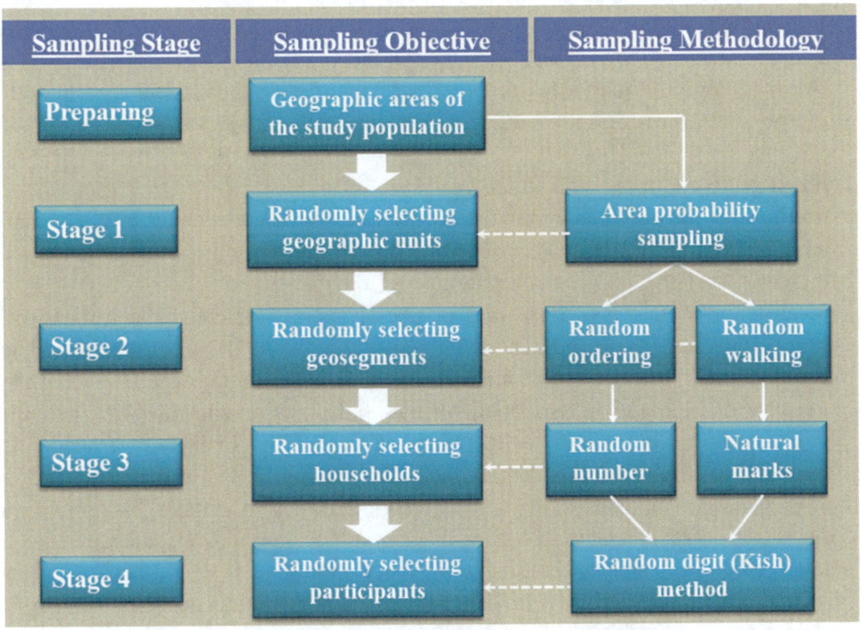

Fig. 3.2 Integrative Four-stage GIS/GPS-assisted probability sampling

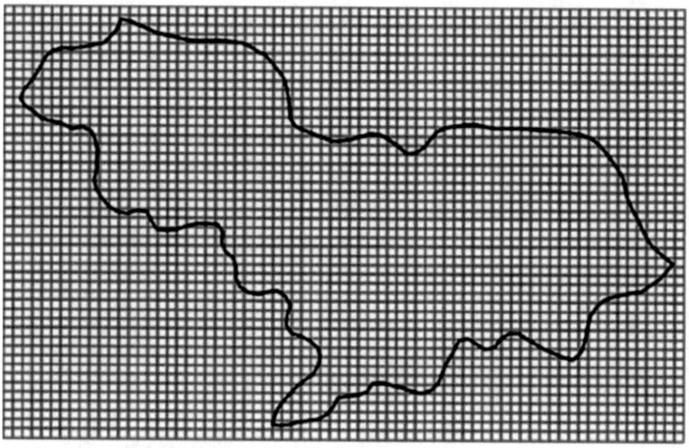

Fig. 3.3 Spatial sampling using a grid network system to divide the targeted study are within the judiciary boundary into mutually exclusive geounits

3.6.2 Stage 1 Sampling: Random Selection of Geographic Units

This stage is also known as spatial sampling. The goal is to generate a set of randomly selected geographic units (geounits for short) with residential housing. Geographic data for locations where the study population resides (often by country or jurisdictions within a country) can be obtained from different sources, mostly free of charge, such as Google Maps and OpenStreetMap (Haklay & Weber, 2008).

After reading the map into computer, we must divide the total areas where the study population reside into mutually exclusive cells, named as geographic units for further sampling. This spatial sampling process is often realized by creating and laying a grid system over the target area (Fig. 3.3).

In Fig. 3.3, the geounits within the geographic boundaries consist of the primary sampling frame (PSF). It is from the PSF, a pre-determined number of geounits will be randomly selected also on computer.

One important task is to determine the size of a geounit to create the grid network system. If the size of a geounit is too large, it will cover a lot of households, which may be beyond our capacity to enumerate all of them for sampling. On the contrary, if the size of a geounit is too small, it may end up with a lot of blank geounits without even one household, or reducing the probability to include a residential household. In traditional spatial sampling, the geounit size A was determined by sampling ratio. For example, if a research determines to sample 10 geounits to cover 0.01% (equivalent to 10^{-4}) of a geographic area with a total area size of 900,000 (9×10^5) km^2, the area size for individual geounit would be A = 9 km^2 ($9 \times 10^5 \times 10^{-4}/10$). A grid with side length = 3 km can thus be used to create the grid network and used to divide the total geographic areas for sampling.

However, more complex approaches are needed to draw geographic samples for population-based survey studies, because A is determined not by sampling ratio but by the probability to include an appropriate number of households and eligible persons for sampling. There is no shortcut to determine the appropriate grid size A. We recommend a pilot study to determine the size by considering two important factors:

1. Density of the study population in the targeted area, and
2. Number of subjects to be recruited from each selected geounit.

For example, when conducting a large-scale survey study targeting the rural-to-urban migrants temporarily living in Wuhan, China, we determined the area size $A = 100 \times 100$ m to ensure 20 eligible participants per geounit. This number was determined through intensive pilot tests in the field. During the pilot study, we used different area size being measured manually using tape rulers and/laser scales in a number of typical regions within the city. We then count the numbers of households and associated with the various sizes of A. Results from our pilot indicated that an area size of $A = 100 \times 100$ m has approximately 80% probability to cover an adequate number of households, ensuring at least 20 subjects per geounit in a city like Wuhan (Chen et al., 2015).

After geounit size A is determine, and the maps of the target population is input into computer, a grid network with size A is created, and overlay it onto the targeted area as having showed in Fig. 3.3. Two methods used for grid network creation and sampling are (1) geographic coordinate systems-based method and (2) side length-based method. Results from the two methods are rather similar if the targeted area is relative small (such as a city, a state with a relative small geographic areas); but the second method is relatively easy to implement. For studies involving very large geographic areas like a very large countries (e.g., Russia, Canada, China, or the United States), multi-countries, continents, or the globe, grid length (distance) defined through an appropriate projection system should be selected.

After the targeted area is divided into mutually exclusive geounits and PSF is constructed with these geounits, a pre-determined number of geounits are then randomly selected from the PSF. Considering large variations in population density across the geographic area, a stratified strategy is thus used to sample geounits with more geounits being allocated to areas with higher population density, following an optimum allocation approach to enhance work efficiency (Cochran, 1977). Also, geounits generated using the grid network have a large chance to cover non-residential areas such as lakes, bridges, highways, and commercial buildings. To overcome this problem and to enhance feasibility while maintaining a probabilistic sampling process, we devised a semi-automatic, computer-assisted, stepwise algorithm with no replacement procedure for implementing the geounit sampling protocol (Fig. 3.4). R codes for the semi-auto procedure is added at the end of this chapter.

With PSF and the automatic algorithm, an immediate question is: How many geounits G are to be sampled? Obviously, G depends on the total sample size N and the average number of persons M per geounit to be sampled. No method has been established to determine G and M (Kondo et al., 2014; Landry & Shen, 2005).

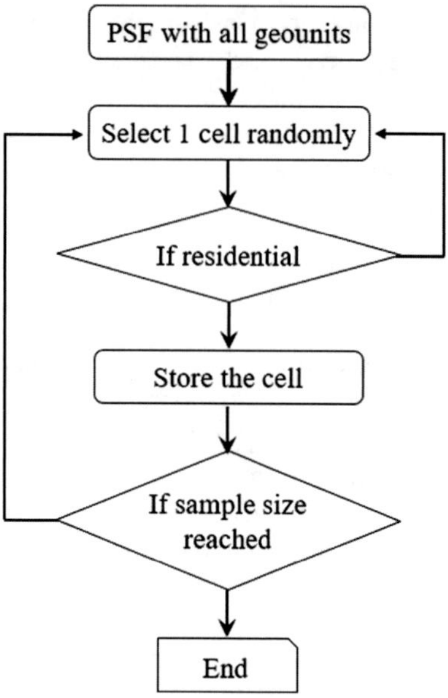

Fig. 3.4 Algorithm for automatic geounit sampling

To overcome this challenge, we proposed to use the same M for all geounits from our own research (Chen et al., 2015, 2018). With our method, researchers will first estimate sample size N through power analysis; and then G can be calculated using the following formula, allowing the M varying from 15 to 25:

$$G = N/M \tag{3.1}$$

For example, if a researcher plan to draw a sample of N = 800 and pilot studies indicate that it is feasible and effective to draw, on average, 20 persons per geounit. Using Eq. 3.1, the number of geounits to be selected: $G = 800/20 = 40$. If you plan to draw 25 subjects per geounits: $G = 800/25 = 32$. Readers can calculate G for M=15. Statistically, a sample selected with smaller number of M and large number of G will be closer to a simple random sample. Experience from our experiences suggest that $M \leq 20$ and $G \leq 20$ can satisfy most survey studies (Chen et al., 2015).

3.6.3 Stage 2 and 3: Random Selection of Geographic Segments and Households

After completion of geographic unit sampling in Stage 1, data for each geounit, including maps, and related information must be uploaded to a GPS receiver. Theoretically any GPS receiver can be used as long as it has the following two functions:

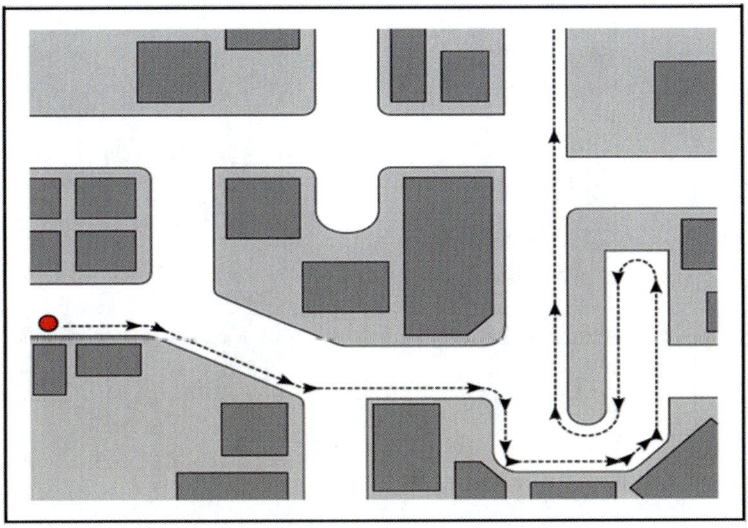

Fig. 3.5 Selection of a geographic segment through random walk. (Source: Bauer J. (2014). Selection error of random route samples *Sociological methods and research* (43)3: 519–544)

1. Upload selected maps for use to guide travel, drive and walk, and
2. Tracking function to mark a geographic area.

We used the GPS receiver (Garmin Oregon 450, Garmin, Ltd) in our previous research.

With the sampled geounits loaded to a GPS receiver, the next stage is to select a segment from each selected geounit and prepare for household selection. Since all geounits are randomly selected, the eligible participants for some households could be greater than M. In this case, we need to select a segment within the selected geounits to have, on average, M subjects.

To avoid bias in segment selection, one method named as *Random Walk* has been widely used (Fig. 3.5). With this method, after a geounit is selected and a map is prepared. Data collectors will locate a start point, often the main entrance to the geounit (like the red dot in Fig. 3.5). Data collector will then start enumerate and recruit participants following the natural paths of the street. The recruitment stops till the pre-determined M participants are recruited.

Research studies have showed that this method does not warrant unbiased sample even with strict instructions in written that are well followed by the data collector (Bauer, 2016). To overcome this limitation, we devised a method named as *Random Ordering method* (Fig. 3.6).

In this method, a set of numbers are randomly casted to the selected geographic unit as showing in the figure. Data collectors will then arrange the households using the number, from small to large, the data collectors then start recruiting participants from the household number 1, then number 2, all the way till the pre-determined

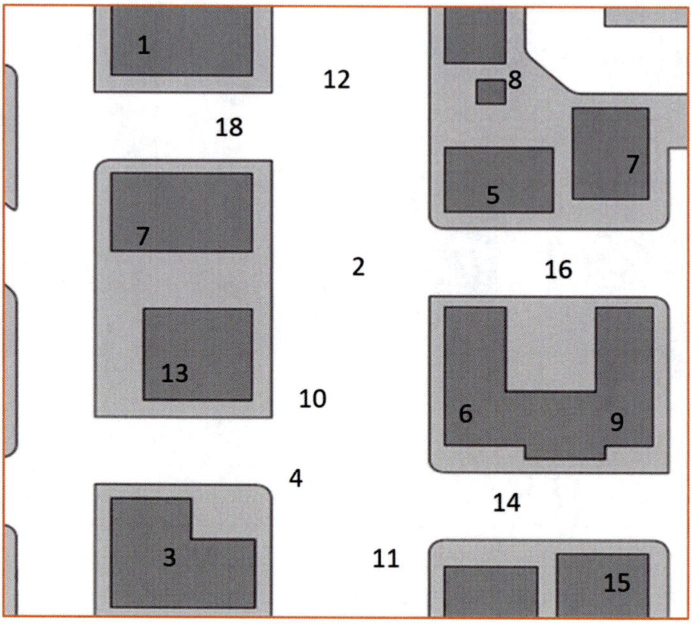

Fig. 3.6 Selection of a geographic segment through random ordering. (Source: Derived from Chen and Hu (2018). *Journal of survey statistics and methodology (2018)5: 182–85*)

number of subjects M is reached. The random numbering process can be achieved either manually or on computer.

3.6.4 *Stage 4: Random Selection of Participants from Households*

In this last step of GIS/GPS-assisted sampling, data collectors will gain access to individual households following either the Random Walk approach or Random Ordering approach. For each household, data collector will first list all individuals in the household and identify the number of eligible individuals. The list of eligible individuals of a household will consist of the secondary sampling frame (SSF) from which individual participants are to be selected.

To ensure independence, only one subject per household will be sampled. For studies involve both male and female, the criterion of *one person per gender per household* can be applied. If only one person is eligible (true in most cases), this person will be included. If more than one person in one household is eligible for participation, one person will be selected randomly using devised sampling methods. The method widely used for sampling individuals from a household is the Kish Table (Kish, 1949).

3.6.5 *Complementary Data Collection*

After completion of household enumeration, participant recruitment and survey data collection for each geounit, data collectors must collect the following complementary information for later use to calculate refusal rate, sampling rate, and sample weights.

1. Data on actual geounit area size Ag for g^{th} geounit. This is the actual area size occupied by the household from which all M participants are recruited. Ag can be determined using GPS receiver recorded tracking data;
2. Total number of households T_g on the selected geounit;
3. Total number of households H_g from which participants are selected;
4. The number of households and the number of eligible subjects who refused to participate.

3.7 Methods to Determine Residential Areas

As we mentioned early in this chapter, the true residential area is conceptually clear but operationally hard to determine as indicated in previous research studies (Kondo et al., 2014; Shannon et al., 2012). Without knowing the true residential area, the geographic and overall sample weight cannot be determined. To overcome this challenge, we have devised two methods for practical use in different settings

3.7.1 *Method 1. Estimate Residential Area with Collected Data*

After completion of sampling and data collection, we will have data on A_g = actual geounit area size for the gth sampled geounit (g = 1,2,...,G). With this data, the total area of G geounits from which the study participants are sampled $B = \sum_g A_g$.

Let R=the total residential area to be estimated, P=total population known to be reside in the targeted area (a district, city, state or a country), Q=the total population covered by all G geounits, which can be estimated by summing up Q_g—the total population covered by g^{th} geounit (see the previous section on Complementary Data Collection).

With both B and Q calculated with data collected from randomly selected G geounits during the sampling, subject recruitment and survey delivery, if G is adequately large (i.e., 20 or more), the ratio of the two will provide an unbiased and reliable estimate of the true ratio of R over P, or mathematically we have:

$$\frac{R}{P} \approx \frac{B}{Q}, \tag{3.2}$$

Therefore the estimated true residential area will be:

$$R = P \times B/Q \tag{3.3}$$

This estimation method relies on the assumption that households in a sampled geounit are associated only with that geounit. In practice, this can be achieved by carefully determine the appropriate grid size for grid network construction often through intensive pilot studies as reported in our previous research (Chen et al., 2015).

3.7.2 *Method 2. Estimate Residential Area with Monte Carlo Method*

To use Method 1 described in the previous part, we need data on total population for the targeted areas, which may not be available in resource-limited countries. To overcome this limitation, we devised another approach to estimate *R* without population data *P*—a Monte Carlo method (Mathews, 1972; Metropolis & Ulam, 1949). In this method, we first obtain the total geographic area size *D* using many GIS software packages. After a map of the targeted area is uploaded to a computer, a large number of *n* points (i.e., several hundred) are randomly casted to the total geographic area. After the points are casted, we will then count the number of points falling in residential areas and non-residential areas.

Let n_r= all points falling on residential areas and n_{nr}= all points falling on non-residential areas, then $n = n_r + n_{nr}$. Since all *n* points are randomly selected, n/n_r provides an unbiased estimate of *R*/*D*. We can easily derive the true residential area *R* using the following equation:

$$R = \frac{n_r}{n_r + n_{nr}} D \tag{3.4}$$

The Monte Carlo method can be completed on computer with aerial imagery maps. To support practical application of this method, R codes to implement this method is also added to the Appendix at the end of this chapter.

3.8 Estimate of Sample Weights

Sample weights are essential for this 4-stage GIS/GPS-assisted sampling method that connecting space with households and individual persons. We proposed the following formula to computer sample weights following the principles for stratified, multistage, and disproportionate probability sampling (Cochran, 1977; Groves et al., 2009; Kish, 1965):

$$W_i = W_g \times W_{gh} \times W_{ghi} \tag{3.5}$$

where

W_i is the sample weight for subject i.

W_g is the geographic sample weight for gth geounit, and it is estimated with R/A_g, where R represents the residential area size (see the two methods to estimate R in Sect. 3.7), and $A_g$is the area size of geounit g.

W_{gh} is the sample weight for household h in geounit g and is computed as T_g/H_g, where T_g is the total number of households in geounit g and $H_g$is the number of households actually sampled in geounit g.

W_{ghi} represents sample weight for individual subject i from household h within geounit g. It equals N_{gh}/n_{gh}, where N_{gh} = total number of eligible persons in household h within geounit g, and n_{gh} = the number of persons sampled from the eligible persons in household h, $n = 1, 2, \ldots, H_g$. If only one person is selected per household, $n_{gh} = 1$. In this case, $W_{ghi} = N_{gi}$.

With the complex design, non-conventional statistical methods are needed to account for variance inflation due to weights and the design effect or correlation among subjects from the same geounit/households. Therefore, when analyzing data collected using this GIS/GPS-assisted sampling design, special statistical methods must be considered, such as the mixed-effects for continuous outcome variables and the generalized linear mixed-effects methods for binary outcome.

3.9 Practical Test of the Method in an NIH Funded Project

We tested the integrative GIS/GPS-assisted sampling method in Wuhan, China when conducting an NIH funded project (R01 MH086322, PI: Chen X) to investigate the relationship between social capital and HIV risk behaviors among rural-to-urban migrants. Wuhan is the capital of Hubei Province with a total population of approximately 10 million and per capita GDP of $12,708 and a large number of rural-top-urban migrants (Statistical Bureau of Wuhan 2012). The field work for sampling and data collection was completed during 2012–2014.

To address the goal of the project, in addition to migrants, non-migrant residents in rural areas from where these migrants come from as well as non-migrant residents in urban area where these migrants live and work were included. Given the fact that many rural migrants do not have a permanent residence in the city and are scattered over almost all areas within the city, we decided to use the GIS/GPS-assisted methodology to select probability samples.

Figure 3.7 illustrates the sampling procedure. The top panel indicates the location of Wuhan within China. In Wuhan, the dark green in the center is the city, and the five bands with 5 km width per band around the city is the rural areas included for sampling. The shortest radius is 50 km and the largest radius is 75 km.

Fig. 3.7 Integrative 4-stage GIS/GPS-assisted sampling

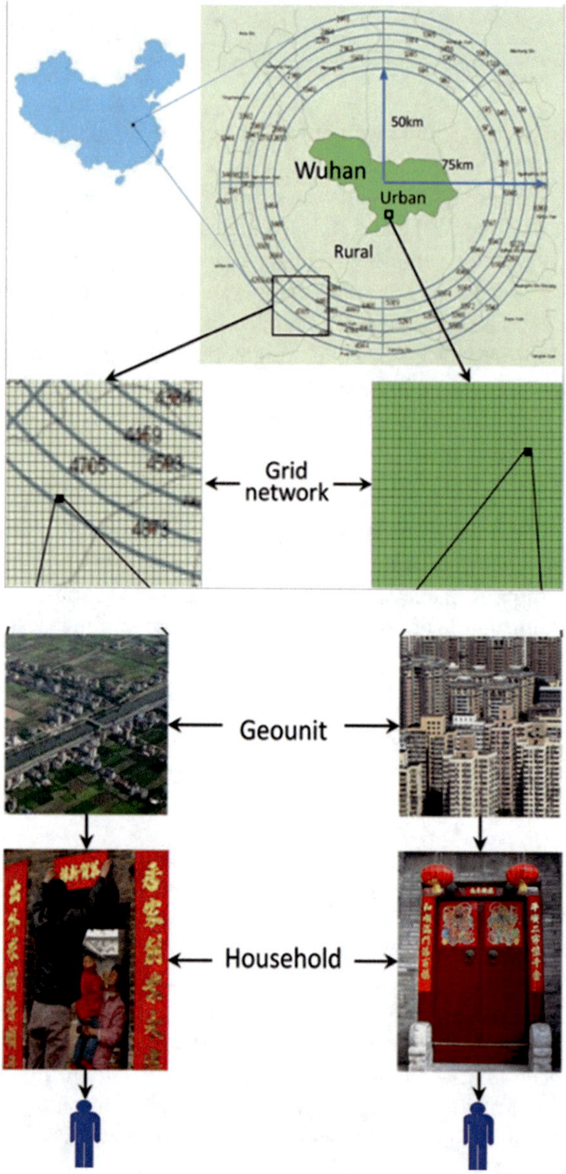

3.9.1 Geographic Sampling Frame and Geounits

Following the procedure described in this study chapter, a district boundary file of Wuhan was obtained using the ArcGIS. Based on pilot studies for field work efficiency, a grid-system with 100 × 100 m cells was created for the urban area and a grid-system with 1 × 1 km was created for rural areas to divide the corresponding

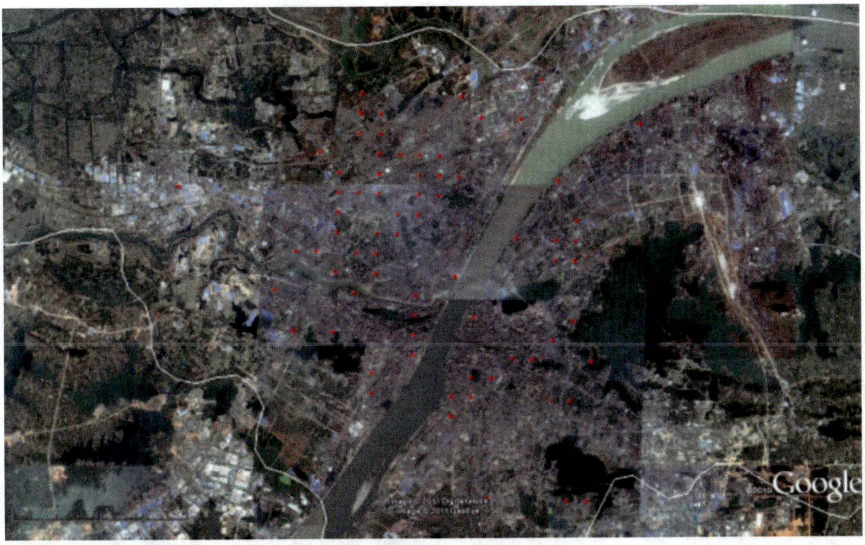

Fig. 3.8 Distribution of the sampled geounits in Wuhan, China

large geographic areas into thousands of small and mutually exclusive cells. These cells were the geounits used to construct the PSF for further sampling.

To determine G, the number of geounits to be samples, we first determined the sample size. According to the study aims and based on results from statistical power analysis, we set N = 1200 subject per group. For sampling in urban area, we set M = 20, the number of subjects to be sampled from each geounit. Using Equation x, G = 1200/20 = 60. This means a total of 60 geounits must be selected from the PSF of Wuhan city. In the field work, data collectors went to each of the 60 randomly selected geounits to recruit the 1200 rural migrants. For effective comparison, the same number of urban residents were also recruited from these geounits to minimize differences in neighborhood conditions. Figure 3.8 showed the distribution of the sampled geounits in Wuhan using a satellite imagery map.

For rural areas, considering the high traveling cost and low feasibility, we set M = 30. With the pre-determined sample size of 1200, G = 1200/30 = 40. Our data collectors travel to each of these 40 randomly selected rural sites to recruit participants and delivery the survey. The field work was very carefully planned such that the subject recruitment and data collection for one site can be completed in one full workday.

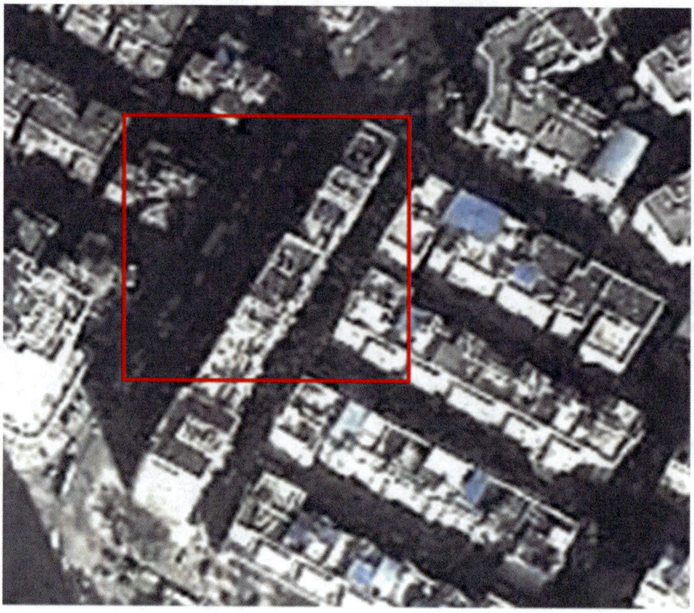

Fig. 3.9 A typical geounit (red square with 100 × 100 m) randomly selected in urban areas with residential houses

3.9.2 *Sampling Geographic Segments, Households and Participants*

The appearance of a sample geounit for rural area can be seen clearly in Fig. 3.7. But a similar geounit for urban area in Fig. 3.7 cannot be directly used for further sampling. Figure 3.9 shows a typical geounit for urban area (included by the red square with the size of 100 × 100 m) we selected in Wuhan for our project. To sample 20 participants in urban area, we used the Random Walk method to select geographic segment in a selected geounit—that is to first identify a main entrance into the selected geounit, starting recruit from the first household on the entrance, and move along the natural path till the required number of participants are reached. We recruited one person per gender per households. For households with more than on eligible subjects, Kish Table was used to select one. When reach to the end of a street, we set the rule to turn right and continue the recruitment process. After completion of recruitment for a geounit, a data collector will collect all the complementary data. In addition to the tracking the area where the households were sampled, the data collector sketched a map showing the location. This map is very useful for accurate determination of the residential area after sampling and data collection.

As an illustration, results from our study indicated that the selected 60 sampled geounits covered 12,016 households in Wuhan. Of these households, 1251 with rural migrants were available and agreed to participate at the time of data collection. A total of 1310 participants were recruited from these households with one participant per gender per household. The total number of households per geounit varied from 30 in least populated areas to 1600 in the most populated areas with a median [quartile 1, quartile 3] of 100 [50, 300] and mean (SD) = 200 (242). The number of households agreed to participate per geounit varied from 12 to 40 with median [quartile 1, quartile 3] of 20 [18, 24] and mean (SD) of 21 (6).

As a verification of the sampling method, applying this method in the study conducted in 2012–2014, we estimated that approximately 58,000 [95% CI: 47000, 68,000] rural-to-urban migrants in Wuhan were MSM with 3650 [95% CI: 2960, 4282] being tested HIV positive (Chen et al., 2015). While official surveillance data from Wuhan indicated that a total of 3408 (primarily MSM) persons living with HIV in 2015 (Wuhan Center for Disease Prevention and Control (CDC) 2016). The observed result is within the estimated 95% CI and the relatively small difference provides some evidence supporting the validity of our method.

Segment and household sampling in rural area are often simpler because each geounit often cover total a complete or a large part of a village. In field work, a whole village was often selected and participants were then selected randomly from individual households.

3.9.3 Determination of Residential Area with Imagery Data and GPS-Tracking File

The residential area can be estimated using the imagery map with the GPS tracking data. Figure 3.10 is a typical example from our study in Wuhan. The red square indicates the sampled geounit, and the yellow trace indicates the order in which households were approached with participants selected. It is worth noting that we started the recruitment outside of the sampling region since there were also migrants on the street. Here the red square serves like an explorer to find migrants. With the map, we determined the residential areas occupied by the households using rectangles (yellow colored) with the line going through half way between the sampled and non-sampled households. The area size can then be correctly calculated either manually or on computer using the actual map scale.

3.10 Strengths and Recommendation

The integrative 4-stage GIS/GPS-assisted probability sampling method introduced in this chapter provides a most updated method for use in different settings to select probability samples for high quality research. It is critical to understanding the strengths of the method and pay attention to key steps in applying the method.

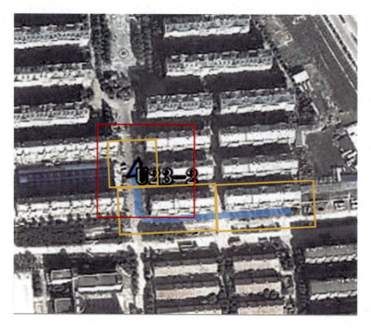

Fig. 3.10 Determination of the residential area from which the households and participants were sampled

3.10.1 Strengths

The integrative GIS/GPS-assisted probability sampling method described in this chapter is based on sound theories for both population and geographic sampling. A major advantage of this method is that it has a minimum data requirement, therefore is particularly useful for global health research to include participating countries and regions with little or even no preliminary data supporting probability sampling or for research studies to access hard-to-reach or hidden populations, such as sex workers, illegal migrants, people living with HIV, etc.

In addition to its high feasibility, researchers can employ the conventionally used stratified sampling strategies in the sampling procedure to optimize geounit allocation to deal with large variations in population density and to increase field-work efficiency (Cochran, 1977). The size of geounits can be determined through pilot testing in the field to ensure an adequate number of households and participants needed for research while taking into account of work efficiency. Both the widely used random walk method (Bauer, 2016) and the random ordering method we introduced in this chapter can be used to ensure an equal probability household sampling.

With our method, many of the sampling tasks can be implemented on computer with open-source software R and free Google imagery data.

Last but not the least, data collected using the integrated 4-stage GIS/GPS-assisted sampling method can be analyzed using many design-based survey methods (Kish, 1965, Cochran, 1977, Lohr 1999, Groves et al., 2009, Heeringa & O'Muircheartaigh, 2010, Valliant, et al. 2013). These methods are widely available in many software packages, including SUDAAN, SAS, STATA (survey module), SPSS, and "survey" package in R.

The integrated 4-stage GIS/GPS-assisted sampling methods can be altered to suit for specific conditions. For example, if a target study population is located in sparsely populated and less developed rural areas, we may just use satellite images to directly identify households for random sampling, such as in the studies reported by Haenssgen (2015), Wampler et al. (2013) and Escamilla et al. (2014).

3.10.2 Recommendations for Application

To maximize the strengths of this sampling method while ensuring the success of applying this method in drawing probability samples, researchers must pay more attention to the following three issues: (1) large variations in population density, (2) determination of the area size of a sampled geounit, and (3) geographic section area and household selection.

Large variations in population density. An innovative mechanism of our method is to connect geographic area with varying population density to households using numerous small geounits for further sampling. We recommend use of the classic stratified sampling strategy to optimize geounit allocation (Cochran, 1977). Our method also offers other possibilities to deal with varying population density issues. For example, instead of using fixed geounit size and sampling grid, with our method researchers can determine the geounit size disproportionate to population density after randomly tossing the pre-determined number of geounits to be selected.

Determination of area size of a geounit. Large sizes have greater probability to cover adequate number of households for sampling. However, if a large-sized geounit is randomly selected in a highly populous area, it will prevent researchers from completing the sampling due to high cost of time and money (Landry & Shen, 2005). We believe that geounit size can be determined if adequate pilot studies are conducted before sampling because pilot study to determine geounit size is not limited by existing data.

Household selection. Although each selected geounit is not large in area size with a relatively fewer number of households, household arrangement can still be complex. In this study, we used the random walk method which is not without problem (Bauer, 2016). The random ordering method appears to be more valid, additional tests are needed to demonstrate its validity.

Appendix 1: R Program Codes for a Semi-automatic, Computer-Assisted, and Step-Wise Algorithm for Geounit Sampling

```
#Required Packages:
#install.packages("rgdal")
#install.packages("Grid2Polygons")
#install.packages("ggmap")
#install.packages("sp")

#Load required packages
library(rgdal)
library(Grid2Polygons)
library(ggmap)
library(sp)

#Download county maps (this file is big so it might take a couple
   of minutes to download)
url<-"http://www2.census.gov/geo/tiger/TIGER2010DP1/
   County_2010Census_DP1.zip"
# specify a location on your computer to save the downloaded
   file, and the default location is "C:/temp/r_temp"
downloaddir<-"C:/temp/r_temp"
destname<-"tiger.zip"
download.file(url, destname)
unzip(destname, exdir=downloaddir, junkpaths=TRUE)

#Get the filenames for the .shp file
filename<-list.files(downloaddir, pattern=".shp",
   full.names=FALSE)
filename<-gsub(".shp", "", filename) #Get rid of the extension
   name

#Read the US county shapefile (NAD83 coordinate system EPSG:
   4269, the file is big and takes some time to read)
uscounty.shp<-readOGR(downloaddir, filename)

# Subset (change the fips code to get the county you want)
shp<-uscounty.shp[substring(uscounty.shp$GEOID10, 1, 5)
   == "12001",]

#re-projection
shp <- spTransform(shp, CRS("+init=epsg:4326")) #WGS84

#Generate grid (lat/long) over a polygon
bb<-bbox(shp) #get bounded box
cs<-c(0.01,0.01) #define cell size 0.01 degree by 0.01 degree
cc<-bb[,1]+(cs/2) #define cell offset

### define SpatialGrid object
cd<-ceiling(diff(t(bb))/cs) #generate number of cells
  per direction
```

```
grd<-GridTopology(cellcentre.offset=cc,cellsize=cs,cells.dim=cd)

sp_grd <- SpatialGridDataFrame(grd,data=data.frame
  (id=1:prod(cd)), proj4string=CRS(proj4string(shp)))

#convert grid to polygon
sp_grd_plys<-Grid2Polygons(sp_grd)

#keep cells that overlay the study area
shp_cell<-sp_grd_plys[shp,]

#plot grid overlaid with the polygon for check up
plot(shp_cell)
plot(shp,add=TRUE)

#overlay on aerial image using Google Map API
shp_cell_fort<- fortify(shp_cell)
shp_fort<-fortify(shp)
centroids <- as.data.frame(getSpPPolygonsLabptSlots(shp))
  #get centroids of alachua county
#centered on centroids of alachua county
qmap(location=c(lon=centroids[1,1],lat=centroids[1,2]),
  zoom = 10,maptype="hybrid") +geom_polygon(aes(x = long,
  y = lat,group=group), data = shp_cell_fort,colour = 'red',
  fill = 'black', alpha = .4, size = .3)   #change the zoom
  to modify the resolution of the map

#define and apply cell id to individual geounits
shp_cell@data[,2]<-c(1:length(shp_cell@data[,1]))
names(shp_cell@data)<-c("z","cellid")

#get centroids of individual geounits (polygons)
centroids <- as.data.frame(getSpPPolygonsLabptSlots(shp_cell))
  #get centroids of polygons
names(centroids)<-c("Longitude","Latitude")

#keep cell id as data for constructing primary sampling frame
cell_id<-shp_cell@data$cellid

########################################
#set up parameters for spatial sampling#
########################################

#create the sampling frame of the cell_id
cell_id_samplefrom<-cell_id

#define number of geounits to be sampled (default = 5)
n.geounits<-5

#define number of geounits with residential area, and set to
  0 as the initial value
n.geounits.res<-0

#create a user input function
```

```
userinput <- function()
{
 n <- readline(prompt="Does this geounit contain residential
  area? If Yes, Enter 1, If No, Enter 0    ")
 return(as.integer(n))
}

#define the output directory (location where the outputted
  .gpx files will be saved)
out<-"C:/temp/"

##the loop using predefined function to complete the sampling
   procedure
while(n.geounits.res<n.geounits){
 #sample one cell
 cell_id.sampled<-sample(cell_id_samplefrom,1)
 #exclude the sampled cell from the sample frame
 cell_id_samplefrom<-cell_id_samplefrom[cell_id_samplefrom!
   =cell_id.sampled]
 #subset the cell
 shp_cell.sampled<-shp_cell[shp_cell@data$cellid==cell_id
   .sampled,]
 #get the centroid of the cell
 centroids.sampled<-centroids[cell_id.sampled,]
 #plot on google map
 shp_cell_fort.sampled <- fortify(shp_cell.sampled)
 print(qmap(location=c(lon=centroids.sampled[1,1],
  lat=centroids.sampled[1,2]), zoom = 16,maptype="hybrid")
  +geom_polygon(aes(x = long, y = lat), data = shp_cell_fort.
  sampled,colour = 'red', alpha = .4, size = .3))
 #ask user to determine if the geounit contain residential
  areas or not
 input<-userinput()
 if(input==1){
  n.geounits.res<-n.geounits.res+1
  line_cell.sampled<-as(shp_cell.sampled,"SpatialLinesDataFrame")
  line_cell.sampled@data$name<-line_cell.sampled@data$cellid
  writeOGR(line_cell.sampled["name"], dsn=paste(out,
   "sampled_geounit", n.geounits.res,".gpx",sep=""),
   layer="tracks", driver="GPX", dataset_options="GPX_USE_
   EXTENSIONS=YES", check_exists=FALSE)
  cat(paste("Geounits Sampled (",n.geounits.res,"/",n.geounits,
  ")",sep=""))
}
if(input==0){
  cat("Geounit not sampled")
}
}
```

Appendix 2: R Program Codes for Monte Carlo Method to Determine Residential Area

```
###### define parameter
n.building<-10000 #number of buildings
mean.area<-600 # mean area of building
sd.area<-150 # sd of building area
min.nh<-1      # minimum number of households
max.nh<-100     # maximum number of households
min.np<-1     # minimum number of people in each household
max.np<-6     # maximum number of people in each household

# Generate Data
set.seed(1)
bid<-c(1:n.building)
area<-rnorm(n.building,mean.area,sd.area)
nh<-sample(min.nh:max.nh,n.building,replace=T)
dat1<-as.data.frame(cbind(bid,area,nh))

# replicate each row by nh
dat2<- dat1[rep(row.names(dat1), dat1$nh),]
rownames(dat2) <- NULL

dat2$hid<-c(1:nrow(dat2))
dat2$np<-sample(min.np:max.np,nrow(dat2),replace=T)

# total population in the study area
(pop.total<-sum(dat2$np))
# total residential area in the study area
(area.total<-sum(dat1$area))

##### Sampling

nbsample<-20 #number of buildings sampled
bid.sample<-sample(1:n.building,nbsample,replace=F)
  #get the sampled building id

res<-matrix(NA,nbsample,5)

for (i in 1:nbsample){
  nh.bid.sample<-dat2[dat2$bid==bid.sample[i],] #get all rows
    where bid=bid.sample
  temp.nh<-nrow(nh.bid.sample) #get total number of households
    in the building
  nsample.nh<-sample(1:temp.nh,1) #determine the number of
    households to sample in the building (randomly select
    "nsample.nh" out of the total number of households)
  hid.sample<-sample(nh.bid.sample$hid,nsample.nh,replace=F)
    #sample "nsample.nh" households from the building
  nh.sample<-nh.bid.sample[nh.bid.sample$hid%in%hid.sample,]
    #get the sampled data
  temp.pop<-sum(nh.sample$np) #obtain the total number of
```

```
    people in all sampled households in the building
  temp.area<-dat1[dat1$bid==bid.sample[i],2] #get the building
    area

  res[i,1]<-bid.sample[i] #store the sampled bid
  res[i,2]<-temp.nh #store the total number of households in
    the sampled building
  res[i,3]<-nsample.nh #store the number of households sampled in
    the sampled bulding
  res[i,4]<-temp.area #store the area of the sampled building
  res[i,5]<-temp.pop #store the total number of people in
    all sampled households in the sampled building
}

colnames(res)<-c("bid","nh","nsample.nh","area","pop")

#mean number of people in sampled households
pop.sample.mean<-sum(res[,5])/sum(res[,3])

#estimated total number of people in sampled building
pop.sample<-pop.sample.mean*sum(res[,2])

# true total number of people in sampled building
true.pop.sample<-sum(dat2[dat2$bid%in%bid.sample,5])

# total residential area in the sampled building
area.sample<-sum(res[,4])

# area ratio
area.r<-area.sample/area.total

# pop ratio
pop.r<-pop.sample/pop.total

cat("Area Ratio=",area.r,", Population Ratio=",pop.r,",
  Difference=",area.r-pop.r)

##### Repeated Sampling
nrsample<-1000 #define sampling number
out<-matrix(NA,nrsample,6)
for (j in 1:nrsample){
  nbsample<-20 #number of buildings sampled
  bid.sample<-sample(1:n.building,nbsample,replace=F)
    #get the sampled building id
  res<-matrix(NA,nbsample,5)
  for (i in 1:nbsample){
  nh.bid.sample<-dat2[dat2$bid==bid.sample[i],]
    #get all rows where bid=bid.sample
  temp.nh<-nrow(nh.bid.sample)
    #get total number of households in the building
  nsample.nh<-sample(1:temp.nh,1) #determine the number
    of households to sample in the building (randomly select
    "nsample.nh" out of the total number of households)
  hid.sample<-sample(nh.bid.sample$hid,nsample.nh,replace=F)
```

```
    # sample "nsample.nh" households from the building
    nh.sample<-nh.bid.sample[nh.bid.sample$hid%in%hid.sample,]
    # get the sampled data
    temp.pop<-sum(nh.sample$np)
    # obtain the total number of people in all sampled households
      in the building
    temp.area<-dat1[dat1$bid==bid.sample[i],2]
    # get the building area
      res[i,1]<-bid.sample[i]
    # store the sampled bid
      res[i,2]<-temp.nh
    # store the total number of households in the sampled building
      res[i,3]<-nsample.nh
    # store the number of households sampled in the sampled bulding
      res[i,4]<-temp.area
    # store the area of the sampled building
      res[i,5]<-temp.pop #store the total number of people in all
        sampled households in the sampled building
    }
  # mean number of people in sampled households
    pop.sample.mean<-sum(res[,5])/sum(res[,3])
  # total number of people in sampled building
    pop.sample<-pop.sample.mean*sum(res[,2])
  # true total number of people in sampled building
    true.pop.sample<-sum(dat2[dat2$bid%in%bid.sample,5])
  # total residential area in the sampled building
    area.sample<-sum(res[,4])
  # compute Ar/Pd
    ratio1<-area.total/pop.total
  # compute population ratio
    ratio2<-area.sample/pop.sample
    out[j,1]<-ratio1
    out[j,2]<-ratio2
    out[j,3]<-ratio1-ratio2
    out[j,4]<-pop.sample
    out[j,5]<-true.pop.sample
    out[j,6]<-pop.sample-true.pop.sample
    cat("Iteration",j,"Done","\n")
  }
  den1<-density(out[,3])
  m1<-mean(out[,3])
  z1=quantile(out[,3],c(0.025,0.975))
  r<-out[,1]/out[,2]
  den2<-density(r)
  m2<-mean(r)
  z2=quantile(r,c(0.025,0.975))
  den3<-density(out[,6])
  m3<-mean(out[,6])
  z3=quantile(out[,6],c(0.025,0.975))
  r2<-out[,4]/out[,5]
  den4<-density(r2)
  m4<-mean(r2)
  z4=quantile(r2,c(0.025,0.975))
```

```
##### plotting
# plot 1
par(mfrow=c(1,2))
plot(den1,type='l',xlab='',main=paste("D, Mean=",round(m1,2)))
abline(v=z1,col='red',lty=3)
abline(v=m1,col='red',lty=1)

plot(den2,type='l',xlab='',main=paste("R, Mean=",round(m2,2)))
abline(v=z2,col='red',lty=3)
abline(v=m2,col='red',lty=1)
par(mfrow=c(1,1))

# plot 2
round(m3,2)
round(m4,2)
par(mfrow=c(1,2))
plot(den3,type='l',xlab='',main=expression(paste(D[P[g]], ",
  Mean=-1.45")))
abline(v=z3,col='red',lty=3)
abline(v=m3,col='red',lty=1)
plot(den4,type='l',xlab='',main=expression(paste(R[P[g]], ",
  Mean=1")))
abline(v=z4,col='red',lty=3)
abline(v=m4,col='red',lty=1)
par(mfrow=c(1,1))

# Plot together
round(m1,2)
round(m2,2)
round(m3,2)
round(m4,2)

par(mfrow=c(2,2))
plot(den3,type='l',xlab='',main=expression(paste(D[P[g]], ",
  Mean=-0.72")))
abline(v=z3,col='red',lty=3)
abline(v=m3,col='red',lty=1)
plot(den4,type='l',xlab='',main=expression(paste(R[P[g]], ",
  Mean=1.00")))
abline(v=z4,col='red',lty=3)
abline(v=m4,col='red',lty=1)
plot(den1,type='l',xlab='',main=expression(paste("D,
  Mean=-0.08")))
abline(v=z1,col='red',lty=3)
abline(v=m1,col='red',lty=1)
plot(den2,type='l',xlab='',main=expression(paste("R,
  Mean=1.00")))
abline(v=z2,col='red',lty=3)
abline(v=m2,col='red',lty=1)
par(mfrow=c(1,1))
```

References

Bauer, J. (2016). Biases in random route survey. *Journal of Survey Statistics and Methodology, 4*(2), 263–287.

Boeuf, P., Drummer, H. E., Richards, J. S., Scoullar, M. J., & Beeson, J. G. (2016). The global threat of Zika virus to pregnancy: Epidemiology, clinical perspectives, mechanisms, and impact. *BMC Medicine, 14*(1), 112. https://doi.org/10.1186/s12916-016-0660-0

Chang, A. Y., Parrales, M. E., Jimenez, J., Sobieszczyk, M. E., Hammer, S. M., Copenhaver, D. J., & Kulkarni, R. P. (2009). Combining Google Earth and GIS mapping technologies in a dengue surveillance system for developing countries. *International Journal of Health Geographics, 8*, 49. https://doi.org/10.1186/1476-072X-8-49

Chen, X. G., & Hu, H. (2018). Rejoinder to the discussion by Steven Heeringa. *Journal of Survey Statistics and Methodology, 6*(2), 182–185. https://doi.org/10.1093/jssam/smy011

Chen, X. G., Hu, H., Xu, X. H., Gong, J., Yan, Y. Q., & Li, F. (2018). Probability sampling by connecting space with households using Gis/Gps technologies. *Journal of Survey Statistics and Methodology, 6*(2), 149–168. https://doi.org/10.1093/jssam/smx032

Chen, X., Yu, B., Zhou, D., Zhou, W., Gong, J., Li, S. Y., & Stanton, B. (2015). Men who have sex with men among rural-to-urban migrants and non-migrant rural and urban residents in China: A GIS/GPS-assisted random sample survey. *PLoS One, 10*(8), e0134712.

Cochran, W. G. (1977). *Sampling techniques* (3rd ed.). Hoboken: Wiley.

Escamilla, V., Emch, M., Dandalo, L., Miller, W. C., Martinson, F., & Hoffman, I. (2014). Sampling at community level by using satellite imagery and geographical analysis. *Bulletin of the World Health Organization, 92*(9), 690–694. https://doi.org/10.2471/Blt.14.140756

Galway, L. P., Bell, N., Al Shatari, S. A. E., Hagopian, A., Burnham, G., Flaxman, A., ... Takaro, T. K. (2012). A two-stage cluster sampling method using gridded population data, a GIS, and Google Earth (TM) imagery in a population-based mortality survey in Iraq. *International Journal of Health Geographics, 11*, 12. https://doi.org/10.1186/1476-072x-11-12

Groves, R. M., Fowler, F. J., Jr., Couper, M. P., Lepkowski, J. M., Singer, E., & Tourangeau, R. (2009). *Survey methodology* (2nd ed.). Hoboken: Wiley.

Haenssgen, M. J. (2015). Satellite-aided survey sampling and implementation in low- and middle-income contexts: A low-cost/low-tech alternative. *Emerging Themes in Epidemiology, 12*, 20. https://doi.org/10.1186/s12982-015-0041-8

Haklay, M., & Weber, P. (2008). OpenStreetMap: User-generated street maps. *Ieee Pervasive Computing, 7*(4), 12–18. https://doi.org/10.1109/Mprv.2008.80

Heckathorn, D. D. (1997). Respondent-driven sampling: A new approach to the study of hidden populations. *Social Problems, 44*(2), 174–199.

Heckathorn, D. D. (2002). Respondent-driven sampling II: Deriving valid population estimates from chain-referral samples of hidden populations. *Social Problems, 49*, 11.

Heeringa, S. G. (2018). Discussion of "probability sampling by connecting space with households using Gis/Gps technologies" by Chen, X.; Xu, X.; Gong, J.; Yan, Y.; Fang, L. *Journal of Survey Statistics and Methodology, 6*(2), 169–181. https://doi.org/10.1093/jssam/smy004

Heeringa, S., & O'Muircheartaigh, C. (2010). Sampling designs for cross-cultural and cross-national survey programs. In J. A. Harkness, M. Baun, B. Edwards, T. P. Johnson, L. E. Lyberg, P. Mohler, B. Pennell, & T. W. Smith (Eds.), *Survey methods in multinational, multiregional and multicultural contexts* (pp. 251–268). New York, NY: Wiley.

Kish, L. (1949). A procedure for objective respondent selection within household. *Journal of American Statistical Association, 44*, 380–387.

Kish, L. (1965). *Survey sampling*. New York: Wiley.

Kondo, M. C., Bream, K. D., Barg, F. K., & Branas, C. C. (2014). A random spatial sampling method in a rural developing nation. *BMC Public Health, 14*, 338. https://doi.org/10.1186/1471-2458-14-338

Landry, P. F., & Shen, M. (2005). Reaching migrants in survey research: The use of the global positioning system to reduce coverage bias in China. *Political Analysis, 13*(1), 1–22.

Lohr, S. L. (1999). Sampling: Design and analysis. Pacific Grove, CA: Duxbury Press.

Mansergh, G., Naorat, S., Jommaroeng, R., Jenkins, R. A., Jeeyapant, S., Kanggarnrua, K., ... Van Griensven, F. (2006). Adaptation of venue-day-time sampling in Southeast Asia to access men who have sex with men for HIV assessment in Bangkok. *Field Methods, 18*(2), 135–152.

Mathews, J. H. (1972). Monte Carlo estimate for pi. *Pi Mu Epson Journal, 5*, 281–282.

Metropolis, N., & Ulam, S. (1949). The Monte Carlo method. *Journal of the American Statistical Association, 44*(247), 335–341.

Murray, J., O'Green, A. T., & McDaniel, P. A. (2003). Development of a GIS database for ground-water recharge assessment of the palouse basin. *Soil Science, 168*(11), 759–768. https://doi.org/10.1097/01.ss.0000100474.96182.51

Pearson, A. L., Rzotkiewicz, A., & Zwickle, A. (2015). Using remote, spatial techniques to select a random household sample in a dispersed, semi-nomadic pastoral community: Utility for a longitudinal health and demographic surveillance system. *International Journal of Health Geographics, 14*, 33. https://doi.org/10.1186/s12942-015-0026-4

Pieterse, J. N. (2015). *Globalization and culture: Global melange* (3rd ed.). Lanham: Rowman & Littlefied.

Schneider, A., Friedl, M. A., & Potere, D. (2009). A new map of global urban extent from MODIS satellite data. *Environmental Research Letters, 4*(4), 044003. https://doi.org/10.1088/1748-9326/4/4/044003

Shannon, H. S., Hutson, R., Kolbe, A., Stringer, B., & Haines, T. (2012). Choosing a survey sample when data on the population are limited: A method using Global Positioning Systems and aerial and satellite photographs. *Emerging Themes in Epidemiology, 9*(1), 5. https://doi.org/10.1186/1742-7622-9-5

Statistical Bureau of Wuhan. (2012). Wuhan statistical yearbook. China statistical press, Beijing.

Tilling, K. (2001). Capture-recapture methods—Useful or misleading? *International Journal of Epidemiology, 30*(1), 12–14.

Tong, T. R. (2005). SARS-CoV sampling from 3 portals. *Emerging Infectious Diseases, 11*(1), 167. https://doi.org/10.3201/eid1101.040645

Valliant, R., Dever, J. A., & Freuter, F. (2013). Practical tools for designing and weighting survey samples, Springer.

Wampler, P. J., Rediske, R. R., & Molla, A. R. (2013). Using ArcMap, Google Earth, and Global Positioning Systems to select and locate random households in rural Haiti. *International Journal of Health Geographics, 12*, 3. https://doi.org/10.1186/1476-072x-12-3

Weyer, J., Grobbelaar, A., & Blumberg, L. (2015). Ebola virus disease: History epidemiology and outbreaks. *Current Infectious Disease Reports, 17*(5), 480. https://doi.org/10.1007/s11908-015-0480-y

Wuhan Center for Disease Prevention and Control (CDC). (2016). Report of HIV/AIDS in Wuhan, china. Wuhan CDC, Hubei Province, China.

Chapter 4
Construal Level Theory Supported Method for Sensitive Topics: Applications in Three Different Populations

Yan Wang and Xinguang Chen

Abstract Social desirability bias is a major threat to data quality for survey studies, particularly studies involving sensitive questions, such as age, income, sexual behaviors, and drug use. In this chapter, we introduced a construal level theory (CLT)-based method we devised to reduce social desirability bias. Construals are our mental constructions of the universe organized in hierarchies along with spatiotemporal and psychosocial distances, with self, here, and now as the reference. Answering sensitive question regarding self is often executed at low construal levels subjected to contextual factors. In this case, the respondent tend to edit the answer to make it socially desirable either to avoid penalty or to enhance reward. In contrast, answering sensitive questions for others is often executed at high construal levels, less likely to subject to contextual factors but more dependent on one's own knowledge, attitudes and beliefs. CLT-based method is a technique based on this theory by asking participants to answer the same questions for 2–3 socially distant others. In this study, we reported our work on building the method through three studies, one with data collected from college students in the US, two with data collected in China, including one sample of urban residents and another sample of rural residents. Four questions (reading newspaper, engaging in physical activity, frequent of sexual intercourse and attitudes toward homosexuality) were used in the college student study conducted in the US; the Brief Sexual Openness Scale (BSOS) was used in the two studies conducted in China. The use of the method and future research are also recommended.

Y. Wang
Department of Epidemiology, University of Florida, Gainesville, FL, USA
e-mail: ywang48@ufl.edu

X. Chen (✉)
Department of Epidemiology, College of Public Health and Health Professions, College of Medicine, University of Florida, Gainesville, FL, USA

Global Health Institute, Wuhan University, Wuhan, China
e-mail: jimax.chen@ufl.edu

X. Chen, (Din) D.-G. Chen (eds.), *Statistical Methods for Global Health and Epidemiology*, ICSA Book Series in Statistics,
https://doi.org/10.1007/978-3-030-35260-8_4

Keywords Sensitive questions · Social desirability bias · Construal-level theory · CLT-based method · Sexual openness

4.1 Introduction

A large part of modern science is built upon survey data, including epidemiology and global health. However, scientists using survey data in research often have to acknowledge the potential for survey responses to be biased as a limitation (Chen, Wang, Li, Gong, & Yan, 2015). Pursuing high quality data is a goal for all disciplines, including epidemiology and global health. However, it remains to be a methodological challenge to obtaining high quality data, particularly data on sensitive topics (Chen et al., 2015; Tourangeau, Lance, & Raninski, 2000; Tourangeau & Yan, 2007).

As being detailed later in this chapter, a variety of methods and techniques have been proposed to enhance the quality of survey data, such as methods to enhance confidentiality, random response and indirect survey methods, and the methods using biomarkers. However, up to date, few of such methods have been frequently employed in research because of technical and practical limitations (e.g., highly complex procedure, low acceptability, and high cost). Sensitive topics are common in epidemiological research and global health, such as mental health, substance abuse, HIV/AIDS, health status, medical insurance, access to healthcare, and patient satisfaction. Novel techniques and methods are needed to collect high quality data with increased efficiency and feasibility.

4.1.1 Factors Affecting the Quality of Survey Data

Quality of the survey data can be affected by a number of factors. Typical examples include errors in defining the study population, errors from random sampling of study participants (Dwyer, 1980), variations in settings for survey delivery, miscomprehension of a survey question (Tourangeau et al., 2000; Tourangeau & Yan, 2007), recall bias in responding to a survey question (Bajunirwe et al., 2014; Tourangeau et al., 2000), and bias from response editing for sensitive survey questions (Steenkamp, De Jong, & Baumgartner, 2010). Response styles are also a factor related to the quality of survey data. Participants often tend to give extreme or neutral answers to multi-choice questions and preference to integers 0, 5, and 10 to questions related to age, income, school grade (Johnson & Bolt, 2010; Meisenberg & Williams, 2008).

4.1.2 Cognitive Censoring and Social Desirability Bias

Among many influential factors, social desirability bias is the most significant and well researched factor. According to the psychology of survey responses, when answering a sensitive question, participants are likely to respond untruthfully to either minimize "harm" or maximize "benefit" (Chen et al., 2015; Tourangeau et al., 2000; Tourangeau & Yan, 2007). Despite provisions to guard privacy and confidentiality, if a true answer is perceived socially undesirable, such as admitting sexually transmitted diseases and disclosing stigmatizing attitudes toward homosexuality, participants may refuse to respond (missing data) or "edit" their response (misreport) to avoid *disclosure threat* (Albaum, Roster, & Smith, 2012; Chen et al., 2015; Krumpal, 2013; Rasinski, Willis, Baldwin, Yeh, & Lee, 1999; Tourangeau et al., 2000; Tourangeau & Yan, 2007). Likewise, if answers to a question are perceived socially desirable, such as being sexually open (a fashion in countries experiencing rapid globalization like China) or stating adherence to prescribed medications by doctors, participants may over-report to seek *disclosure rewards* (Bockenholt, 2014; Cordero-Coma & Breen, 2012; Paulhus, Harms, Bruce, & Lysy, 2003; Yuen et al., 2013). Therefore, a participant's perception, appraisal, and responding work together like a "*cognitive censoring system*", leading to untruthful answers to different types of survey questions (Bond, Ramsey, & Boddy, 2011; Chen et al., 2015).

4.1.3 Existing Methods to Reduce Social Desirability Bias

A review of published studies reveals a long list of methods and techniques developed to reduce social desirability bias in survey studies. These methods can be categorized into three groups. Methods in *Group I* include indirect measurement by asking participants to assess peers (Bond et al., 2011; Fisher & Tellis, 1998; Jo, 2000), application of lie-detection scales (Crowne & Marlowe, 1960; Paulhus, 1984), random response method (Gupta, Gupta, & Singh, 2002; Warner, 1965) and its derivatives (Bockenholt, 2014; Bockenholt & van der Heijden, 2007; Himmelfarb, 2008), multi-group item randomized response method (de Jong, Pieters, & Stremersch, 2012; Himmelfarb, 2008), and computer/smartphone/online digital encrypt methods that mask data but preserve the statistical relationships (Pei, Chen, Xiao, & Wu, 2015; Wu, Chen, Burr, & Zhang, 2016). A primary goal of these methods is to enhance privacy and confidentiality, which has showed limited effect (Gueguen, 2015; Holbrook & Krosnick, 2010). Furthermore, the indirect method is still subject to over-reporting socially undesirable behaviors and under-reporting socially desirable behaviors (Bond et al., 2011; Fisher & Tellis, 1998; Ostapczuk & Musch, 2011).

Methods in *Group II* include the use of biomarkers (Dasgupta, 2015; Tavakoli, Hull, & Okasinski, 2011), biosensors (Robles et al., 2011; Selvam, Muthukumar, Kamakoti, & Prasad, 2016), audio and video records, and mobile devices as objective data or digital markers (Chen, Wang, Leeman, Li, & Zhao, 2018; Robinson, Hensel, Morabito, & Roundtree, 2015) or measurement instrumentations (Sakai, Mikulich-Gilbertson, Long, & Crowley, 2006; Selvam et al., 2016). However, these methods are often intrusive, expensive, and practically less feasible. More problematic than feasibility issues is that many of these measures are not always a good proxy of behaviors, therefore often insufficient for research (Pollack, 2012; Selvam et al., 2016; Tavakoli et al., 2011). For example, biomarkers of substance use from urine or blood at specific point in time, although objective, are inadequate to describe the complex dynamics of substance use behavior. Therefore, these measures are often used to verify self-reported data on protective and risk health behaviors. In addition, methods for biomarkers are also subject to errors from sample collection, storage, process, and lab detection.

Methods in *Group III* involve the use of data from multiple informants—persons who have close contact with the participants and are therefore, to a certain extent, able to provide information on the study questions (Achenbach & Ruffle, 2000; Penney, McMaster, & Wilkie, 2014). For example, when collecting data on performance and behaviors among students, relevant informants might be classmates, teachers and parents. This method enhances data quality by incorporating information from multiple informants using advanced psychometric methods such as a bifactor or tri-factor analysis (Achenbach & Ruffle, 2000; Bauer et al., 2013; Penney et al., 2014). Although very promising, challenges remain to implement the multi-informant method. It is often difficult to locate appropriate informants for non-student populations. Furthermore, recruiting and collecting data from multiple informants increase the work burden and complicate the already complex process for human subject protection.

4.2 Theoretical and Analytical Foundations

The method we introduced in this chapter is rooted deeply on construal-level theory, the measurement modeling theory and complex factor modeling analysis. Understanding these theories and models are essential to understand the new method.

4.2.1 Construal-Level Theory and Social Desirability Bias

In a previous study, we tested a method to minimize social desirability bias in collecting survey data on sensitive questions (Chen et al., 2015), guided by construal level theory (CLT) (Liberman & Trope, 2008; Trope & Liberman, 2010). Construals are our mental constructions of the universe organized in hierarchies according to spatiotemporal and psychosocial distances, with self, here, and now as the reference (Liberman & Trope, 2008; Trope & Liberman, 2010). According to the CLT, responses to sensitive questions will be less error-prone if a participant is asked to assess socially distant others rather than oneself (Wright, 2012). This phenomenon occurs because self-assessment is processed at lower construal levels with close reference to social context (Liberman & Trope, 2008; Liberman, Trope, & Stephan,

2007; Liberman, Trope, & Wakslak, 2007; Trope & Liberman, 2010; Yaacov Trope & Liberman, 2012), and often coupled with the cognitive censoring (Fisher & Tellis, 1998).

However, activation of the cognitive censoring system will be less likely if a person is asked to assess socially distant others, because such assessment is often made based on one's own knowledge and beliefs that are stored at higher construal levels and they are less likely to be affected by contextual factors (Fisher & Tellis, 1998). Social distance thus acts as a mechanism to manipulate construal levels, reducing the sensitivity of a question for quality data (Kim, Schnall, Yi, & White, 2013; Liberman & Trope, 1998; Steenkamp et al., 2010; Wright, 2012).

4.2.2 The Measurement Theory Underpinning of CLT-Based Survey

Guided by the latent variable theory (Bollen, 2002; Borsboom, Mellenbergh, & van Heerden, 2003), we developed a method to deal with the sensitivity of a survey question by analytically linking the responses to a specific question across various construal levels to one latent construct (Chen et al., 2015). For example, from the previous discussion regarding the concept of construal level and social desirability, a participant's self-assessment of a question (e.g., if same-sex marriage is acceptable or not) and his/her assessments of the same question for socially distant others such as family members, friends, acquaintances, and strangers, are hypothesized to be determined by one latent construct—this participant's knowledge, attitude and belief about the question. In measurement theory, this latent construct functions as a factor determining the response of a survey participant to the question for him/herself, and socially distant others.

This phenomenon of construing others' behaviors and attitudes with reference to oneself has been documented in published studies in the literature as *false consensus effect* (Dunn, Thomas, Swift, & Burns, 2012; Ross, Greene, & House, 1977). For example, individuals who are more open toward sex are more likely to believe that others are also sexually open (Sieving, Eisenberg, Pettingell, & Skay, 2006); individuals who use drugs tend to believe that many others use drug users, too (Dunn et al., 2012); and individuals who are rich may also believe that many others are rich (Dawtry, Sutton, & Sibley, 2015). However, this principle has not been used in survey studies to improve the reliability of self-reported data.

Connecting the CLT with latent variable theory creates the foundation supporting the use measurement modeling techniques to assess the new method we developed to improve data quality for sensitive topics. We term this approach as *CLT-based Measurement Modeling*, in which self-assessment and assessments of socially distant others on a sensitive topic are treated as separate items or subconstructs determined by one single latent construct—the participant's own behavior or attitude. With this CLT-based modeling approach, survey items assessing targets at different social distances from self to more distant others can be integrated as indicators of their shared determinant factor—the latent construct of individual participants. The CLT-Based Measurement Modeling thus enables extraction of the common variance representing the latent factor (knowledge, attribute, and behavior) of individual participants, and factor loadings representing contributions of individual items or subconstructs to the common factor.

4.2.3 Statistical Modeling of CLT-Based Survey Data

The CLT-based Measurement Modeling described in the previous section resembles, to a large extent, the essence of multiple informant approach in data collection. Multiple informant method, as proposed in the multitrait and multimethod (MTMM) model (Campbell & Fiske, 1959) is a method in which ratings from multiple resources (such as parents, teachers, and peer) are added to children's self-ratings to improve data quality for assessing the characteristics or behaviors of the child. This approach has been accepted as the optimal method for data quality improvement in child behavior research (Achenbach, Mcconaughy, & Howell, 1987; Bauer et al., 2013).

Instead of depending on multiple informants that are often financially expensive and practically challenging to implement, the CLT-based method asks individual participants to rate a sensitive topic for a series of socially distant groups in addition to self-rating. While the multi-informant method improves data quality by including knowledge beyond the participants, CLT-based method does so by tapping the knowledge of only the participants'. Nevertheless, the two methods share one mechanism in common: using additional information from diverse sources (e.g., different informants or different social groups) to "triangulate" a latent construct for more accurate measurement (Chen et al., 2015; Kraemer et al., 2003). By applying this principle, CLT-based scales can be developed to address specific research questions that are sensitive and therefore subject to social desirability bias.

4.2.4 Bifactor and Tri-factor Modeling Analysis of CLT-Based Data

The similarity between the CLT-based method and MTMM makes it possible to apply existing measurement modeling methods for data analysis. Two methods that are particularly relevant for analyzing CLT-based data are bifactor model (Cai, Yang, & Hansen, 2011; Gibbons et al., 2007; Holzinger & Swineford, 1937) and tri-factor model (Bauer et al., 2013). These two analytical methods have been well-established in education research. We have adapted them to model CLT-base data. With these psychometric modeling techniques, the reliability of any CLT-based scale can be evaluated and reliable data be derived to minimize social desirability bias.

Specifically, with either the bifactor or the tri-factor model, a common factor for the hypothetic latent variable can be extracted with data from the multiple assessments of different targets. In other words, variances of a participant's *perspective* for him/herself and socially distant others and variances due to *heterogeneity* in individual survey items can be analytically separated from the common factors. Factor score for the common latent factor provides a "true" measure of a participant's answer to a sensitive question; factor scores for the factor of participants' self-perspective provide a measure of bias or misreport; while factor scores for perspective factors of socially distant others provide a measure of participants' knowledge of these people.

4.3 Detecting the Sensitive of a Question Using CLT-Based Method

As an introduction, in this section, we introduce the application of CLT-based method in assessing if a study question is sensitive.

4.3.1 Participants and Procedures

A convenience sample of college students (n = 401) were recruited from a university campus. An online survey was conducted using the REDCap software. The study was approved by IRB at the University of Florida. To assess the sensitivity of various survey topics, data for the following four behaviors were analyzed:

1. Reading newspapers and magazines;
2. Engaging in physical activities;
3. Frequency of having sex; and
4. Attitudes toward homosexuality (sex with the same-gender persons).

According to the principle of CLT-based method, these four questions were measured in three targets: participants themselves, classmates, and school mates. Using the first question as an example, in this CLT-based survey, participants were asked to answer the following three questions:

1. How often do you read newspapers and magazines (response option: "none", "sometimes", "often", "daily", and "several times a day")?
2. How many of your classmates do you think read newspapers and magazines (responses include "none", "less than a half", "about a half", "more than a half", "everyone")?
3. How many students in the current university of yours do you think read newspapers and magazines (responses include "none", "less than a half", "about a half", "more than a half", "everyone")?

With this CLT-based survey design, each of the four study questions was measured using three survey items, forming a CLT-based scale. According to this method, a participant response to the same question for him/herself, classmates and school mates were determined by one latent construct in the brain of the participants. If the CLT-based method is valid, the three items will form a reliable scale for sensitive questions (e.g., attitude toward homosexuality); otherwise, no reliable scale will be formed (e.g., reading newspapers and magazines).

4.3.2 *Statistical Analysis and Results*

Descriptive statistics including mean and standard deviation were used to assess individual survey items, correlation analysis, item-response theory (IRT)-based analysis and measurement modeling with confirmatory factor analysis (CFA) were used to assess the validity of the CLT-based method and sensitivity levels of the four questions.

Table 4.1 summarizes the main results assessing item responses. These items captured information from the individual participants with distribution very close to normal. The mean scores for all items were also close to 3.00, the theoretical value of the rating scale with SD much smaller than the mean.

Table 4.1 Mean, SD, and response distribution (%) of individual items

Item/social	Mean (SD)	1	2	3	4	5
Reading						
Self	2.75 (0.95)	3.74	48.63	35.41	11.72	0.50
Classmates	2.84 (0.71)	1.75	28.93	53.62	15.21	0.50
Schoolmates	2.97 (0.74)	1.75	23.44	51.62	22.69	0.50
Physical						
Self	2.94 (0.68)	0.25	24.19	58.10	15.96	1.50
Classmates	2.90 (0.70)	0.50	27.43	53.62	17.96	0.50
Schoolmates	3.00 (0.68)	0.25	21.45	56.86	20.70	0.75
Sex						
Self	2.87 (1.11)	9.98	26.68	39.15	17.71	6.48
Classmates	2.59 (0.77)	5.24	41.90	41.90	11.22	0.25
Schoolmates	2.64 (0.74)	2.74	42.89	43.39	9.73	1.25
Homosexual						
Self	2.61 (0.79)	6.48	39.15	41.90	12.22	0.25
Classmates	2.68 (0.83)	4.49	42.14	35.91	16.71	0.75
Schoolmates	2.71 (0.74)	2.74	37.41	46.13	13.47	0.25

Note: 1(*none*), 2 (*sometimes*) for self and (*less than a half*) for the other two target groups; 3 (*often*) for self and (*about s half*) for other two; and 4 (*about daily*) for self and (*more than a half*) for other two; and 5 (*more than daily*) for self and (*everyone*) for other two

Table 4.2 Psychometric assessment of responses to four questions for self-assessment and assessments of two socially distance groups (classmates and schoolmates)

Social distance	Reading newspaper	Physical activity	Frequency of sex	Attitude to homosexuality
Item-total correlation				
Self	0.0120	0.2761	0.3857	0.5118
Classmate	0.3343	0.3286	0.4808	0.5907
School mates	0.2780	0.3344	0.4674	0.6129
Slope (information)				
Self	0.3808	2.3420	0.1108	1.5820
Classmate	2.3642	−0.0924	1.4459	2.4145
School mates	2.0989	−0.1522	1.4550	2.8918
Alpha	0.33	0.50	0.62	0.74

The results from correlation and IRT analysis are presented in Table 4.2. In the table, the four behaviors were assessed as four separate measurement scales of the four behaviors each as an independent measurement scale. Results from correlation analysis revealed the item-total correlation was the lowest for the reading behavior the highest for the measure of attitude toward homosexuality. In addition, the item-total correlation increased from the smallest for self-assessment to the highest for the assessment of school mates with the value for classmates in between.

The slope estimated through IRT analysis provides a measure of information by individual items to the total scale if the scale is correct. The estimated slope did not show any systematic pattern for the reading behavior and physical activity but showed a pattern similar to the item-total correlation for the two sex-related measures.

Lastly, as a measure of scale reliability the estimated Cronbach alpha = 0.33, the smallest and not acceptable as a scale to measure reading behavior; it reached 0.74, the largest and acceptable as a scale to measure attitudes toward homosexuality. The alpha estimates for the other two behaviors was in between the two.

Results from CFA of the four CLT-based measures in Fig. 4.1 provide additional evidence supporting the findings presented in Table 4.2. The data-model fit was the worst (e.g., CFI = 0) for the scale measuring reading behavior, and the best (CFI = 0.87) for the scale measuring attitudes toward homosexuality.

4.3.3 Summary

In this study, we purposely selected four questions, from less sensitive (i.e., reading newspapers and magazines) to more sensitive (i.e., attitudes toward homosexuality). A comparison of the results from correlation, IRT and CFA analyses of the four measures suggests: CLT-based method works for measuring sensitive questions.

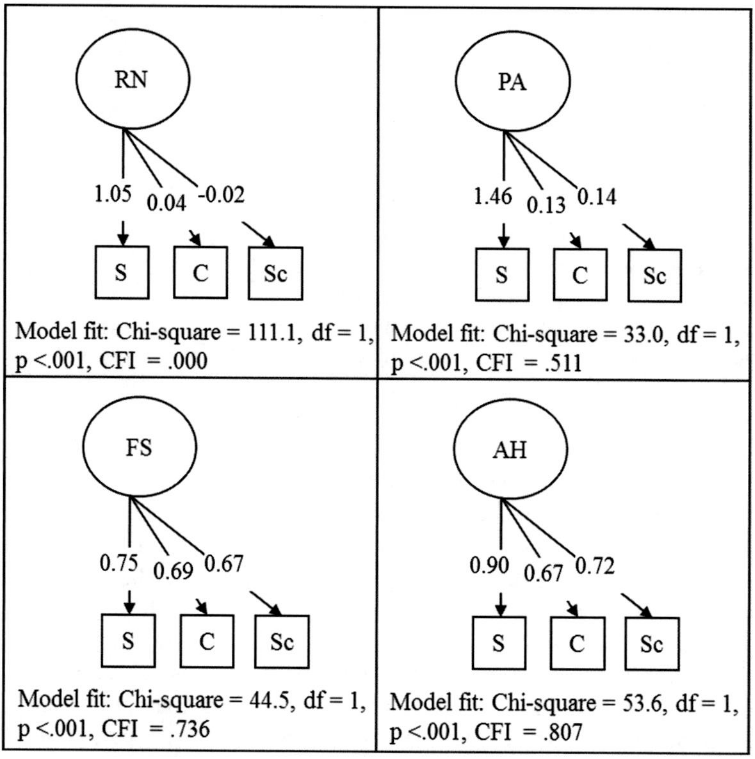

Fig. 4.1 CFA model results for the CLT-based measures. Note. *RN* Reading newspaper, *PA* Physical activity, *FS* Frequency of sex, *AH* Attitude to homosexuality, *S* Self, *C* Classmates, *Sc* School mates

Among the four behaviors included in this study, the reliability of CLT-based measure increases with the sensitivity level of a question.

As a byproduct of this analysis, CLT-based method may be used to quantitatively assess the sensitivity level of a study question.

4.4 Application of CLT-Based Method in an Urban Population

Findings presented in Sect. 4.3 provided empirical data supporting the validity of CLT in guiding the new method we proposed to assess sensitive topics for quality data. In this section, we systematically evaluated the CLT-based survey method based on the principles and findings from the previous sections.

4.4.1 *Participants and Procedures*

Data were derived from the urban sample of a large project funded by the National Institute of Health (R01 MH086322). Participants (18–45 years old) were urban residents in Wuhan, a provincial capital city of Hubei Province with a population of approximately ten million and per capita GDP of $10,355 (Statistical Bureau of Wuhan, 2012); they were randomly selected using a GIS/GPS-assisted method (Chen et al., 2018). Data were collected using audio computer-assisted self-interview (ACASI) technique in 2010–2013. Institutional Review Board (IRB) approvals were obtained from multiple agencies for data collection and analysis.

4.4.2 *Conventional and CLT-Based Brief Sexual Openness Scale*

The Brief Sexual Openness Scale (BSOS) was originally devised as a conventional instrument to assess sexual openness from five aspects using the following five questions:

1. "It doesn't matter to have sex with many people."
2. "It is totally acceptable to have sex with boy/girlfriend before marriage."
3. "One can have sex with others in addition to spouse as long as it does not jeopardize his/her own family."
4. "We should understand and accept those who have sex with the same-sex persons."
5. "In special situations, such as long-term separation with spouse due to work or business trip, it is okay to have sex with sex workers."

Individual items were assessed using a five-point Likert scale, varying from 0 (*strongly disagree*) to 4 (*strongly agree*).

Since sexually related topics are sensitive, we expanded the conventional scale into the CLT-Based BSOS to obtain more reliability data. In the CLT-Based BSOS, participants answer the five questions first, and then move to the same questions for two socially distant groups: the non-migrant urban residents and the non-migrant rural residents in general. Instead of asking for "agree" or "disagree", participants were instructed to estimate how many of people in a group may agree or disagree with options of 0 (*none or a few*), 1 (*less than a half*), 2 (*about a half*), 3 (*more than a half*), and 4 (*everyone*).

The full CLT-based BSOS consisted consists of a total of 15 items with 5 for self-assessment, and 5 for urban and 5 for rural residents respectively. These items can be used for two measurement purposes: (1) Using the three items for each question to construct five single-question CLT-based scales and (2) using all 15 items to construct a multi-item scale. These two types of scales are useful for research.

4.4.3 Variable for Predictive Validity Analysis

1. Sexual desire: Measured using the Brief Sexual Desire Scale (BSDS) (Chen et al., 2015); and it uses four items to assess the frequencies of "thinking of sex during free time", "having strong drive for sex", "talking about sex with others", and "noticing sexually attractive persons around". Cronbach alpha = 0.93. Mean scores were computed over the four items with response options 1 (*never*), 2 (*occasionally*), 3 (*not every day but at least once a week*), 4 (*one or more times per day*), 5 (*several times per day*).
2. Lifetime number of sexual partners: Measured based on participants' response to the question: "Up to now, with how many people have you had sexual intercourse, including your spouse, lovers, and strangers?" The reported number was used for analysis.
3. Unplanned pregnancy (yes/no): After a series of questions regarding sex and pregnancy, participants were asked, "Have you ever become pregnant (or got others pregnant for males) without planning to do so?" Participants who responded positively to this question were coded as having had an unplanned pregnancy.
4. Sexually transmitted diseases (STD, yes/no): Measured using the cognitive interviewing techniques (Nguyen et al., 2015; Willis, 2015) by first asking: "Have you ever had sexually transmitted diseases?" For those who responded positively, their answer was further confirmed with two follow-up questions: (a) "Please indicate the type of sexually transmitted diseases?" with a checklist of STDs commonly reported locally; and (b) "How did you know that you had the disease?" with answer options (doctor's diagnosis, self-assessment, told by others, and other methods).

In addition to the four outcome variables, demographic and socioeconomic factors were included, such as age (in years), sex (male vs. female), marital status (married and not married), education (primary school or less, middle school, high school, college or more), having children (yes/no), and monthly income (in US dollar). In addition to describing the study sample, some of these variables were used as covariates in predictive validity analysis.

4.4.4 Statistical Analysis

Data from participants self-assessments were analyzed conventionally, including correlation and IRT analysis to assess item response, internal consistency, item information, scale reliability and scale information. IRT analysis for CLT-based data was conducted using a two-parameter polytomous response model with model parameters estimated using the generalized partial credit (GPC) method (Verhelst & Verstralen, 2008), considering the potential local correlations between self-assessment and assessment of socially distant others. After IRT modeling analysis, item difficulty was manually computed as the mean of the estimated step parameters.

Item and scale reliability were estimated using the Bayes model estimate (BME) method (Nicewander & Thomasson, 1999).

The structural validity of the CLT-based BSOS was assessed first using a two-level second-order CFA, followed by a tri-factor modeling analysis (Bauer et al., 2013). (1) The CFA was used to test the structure validity that participants' self-assessment and their assessments of socially distant others were the three level-1 subconstructs, which were determined by one level-2 sexual openness construct. (2) The tri-factor analysis was used to (a) separate participants' perspectives of themselves and of the two socially distant groups from their own "true" sexual openness, and (b) item-level disturbances for the five sexual attitudes/behaviors.

There are some differences in using the *tri-factor* model to analyze CLT-based data than the MTMM data (Bajtelsmit, 1979; Campbell & Fiske, 1959). The main differences include: (1) MTMM data are collected from different participants while CLT-based data are collected from the same participants; as a result, (2) CLT-based data might be locally dependent while MTMM data are locally independent. Fortunately, the tri-factor model makes it possible to handle the local dependence (Bauer et al., 2013). In all factor analyses, the following data-model fitting criteria were used: Comparative fitting index (CFI) >0.90, Tucker-Lewis Index (TFI) >0.90, and root mean square error of approximation (RMSEA) <0.05 (Kline, 2005).

After tri-factor analysis, scale scores were calculated, including the common factor scores measuring CLT-based BSOS and scores for the three perspective factors, one for self-assessment and two for assessing the two socially distant groups. The computed perspective factors scores were associated with the conventional BSOS scores to test our study hypotheses that (1) the conventional BSOS scores are biased because such assessment is based on information at the lower construal levels that are less stable and more likely to be shaped by social contextual factors; and the (2) when assessing socially distant others, participants depend primarily on their own knowledge and beliefs stored at higher construal levels that are more stable and less likely to be shaped by contextual factors.

Multivariate regression was used to assess concurrent predictive validity with the following two hypotheses:

1. a CLT-based measure will perform better than a conventional measure in predicting well-assessed outcome measures, including the highly reliable sexual desire measure, the unplanned pregnancy assessment that is less error-prone (Brener et al., 2002), and the STD assessment that was verified through cognitive interview (Nguyen et al., 2015; Willis, 2015).
2. CLT-based measures will perform less well than the conventional measure in predicting reported number of sex partners because the reported number of sex partners is subject to over-report by males and under-report by females (Jonason & Fisher, 2009).

Second-order factor analysis and *tri-factor* analysis were conducted using the software Amos of IBM SPSS Statistics for Windows v. 22 (IBM Corp. Armonk, NY). Other statistical analyses were conducted using the software SAS v. 9.4 (SAS Institute, Cary, NC).

Table 4.3 Characteristics of the study sample

Variable	Female no. (% row)	Male no. (% row)	Total no. (% row)
Total sample, N (%)	683 (54.64)	567 (45.36)	1250 (100.00)
Age (in years)			
Range	18–45	18–45	18–45
Mean (SD)	35.27 (7.48)	34.85 (7.62)	35.08 (7.54)
Education			
Primary school or less	28 (53.85)	24 (46.15)	52 (4.16)
Middle school	144 (54.14)	122 (45.86)	266 (21.28)
High school	239 (53.95)	204 (46.05)	443 (35.44)
College or more	272 (55.64)	217 (44.38)	489 (39.12)
Marital status			
Married	571 (57.50)	422 (42.50)	993 (79.44)
Unmarried	112 (43.58)	145 (56.42)	257 (20.56)
Having children			
Yes	532 (58.21)	382 (41.79)	914 (73.12)
No	151 (44.94)	185 (55.06)	336 (26.88)

4.4.5 Sample Characteristics

Among the 1249 participants, 54.64% were female with a mean age of 35.08 (SD = 7.54), 79.44% were married and 73.12% had children. More details about the study sample are presented in Table 4.3.

4.4.6 Performance of the BSOS as a Conventional Scale

Results in Table 4.4 indicate that BSOS as a conventional scale is good. The mean item scores varied from 1.64 (SD = 0.99) to 2.63 (1.22), toward the middle of the score range (0–4); the item-total correlation varied from 0.46 to 0.67, all statistically significant at $p < 0.01$ and the Cronbach alpha = 0.79 for the total sample and males and 0.73 for females. Results from IRT analysis indicated some variations in item information with the least information for the item assessing premarital sex and most for the item assessing extramarital sex. There were also a sex differences with males scoring higher than females on all five items ($p < 0.05$ or 0.01).

The conventional BSOS data fit the five-level polytomous IRT model satisfactorily as indicated by the item characteristic curves (ICC) for individual items and the measurement scale information curves in Fig. 4.2. Based on the scale information, BSOS has 80% or greater reliability to assess sexual openness trait within a large range of −0.2 to 3.1 standard deviations.

As expected, all the results presented in Table 4.4 and Fig. 4.2 above suggest that as a conventional tool, the BSOS performed good, but not excellent.

Table 4.4 Brief sexual openness scale and its performance among urban residents in Wuhan, China—conventional measurement approach

Parameter	Multiple sex-partner	Premarital sex	Extramarital sex	Homo-sexuality	Commercial sex
Total sample, n = 1249					
Mean (SD)	1.78 (1.08)	2.63 (1.22)	1.69 (1.01)	2.08 (1.15)	1.64 (0.99)
Item-total r	0.57	0.53	0.67	0.46	0.64
Cronbach α if deleted	0.75	0.76	0.72	0.79	0.73
Difficulty	1.35	0.58	1.26	1.36	1.39
Information	1.5	0.9	4.2	0.6	2.4
Reliability	60%	47%	81%	38%	71%
Male, n = 566					
Mean (SD)	2.15 (1.17)	3.00 (1.22)	2.04 (1.12)	2.16 (1.17)	2.02 (1.09)
Item-total r	0.57	0.54	0.64	0.50	0.63
Cronbach α if deleted	0.76	0.77	0.74	0.78	0.74
Difficulty	0.98	0.13	0.96	1.11	1.05
Information	1.3	0.7	2.5	1.5	1.8
Reliability	57%	41%	71%	60%	64%
Female, n = 683					
Mean (SD)	1.47 (0.89)	2.32 (1.13)	1.40 (0.79)	2.02 (1.14)	1.33 (0.76)
Item-total r	0.46	0.44	0.62	0.47	0.53
Cronbach α if deleted	0.69	0.71	0.64	0.69	0.67
Difficulty	1.93	1.22	1.66	1.45	1.85
Information	1.1	0.4	5.1	0.5	2.0
Reliability	52%	29%	84%	33%	67%

Note: The Cronbach alpha = 0.79 for the total sample, 0.79 for males and 0.73 for females

4.4.7 Performance of the CLT-Based Method for Assessing Single Questions

When the 15 items were constructed as five single-question CLT-based measures, results in Table 4.5 show the psychometric characteristics of these scales in assessing the five sexual attitudes and behaviors individually. The information-based reliability for the scales varied from 85 to 91%. The scale scores (SD) varied from 1.90 (1.04) for commercial sex, to 2.38 (1.17) for premarital sex. The difficult index was always greater for participants' self-assessment than their assessment of urban and rural residents, indicating under-report of self-assessment. Opposite to difficult index, the information and reliability increased from participants' self-assessment to their assessment of the two socially distant groups.

Data for the five single-question CLT-based scales also fit the five-level polytomous IRT model satisfactorily as indicated by the item characteristic curves (ICC) for individual items and the measurement scale information curves in Fig. 4.3.

Based on the results in Table 4.5 and Fig. 4.3, we can conclude that CLT-based method can be constructed and used to assess single sensitive questions related to

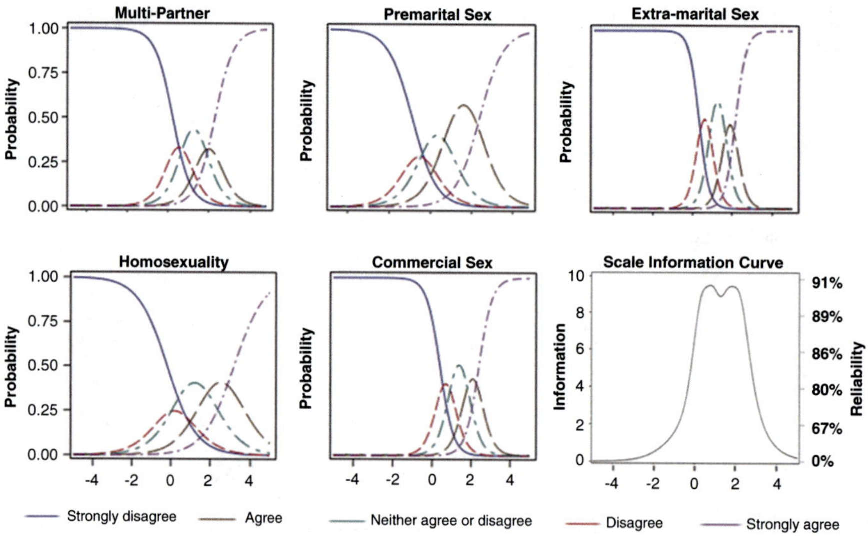

Fig. 4.2 Item-characteristic curve and measurement information curve of BSOS

sex related attitudes and behaviors to obtain more reliable data. Further research is needed to assess the utility of this CLT-based method in assessing other sensitive topics for global health and epidemiological research.

4.4.8 Construct Validity of CLT-Based Method as a Multi-contents Instrument

When data for all 15 items were organized as a second order multi-content measure, it can help us achieve three goals: (a) Assessing the structural validity of this complex CLT-based method, (b) assess the bias in reported data, and (c) derive "true" measurement scores.

Results from CFA indicate good fit of the 15-item data to the two-level structure of CLT-BSOS scale with CFI = 0.94, TLI = 0.93, and RMSEA = 0.09 (no item-level covariance added). The modeling results in Fig. 4.4 indicate that all freely estimated factor loadings were statistically significant at $p < 0.01$ level. Participants' self-assessment and their assessments of the two socially distant groups formed three independent subcontructs, which in turn formed the common construct sexual openness. The free-estimated factor loadings from the three first-level factors to the common factor were 0.27 for self-assessment, 0.80 for assessing rural residents and 1.00 (freely estimated) for assessing urban residents.

Table 4.5 CLT-based openness to five specific sexual attitudes/behaviors by incorporating information from two socially distant groups

	Item-level character			
Trait/parameter	Self-assessment	Assessment of urban residents	Assessment of rural residents	Scale
Multi-partners				
Mean (SD)	1.78 (1.08)	2.27 (1.20)	2.02 (1.05)	2.02 (1.11)
Difficulty	3.76	0.81	0.99	n/a
Information	0.1	3.8	2.0	5.5
Reliability	9%	79%	67%	85%
Premarital sex				
Mean (SD)	2.63 (1.22)	2.37 (1.24)	2.13 (1.05)	2.38 (1.17)
Difficulty	1.75	0.90	0.63	n/a
Information	0.1	3.6	3.8	6.8
Reliability	9%	78%	79%	87%
Extramarital sex				
Mean (SD)	1.69 (1.01)	1.97 (0.99)	2.11 (1.15)	1.92 (1.05)
Difficulty	3.98	1.02	0.84	n/a
Information	0.2	5.3	4.6	9.7
Reliability	17%	84%	82%	91%
Homosexuality				
Mean (SD)	2.08 (1.15)	1.94 (1.08)	1.86 (0.96)	1.96 (1.06)
Difficulty	3.10	1.15	0.98	n/a
Information	0.1	4.1	6.9	10.4
Reliability	9%	80%	87%	91%
Commercial sex				
Mean (SD)	1.64 (0.99)	2.11 (1.15)	1.96 (0.99)	1.90 (1.04)
Difficulty	3.30	1.05	0.85	n/a
Information	0.2	4.6	5.8	10
Reliability	17%	82%	85%	91%

4.4.9 Separation of Three Factors Based on CLT-Based Data

By modeling the CLT-based data with 15 items in two levels and three subconstructs with tri-factor analysis model, we can separate the common factor (for assessing "true" scores), perspective factors and item heterogeneity factors. Results from our analysis indicate a satisfactory fit of the data to the tri-factor model with CFI = 0.94, TLI = 0.92, and RMSEA = 0.09 (no item-level covariance was added).

Figure 4.5 presents the tri-factor analysis results. The common factor O on the top provides the true measure of sexual openness. Factor loadings to O were in general the largest for participants' assessment of other urban residents (>0.7 for all), followed by their own assessment (0.46–0.65) and their assessment of rural residents (0.39–0.49).

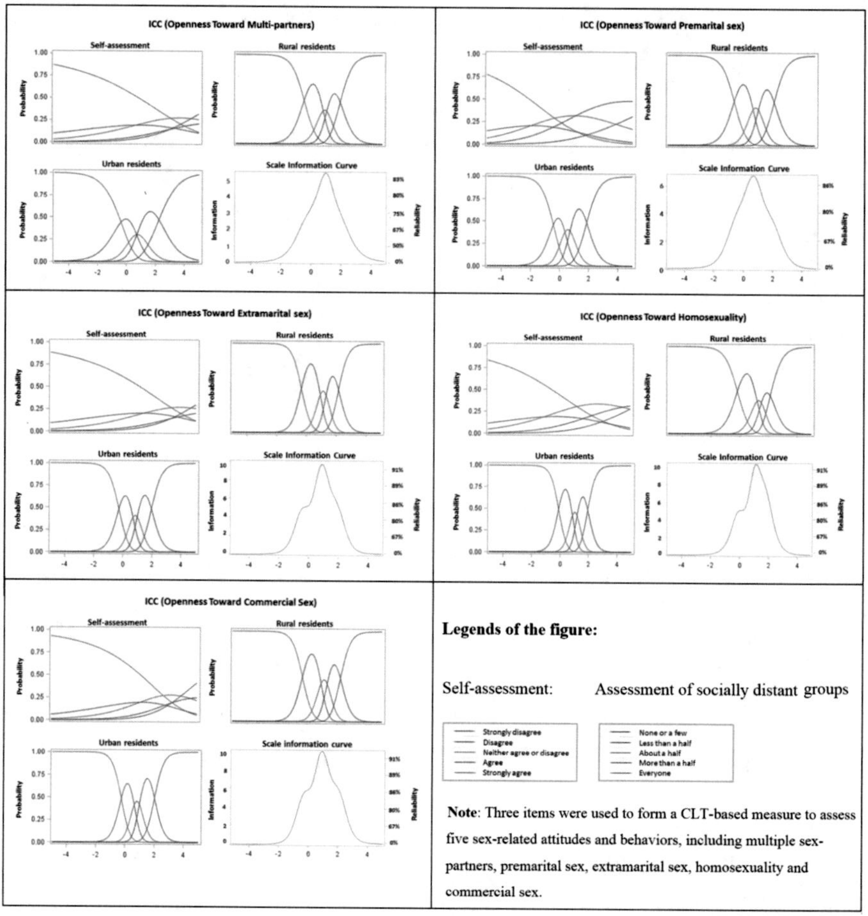

Fig. 4.3 Item characteristic curve (ICC) and measurement information curve of five CLT-based measure of sex-related attitudes and behavior, n = 1249. Note: Three items were used to form a CLT-based measure to assess five sex-related attitudes and behaviors, including multiple sex-partners, premarital sex, extramarital sex, homosexuality and commercial sex

The perspective factor S provide a measure of bias by participants who might have cognitively *edited* their answers according to social context. Perspective factors U and R provide a measure of participants' observation, knowledge or stereotypic about the other urban and the rural residents respectively.

The five item-level factors corresponding to the five survey questions suggest item-level disturbance, although the factor loadings were relatively small for all.

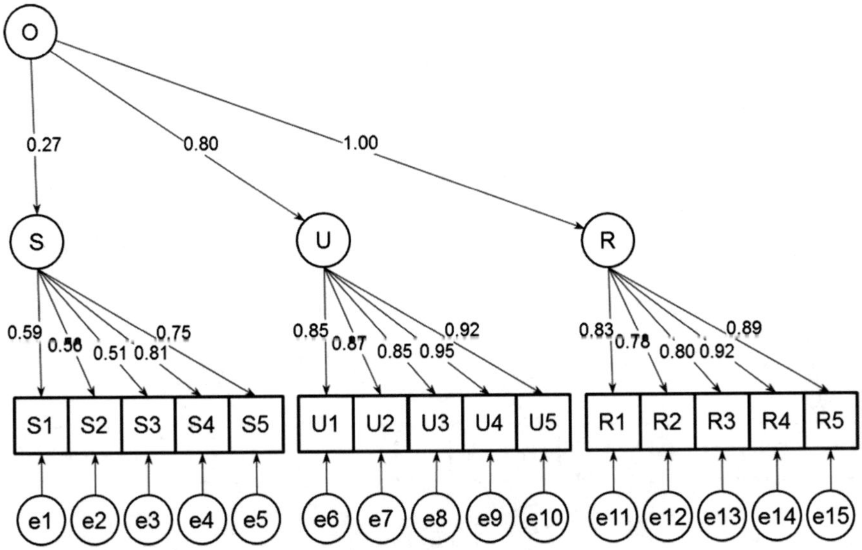

Fig. 4.4 Second-order modeling of the CLT-based BSOS measure. Note. *O* The second-order factor of latent sexual openness, *S* Self-assessment, *U* Assessment of urban residents, *R* Assessments of rural residents. Model fit: CFI = 0.94, TLI = 0.93, and RMSEA = 0.09. No covariance between any two items was added

4.4.10 Bias Assessment

If we suspect that the score from the conventional BSOS are biased, results from tri-factor analysis provide an opportunity to assess the bias in survey responses. Figure 4.6 depict the relationship between the standardized conventional BSOS scores (mean = 0, SD = 1) and the CLT-based perspective factor scores of (a) themselves and (b) urban and (c) rural residents. The conventional BSOS score would *not* be associated with the three perspective scores, if there was no response bias. However, results in Fig. 4.6a indicated a significant and positive relationship between the two (intercept = 0.000, p > 0.05; b = 0.793, p < 0.01, and $R^2 = 0.69$), suggesting a large positive response bias in answering the five sex-related questions. Furthermore, the majority of the data points were located within ±1 SD range, indicating a relatively even over-reporting across the five points of the Likert scale. The R^2 value indicated that despite the adequate reliability of the conventional BSOS (alpha = 0.79), reported error (information bias) could be as big as 69%.

Results in Fig. 4.6b, c indicate a weak but negative association between the conventional BSOS scores and perspective scores for urban (intercept a = −0.000, p > 0.05; b = −0.129, $p < 0.001$; and $R^2 = 0.04$) and rural (a = −0.000, p > 0.05; b = −0.107, p < 0.01, and $R^2 = 0.02$) residents. The negative b's indicate that participants did not believe that these two socially distant groups were sexually as open as they were, although the difference was relatively small.

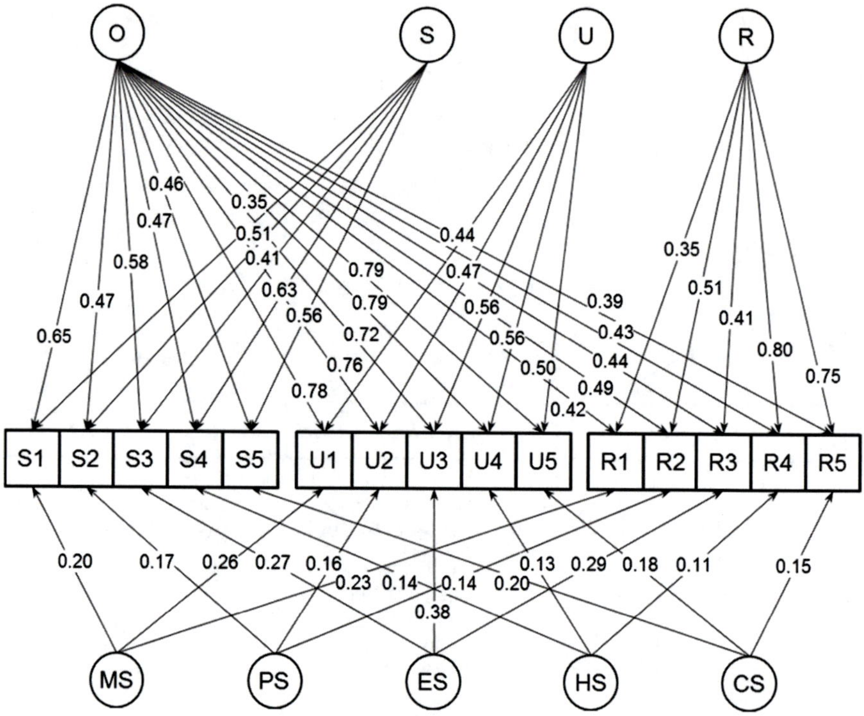

Fig. 4.5 Trifactor modeling of the CLT-based BSOS measure. Note. *O* The common factor, *S* the perspective factor of urban residents themselves, *U* the perspective factor of urban residents, *R* the perspective factor of rural residents, *MS* the latent factor assessing the item multi-partners, *PS* the latent factor assessing the item premarital sex, *MS* the latent factor assessing the item multiple sexual partners, *HS* the latent factor assessing the item homosexuality, *CS* the latent factor assessing the item commercial sex. Model fit: CFI = 0.94, TLI = 0.92, and RMSEA = 0.09. No covariance between any two items was added

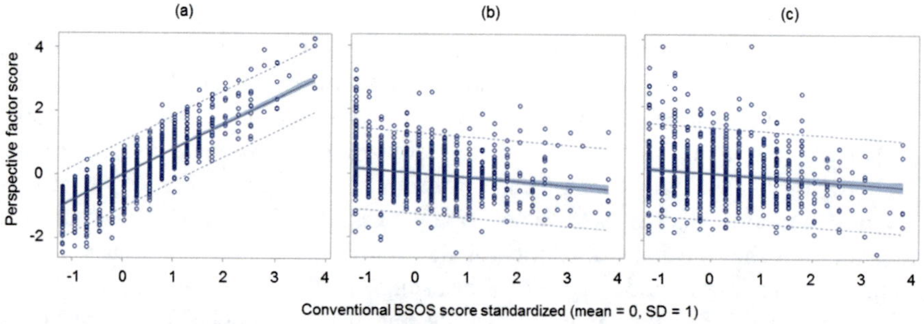

Fig. 4.6 Relationship between the mean BSOS scores and the perspective scores for participants themselves (**a**), urban (**b**) and rural residents (**c**)

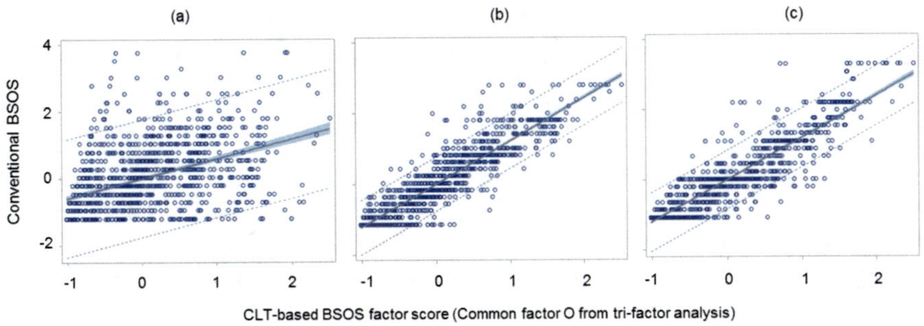

Fig. 4.7 Relationship between CLT-based and conventionally-based BSOS. (**a**) Participants themselves. (**b**) Urban residents. (**c**) Rural residents

Figure 4.7a plots the CLT-based O factor score with conventional BSOS score. If no bias, all the data points were be on the diagonal with intercept = 0 and slope = 1. Results in the figure show that intercept a = 0.000, $p > 0.05$; b = 0.589, $p < 0.01$ ($R^2 = 0.19$). The estimated b < 1.0, indicating systematically underreport with the conventional measure.

Figure 4.7b, c demonstrate to what extent participants rated the two socially distant groups based on their own openness. There was a strong and positive relation between participants' *true* sexual openness and their assessment of the other urban residents (intercept a = −0.000, $p > 0.05$; b = 1.219, $p < 0.01$; $R^2 = 0.85$) and the rural residents (a = −0.000, $p > 0.05$; b = 1.199, $p < 0.01$; and $R^2 = 0.82$). The R^2 indicates that greater than 80% of the assessments of the two socially distant groups was based on participants own beliefs.

4.4.11 Predictive Validity

Table 4.6 summarizes the results from the validity analysis of different sexual openness measures in predicting the four selected outcomes. Overall, CLT-based measures consistently predicted the four outcome variables with greater standardized regression coefficients or odds ratio (OR).

4.4.12 Summary

This section provides the most comprehensive introduction to the CLT-based method using an empirical example. It covers the theory, application and verification of the method with the hope to assist readers in understanding the method and applying the method in solve their own research questions.

Table 4.6 Predictive validity of CLT-based and conventional BSOS, overall and by single items

	Linear regression standard b (R^2)		Logistic regression OR (95% CI)	
Predictor	Sexual desire	# sex partners	Unplanned pregnancy	Cognitively verified STD
Scale scores				
CLT-BSOS	0.339 (0.315) **	0.220 (0.119) **	1.90 (1.56, 2.31)**	2.89 (1.51, 5.55)**
BSOS	0.300 (0.285) **	0.248 (0.127) **	1.44 (1.24,1.67)**	1.58 (1.01, 2.48)*
Multi-partner				
CLT-based	0.297 (0.292) **	0.189 (0.108) **	4.83 (2.63, 8.87)**	20.69 (2.92, 146.5)**
Single question	0.229 (0.255) **	0.228 (0.120) **	1.41 (1.24, 1.61)**	1.26 (0.80, 1.97)
Pre-marital sex				
CLT-based	0.275 (0.281) **	0.153 (0.096) **	8.71 (4.07, 18.64)**	47.23 (4.21, 530.4)**
Single question	0.206 (0.246) **	0.199 (0.109) **	1.35 (1.18, 1.54)**	1.36 (0.90, 2.06)
Extra-marital sex				
CLT-based	0.239 (0.264) **	0.093 (0.082) **	2.74 (1.42, 5.25)**	15.05 (2.12, 106.9)**
Single question	0.148 (0.229) **	0.122 (0.088) **	1.21 (1.06 1.37)**	1.15 (0.75, 1.78)
Homosexuality				
CLT-based	0.292 (0.291) **	0.148 (0.095) **	7.56 (3.69, 15.51)**	30.93 (3.37, 283.9)**
Single question	0.255 (0.267) **	0.138 (0.091) **	1.206 (1.05, 1.39)**	1.63 (1.09, 2.43)**
Commercial sex				
CLT-based	0.297 (0.292)**	0.189 (0.108) **	4.83 (2.63, 8.87)**	20.69 (2.92, 146.5)**
Single question	0.229 (0.254)**	0.187 (0.105) **	1.15 (0.99, 1.33)	1.50 (0.98, 2.30)

Note: Predictive validity of the CLT-based BSOS was assessed using tri-factor modeling method, the predictive validity for the conventional BSOS was assessed using the one-factor modeling method, and the predictive validity for individual attitudes/behavior was assessed using linear or logistic regression method. Age, gender and marital status were included in all predictive models as covariates. Standard coefficients were reported for linear regressions. Odds ratios were reported for logistic regressions. * $p < 0.05$ and ** $p < 0.01$

4.5 Application of the CLT-Based Method in an Rural Sample

4.5.1 Data Sources and Participants

Data and variables used for this study were the same as those described in Sect. 4.4 for urban resident sample except that the study participants were rural residents. These participants were randomly sampled from a band region 25 km wide 50 km away from and surrounding Wuhan, the capital city of Hubei Province, China.

4.5.2 BSOS as Conventional and CLT-Based Scale

The same BSOS as used in Sect. 4.4 was used here as a conventional instrument to assess the openness of rural residents in China, including five items to assess attitudes toward (1) premarital sex, (2) multiple sexual partners, (3) homosexuality, (4) extramarital sex, and (5) commercial sex. To illustrate the CLT-based survey, we only used the first three questions to form a brief scale.

To construct the CLT-based scale, three socially distant groups were used: (1) rural-to-urban migrants (close), (2) urban residents (far), and (3) foreigners (farthest). This selection utilized the natural social distance sequence in Chinese society defined by social mobility from rural to urban to foreign countries. With three socially distant groups and three sexual openness question, the constructed CLT scale consists of 12 items.

4.5.3 Variables for Validity Assessment

1. *Ever had sex in lifetime* (Yes/No): This variable was assessed based on response to the question: "Please recall from the time when you can recall till today. During this period, have you ever had sex with anyone, including with the same gender and any sexual behavior through vagina, anus or mouth?"
2. *Premarital sex* (*Yes/No*): Premarital sex was measured by the question: "Did you have your first sex before getting married?"
3. *Multiple sexual partners* (*Yes/No*): All participants were asked, "Up to now, with how many persons have you had sexual intercourse, including your spouse, lovers, and strangers?" Participants who reported having two or more partners were coded as "Yes"; otherwise, their responses were coded as "No".

4.5.4 Statistical Analysis

Since the psychometric modeling analyses have been covered in detail in Sect. 4.4, we only focused on two analyses: (1) Tri-factor modeling of the simplified 3-question CLT-based BSOS and (2) the predictive validity of this CLT-based measure relative to the conventional measure. In predictive validity analysis, multiple logistic regression models were used to assess the predictive validity. Four types of BSOS scores were used, the simple summary scores over the total 12 items, plus the latent scale scores for the second-order and tri-factor latent scale scores. For each of the four outcome variables, four logistic regression models, one for each of the four BSOS scores were used.

Data processing and general statistical analyses were completed using the commercial software SAS version 9.3 (SAS Institute Inc., Cary, NC). The measurement modeling analyses were conducted using the software AMOS 22.0 (IBM Corp., Armonk, NY).

4.5.5 Sample Characteristics

Data for a sample of 1143 participants were analyzed after an exclusion of 147 who claimed that their answers to the survey were either "not truthful at all" or "mostly not truthful". Among the total 1143 participants, 50.7% were male, with a mean age of 35.9 (SD = 7.7), 99.6% Han, 89.5% married, 71.5% with middle school or more education, and a mean family annual income between \$1626 and \$3250. The sample characteristics are summarized in Table 4.7.

4.5.6 Results from Tri-factor Analysis

The three-question CLT-based data fit the tri-factor well with CFI = 0.94, TLI = 0.92, and RMSEA = 0.09 (no item-level covariance was added). The modeling results were presented in Fig. 4.8. Factor loadings to O were in general the largest for participants' assessment of other urban residents and foreigners (>0.65 for all), followed by their assessment of rural-to-urban migrants (0.53–0.65), and were smallest for their own assessment (0.31–0.63). The loadings for perspective factors (S, M, U, F) were moderate (0.33–0.59). The three item-level

Table 4.7 Characteristics of the study sample

Variable	Female no. (% row)	Male no. (% row)	Total no. (% row)
Total sample, N (%)	564 (49.34)	579 (50.66)	1143 (100.00)
Age (in years)			
Range	18–45	18–45	18–45
Mean (SD)	35.27 (7.48)	34.85 (7.62)	35.95 (7.71)
Education			
Primary school or less	235 (41.67)	91 (46.15)	326 (28.52)
Middle school	272 (48.23)	348 (60.10)	620 (54.24)
High school	55 (9.75)	122 (21.07)	177 (15.49)
College or more	2 (0.35)	18 (3.11)	20 (1.75)
Marital status			
Married	536 (95.04)	488 (84.28)	1024 (89.59)
Unmarried	28 (4.96)	91 (15.72)	119 (10.41)
Having children			
Yes	530 (93.97)	483 (83.42)	1013 (88.63)
No	34 (6.03)	96 (16.58)	130 (11.37)

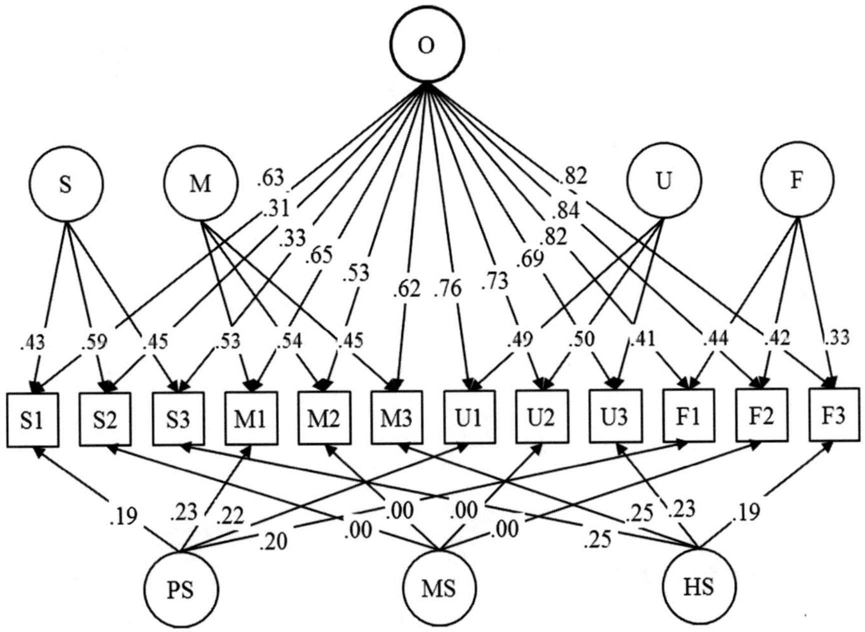

Fig. 4.8 Trifactor modeling of the CLT-based Brief Sexual Openness Scale. *Note. O* The common factor, *S* the perspective factor of rural residents themselves, *M* the perspective factor of rural-to-urban migrants, *U* the perspective factor of urban residents; and *F* the perspective factor of foreigners, *PS* the latent factor assessing the item premarital sex, *MS* the latent factor assessing the item multiple sexual partners, *HS* the latent factor assessing the item homosexuality. Data-model fit: Chi-square = 582.81, df = 49, CFI = .93, TLI = .90, RSMEA = .10. No covariance between any two items was added

factors were relatively small (0.00–0.25), suggesting item-level disturbance were relatively small for all.

4.5.7 Predictive Validity

Results in Table 4.8 indicate that the three-item BSOS significantly predicted three of the four outcome variables regardless of the scoring methods. Among the three scoring method, the odds ratio for the simple summary scores of the 12 items and the tri-factor latent scale scores appeared to be higher than that of the second-order latent scale scores.

Table 4.8 Predictive Validity (Odds Ratio) of the CLT-Based BSOS

Sexual openness	Ever had sex (414 = yes)	Premarital sex (214 = yes)	Multiple partners (102 = yes)
Total (N = 1143)			
Conventional scale score	2.01***	2.50***	2.54***
Second-order factor score	1.69***	1.91***	1.85***
Tri-factor score	2.02***	2.48***	2.28***
Male (n = 579)			
Conventional scale score	2.29***	2.41***	2.15*
Second-order factor score	1.88***	1.87***	1.68***
Tri-factor score	2.25***	2.25***	2.01***
Female (n = 564)			
Conventional scale score	1.65***	2.20***	2.53***
Second-order factor score	1.46***	1.77***	1.91*
Tri-factor score	1.73***	2.23***	2.21*

Note. * $p < .05$, ** $p < .01$, *** $p < .001$

4.5.8 Summary

In this section, we applied the same method in assessing sexual openness for rural residents with the CLT-Based BSOS slightly modified. The purpose is to show that the CLT-based method can be used to adapt published instruments for different populations.

4.6 Discussion and Conclusions

In this chapter, we reported one of our research efforts in attempting to collect reliable data for sensitive questions by reducing SDB. This method is theory-based, supported by rigorous psychometric testing with empirical data collected from different populations. The method is simple, noninvasive, and easy to use in any survey studies. In addition to obtaining high quality data, the method can be used to test sensitivity levels of a survey question and can be used to assess SDB for a survey question.

4.6.1 Theoretical Framework of the CLT-Based Method

Our confidence in the novel CLT-based method is stemmed first from its strong and relevant theoretical foundations. In addition to the psychology of survey responses as its theoretical foundation (Schwarz, 2007; Tourangeau et al., 2000), this method is built upon the one decade work of construal level theory (Liberman & Trope, 2008;

Liberman, Trope, & Stephan, 2007), the century long development of psychometric theories in general (Bollen, 2002; Borsboom et al., 2003; Raykov & Marcoulides, 2011; Spearman, 1904, 1931) and recent advancement in measurement modeling in particular (Bauer et al., 2013; Cai et al., 2011; Gibbons et al., 2007; Holzinger & Swineford, 1937). The cognitive mechanism of survey response has been extensively studied and this body of work serves as the foundation that provides the basic principles to improve reliability and validity of survey response (Schwarz, 2007; Tourangeau et al., 2000). Prior research indicates that deliberate editing is a major source of unreliable survey response, suggesting the reduction of editing may be one of the most important tasks in improving data quality for survey research (Holtgraves, 2004; Paulhus, 1984, 1991; Tourangeau & Yan, 2007).

Different from previous attempt for better quality data by circumventing the cognitive process involved in survey responses, our method directly works on the cognitive process with the guidance the construal level theory (Liberman, Trope, & Stephan, 2007). Our method works by simply asking participants, in addition to self-assessment, to assess 2–3 socially distant groups. Since the assessment of socially distant others are less likely to be affected by contextual factors, the assessments of socially distant others provide another data source to correct SDB (Cai et al., 2011; Liviatan, Trope, & Liberman, 2008; Rim, Trope, Liberman, & Shapira, 2013; Ross et al., 1977; Trope & Liberman, 2010). With several analytical methods based on the powerful latent variable theory (Bollen, 2002; Borsboom et al., 2003) and factor-analytic theory (Spearman, 1904, 1931), we can integrate the data from self-assessment and assessments of socially distant others to derive quality data.

4.6.2 Empirical Support for the CLT-Based Method

Findings of this study provide solid data supporting validity of the CLT-based method. The first piece of supportive evidence was the fact that only sensitive questions can form a latent construct using the CLT-based method as show in the first study. According to the psychology of survey responses, in answering a sensitive or intrusive question, participants may edit their responses to minimize harm and to maximize benefit (Krumpal, 2013; Tourangeau & Yan, 2007). This mechanism will not be activated when answering non-sensitive questions. In another word, if participants' self-assessment and their assessments of 2–3 socially distant others can form a "reliable" scale, the question is sensitive; otherwise, may not be sensitive.

The second piece of supportive evidence was the improvement in data reliability with the CLT-based method, compared to a conventional measure. Findings of this study indicate substantial improvement in the reliability of BSOS if the CTL-based method was used (Cronbach alpha increased from .78 to .96) for rural residents in the third study presented in this chapter and rural-to-urban migrants (from .81 to .96) in a published study (Chen et al., 2015). Furthermore, the increase has little to do with the increase in measurement items as demonstrated with Spearman-Brown prophecy formula (Brown, 1910; Spearman, 1910).

The third piece of supportive evidence came from the existence of a latent common factor as revealed from the factor modeling analyses. Successful extraction of the common factor from the multiple assessments provided by the same participant for different social groups supported the latent construct hypothesis we proposed that the assessments of different targets including self and socially distant others are determined by one latent construct—participant's own knowledge, attitudes and beliefs.

The fourth piece of supportive evidence was the improved predictive validity of a CLT-based measure. In the study presented in this chapter, sexual openness measured using the CLT-based method is more reliable and valid because it better predicted outcome variables measured in samples selected from three different populations—urban residents in the second study, rural residents in the third study and rural-to-urban migrants in a published study (Chen et al., 2015).

4.6.3 Recommendations and Future Research

The CLT-based method is easy to use. If your research needs to address a sensitive question as the main outcome or predictor, compose a question in your survey, and ask all participants to provide answer for themselves and for two to three socially distant groups. After data collection, using factor modeling analysis to derive the CLT-based scores as data.

However, one question remained on how to select the socially distant groups. As a recommendation to using the method, a rule of thumb would be to choose socially distant groups that are not too close or too distant. For example, for any participants as the target, family members would be too close to consider as a socially distant groups. For students, classmates and school mates consist of two good socially distant groups; while friends and classmates do not. In our study of rural residents in this chapter, the rural-to-urban migrants and the urban residents represent two suitable socially distant groups. In the published study of rural-to-urban migrants, the rural residents and the urban residents present two suitable socially distant groups (Chen et al., 2015).

To ensure successful use of CLT-based method, a pilot-test is highly recommended (1) to determine socially distant groups, (2) to improve the statement of the questions, and (3) even to test the order of self-assessment and the assessments of socially distant others. With regarding the last point in pilot testing, in our previous studies, we present the question along with the social distance with self-assessment first, and the most distant assessment last. We do not know if this is the best relative to other alternatives, such as reverse-order of random order.

References

Achenbach, T. M., Mcconaughy, S. H., & Howell, C. T. (1987). Child adolescent behavioral and emotional-problems - implications of cross-informant correlations for situational specificity. *Psychological Bulletin, 101*(2), 213–232. https://doi.org/10.1037//0033-2909.101.2.213

Achenbach, T. M., & Ruffle, T. M. (2000). The Child Behavior Checklist and related forms for assessing behavioral/emotional problems and competencies. *Pediatrics in Review, 21*(1), 265–271.

Albaum, G., Roster, C. A., & Smith, S. M. (2012). A cross national study of topic sensitivity: Implications for web-based surveys. *Journal of Marketing Development and Competitiveness, 6*(5), 71–82.

Bajtelsmit, J. W. (1979). Convergent and discriminant validation of chartered life underwriter (Clu) examinations by the multitrait-multimethod matrix. *Educational and Psychological Measurement, 39*(4), 891–896. https://doi.org/10.1177/001316447903900422

Bajunirwe, F., Haberer, J. E., Boum, Y., 2nd, Hunt, P., Mocello, R., Martin, J. N., ... Hahn, J. A. (2014). Comparison of self-reported alcohol consumption to phosphatidylethanol measurement among HIV-infected patients initiating antiretroviral treatment in southwestern Uganda. *PLoS One, 9*(12), e113152. https://doi.org/10.1371/journal.pone.0113152

Bauer, D. J., Howard, A. L., Baldasaro, R. E., Curran, P. J., Hussong, A. M., Chassin, L., & Zucker, R. A. (2013). A Trifactor model for integrating ratings across multiple informants. *Psychological Methods, 18*(4), 475–493. https://doi.org/10.1037/a0032475

Bockenholt, U. (2014). Modeling motivated misreports to sensitive survey questions. *Psychometrika, 79*(3), 515–537. https://doi.org/10.1007/s11336-013-9390-9

Bockenholt, U., & van der Heijden, P. G. M. (2007). Item randomized-response models for measuring noncompliance: Risk-return perceptions, social influences, and self-protective responses. *Psychometrika, 72*(2), 245–262. https://doi.org/10.1007/s11336-005-1495-y

Bollen, K. A. (2002). Latent variables in psychology and the social sciences. *Annual Review of Psychology, 53*, 605–634. https://doi.org/10.1146/annurev.psych.53.100901.135239

Bond, D., Ramsey, E., & Boddy, C. R. (2011). Projective techniques: Are they a victim of clashing paradigms? *Munich Personal RePEc Archive*. Retrieved from http://mpra.ub.uni-muenchen.de/33331/

Borsboom, D., Mellenbergh, G. J., & van Heerden, J. (2003). The theoretical status of latent variables. *Psychological Review, 110*(2), 203–219.

Brener, N. D., Kann, L., McManus, T., Kinchen, S. A., Sundberg, E. C., & Ross, J. G. (2002). Reliability of the 1999 youth risk behavior survey questionnaire. *The Journal of Adolescent Health, 31*(4), 336–342.

Brown, W. (1910). Some experimental results in the correlation of mental abilities. *British Journal of Psychology, 1904–1920, 3*(3), 296–322. https://doi.org/10.1111/j.2044-8295.1910.tb00207.x

Cai, L., Yang, J. S., & Hansen, M. (2011). Generalized full-information item bifactor analysis. *Psychological Methods, 16*(3), 221–248. https://doi.org/10.1037/A0023350

Campbell, D. T., & Fiske, D. W. (1959). Convergent and discriminant validation by the multitrait-multimethod matrix. *Psychological Bulletin, 56*(2), 81–105.

Chen, X., Wang, Y., Li, F., Gong, J., & Yan, Y. (2015). Development and evaluation of the Brief Sexual Openness Scale-A construal level theory based approach. *PLoS One, 10*(8), e0136683. https://doi.org/10.1371/journal.pone.0136683

Chen, X., Hu, H., Xu, X., Gong, J., Yan, Y. Q., & Li, F. (2018). Probability sampling by connecting space with households using Gis/Gps technologies. *Journal of Survey Statistics and Methodology, 6*(2), 149–168. https://doi.org/10.1093/jssam/smx032

Chen, X., Wang, Y., Leeman, R. F., Li, F., Zhao, J., & Bruijnzeel, A. W. (2018). Videoassisted topographical measurement of cigarette smoking: Exploration of an objective approach to evaluate nicotine dependence. *Tobacco Prevention & Cessation, 41*, 21. https://doi.org/10.18332/tpc/90821.

Cordero-Coma, J., & Breen, R. (2012). HIV prevention and social desirability: Husband-wife discrepancies in reports of condom use. *Journal of Marriage and Family, 74*(3), 601–613.

Crowne, D. P., & Marlowe, D. (1960). A new scale of social desirability independent of psychopathology. *Journal of Consulting Psychology, 24*(4), 349–354. https://doi.org/10.1037/h0047358

Dasgupta, A. (2015). *Alcohol and its biomarkers: Clinical aspects and laboratory determination*. New York: Elsevier.

Dawtry, R. J., Sutton, R. M., & Sibley, C. G. (2015). Why wealthier people think people are wealthier, and why it matters: From social sampling to attitudes to redistribution. *Psychological Science, 26*(9), 1389–1400. https://doi.org/10.1177/0956797615586560

de Jong, M. G., Pieters, R., & Stremersch, S. (2012). Analysis of sensitive questions across cultures: An application of multigroup item randomized response theory to sexual attitudes and behavior. *Journal of Personality and Social Psychology, 103*(3), 543–564. https://doi.org/10.1037/A0029394

Dunn, M., Thomas, J. O., Swift, W., & Burns, L. (2012). Elite athletes' estimates of the prevalence of illicit drug use: Evidence for the false consensus effect. *Drug and Alcohol Review, 31*(1), 27–32. https://doi.org/10.1111/j.1465-3362.2011.00307.x

Dwyer, J. H. (1980). Measurement models. In J. H. Dwyer (Ed.), *Statistical models for the social and behavioral sciences*. New York: Oxford University Press.

Fisher, R. J., & Tellis, G. J. (1998). Removing social desirability bias with indirect questioning: Is the cure worse than the disease? *Advances in Consumer Research, 25*, 563–567.

Gibbons, R. D., Bock, R. D., Hedeker, D., Weiss, D. J., Segawa, E., Bhaumik, D. K., ... Stover, A. (2007). Full-information item bifactor analysis of graded response data. *Applied Psychological Measurement, 31*(1), 4–19. https://doi.org/10.1177/0146621606289485

Gueguen, N. (2015). Similarity and sensitive topics survey: When similarity elicits answers to intimate questions in survey research. *Current Psychology, 34*(1), 58–65. https://doi.org/10.1007/s12144-014-9240-7

Gupta, S., Gupta, B., & Singh, S. (2002). Estimation of sensitivity level of personal interview survey questions. *Journal of Statistical Planning and Inference, 100*(2), 239–247. https://doi.org/10.1016/S0378-3758(01)00137-9

Himmelfarb, S. (2008). The multi-item randomized response technique. *Sociological Methods & Research, 36*(4), 495–514. https://doi.org/10.1177/0049124107313900

Holbrook, A. L., & Krosnick, J. A. (2010). Measuring voter turnout by using the randomized response technique: Evidence calling into question the method's validity. *Public Opinion Quarterly, 74*(2), 328–343.

Holtgraves, T. (2004). Social desirability and self-reports: Testing models of socially desirable responding. *Personality and Social Psychology Bulletin, 30*(2), 161–172. https://doi.org/10.1177/0146167203259930

Holzinger, K. J., & Swineford, F. (1937). The bi-factor method. *Psychometrika, 2*(1), 41–54. https://doi.org/10.1007/Bf02287965

Jo, M.-S. (2000). Controlling social-desirability bias via method factors of direct and indirect questioning in structural equation models. *Psychology & Marketing, 17*(2), 137–148. https://doi.org/10.1002/(sici)1520-6793(200002)17:2<137::aid-mar5>3.0.co;2-v

Johnson, T. R., & Bolt, D. M. (2010). On the use of factor-analytic multinomial logit item response models to account for individual differences in response style. *Journal of Educational and Behavioral Statistics, 35*(1), 92–114.

Jonason, P., & Fisher, T. (2009). The power of prestige: Why young men report having more sex partners than young women. *Sex Roles, 60*(3–4), 151–159. https://doi.org/10.1007/s11199-008-9506-3

Kim, H., Schnall, S., Yi, D. J., & White, M. P. (2013). Social distance decreases responders' sensitivity to fairness in the ultimatum game. *Judgment and Decision making, 8*(5), 632–638.

Kline, R. B. (2005). *Principles and practice of structural equation modeling* (2nd ed.). New York: Guilford Press.

Kraemer, H. C., Measelle, J. R., Ablow, J. C., Essex, M. J., Boyce, W. T., & Kupfer, D. J. (2003). A new approach to integrating data from multiple informants in psychiatric assessment and research: Mixing and matching contexts and perspectives. *American Journal of Psychiatry, 160*(9), 1566–1577. https://doi.org/10.1176/appi.ajp.160.9.1566

Krumpal, I. (2013). Determinants of social desirability bias in sensitive surveys: A literature review. *Quality & Quantity, 47*(4), 2025–2047. https://doi.org/10.1007/s11135-011-9640-9

Liberman, N., & Trope, Y. (1998). The role of feasibility and desirability considerations in near and distant future decisions: A test of temporal construal theory. *Journal of Personality and Social Psychology, 75*(1), 5–18. https://doi.org/10.1037/0022-3514.75.1.5

Liberman, N., & Trope, Y. (2008). The psychology of transcending the here and now. *Science, 322*(5905), 1201–1205. https://doi.org/10.1126/science.1161958

Liberman, N., Trope, Y., & Stephan, E. (2007). Psychological distance. In A. W. Kruglanski & E. T. Higgins (Eds.), *Social psychology: Handbook of basic principles*. New York: Guilford Press.

Liberman, N., Trope, Y., & Wakslak, C. (2007). Construal level theory and consumer behavior. *Journal of Consumer Psychology, 17*(2), 113–117. https://doi.org/10.1016/S1057-7408(07)70017-7

Liviatan, I., Trope, Y., & Liberman, N. (2008). Interpersonal similarity as a social distance dimension: Implications for perception of others' actions. *Journal of Experimental Social Psychology, 44*(5), 1256–1269. https://doi.org/10.1016/j.jesp.2008.04.007

Meisenberg, G., & Williams, A. (2008). Are acquiescent and extreme response styles related to low intelligence and education? *Personality and Individual Differences, 44*(7), 1539–1550. https://doi.org/10.1016/j.paid.2008.01.010

Nguyen, B. H., Nguyen, C. P., McPhee, S. J., Stewart, S. L., Bui-Tong, N., & Nguyen, T. T. (2015). Cognitive interviews of Vietnamese Americans on healthy eating and physical activity health educational materials. *Ecology of Food and Nutrition, 54*(5), 455–469. https://doi.org/10.1080/03670244.2015.1015119

Nicewander, W. A., & Thomasson, G. L. (1999). Some reliability estimates for computerized adaptive tests. *Applied Psychological Measurement, 23*(3), 239–247. https://doi.org/10.1177/01466219922031356

Ostapczuk, M., & Musch, J. (2011). Estimating the prevalence of negative attitudes towards people with disability: A comparison of direct questioning, projective questioning and randomised response. *Disability and Rehabilitation: An International, Multidisciplinary Journal, 33*(5), 399–411. https://doi.org/10.3109/09638288.2010.492067

Paulhus, D. L. (1984). Two-component models of socially desirable responding. *Journal of Personality and Social Psychology, 46*(3), 598–609. https://doi.org/10.1037/0022-3514.46.3.598

Paulhus, D. L. (1991). Measurement and control of response bias. In J. P. Robinson, P. R. Shaver, & L. S. Wrightsman (Eds.), *Measures of personality and social psychological attitudes* (pp. 17–59). San Diego, CA, US: Academic.

Paulhus, D. L., Harms, P. D., Bruce, M. N., & Lysy, D. C. (2003). The over-claiming technique: Measuring self-enhancement independent of ability. *Journal of Personality and Social Psychology, 84*(4), 890–904. https://doi.org/10.1037/0022-3514.84.4.890

Pei, Q.L., Chen, S., Xiao, Y., & Wu, S.S. (2015). A noval prevacy preseveing method for data collection and sharing in HIV survey studies. *Current HIV Research*, Accepted (invited mansucript).

Penney, S. R., McMaster, R., & Wilkie, T. (2014). Multirater reliability of the historical, clinical, and risk management-20. *Assessment, 21*(1), 15–27. https://doi.org/10.1177/1073191113514107

Pollack, A. Z. (2012). *Metals, reproductive hormones, and oxidative stress in women and consideration of correlated biomarker measurement error* (Vol. 72, pp. 5850–5850). Ann Arbor: University microfilms.

Rasinski, K. A., Willis, G. B., Baldwin, A. K., Yeh, W. C., & Lee, L. (1999). Methods of data collection, perceptions of risks and losses, and motivation to give truthful answers to sensitive survey questions. *Applied Cognitive Psychology, 13*(5), 465–484. https://doi.org/10.1002/(Sici)1099-0720(199910)13:5<465::Aid-Acp609>3.0.Co;2-Y

Raykov, T., & Marcoulides, G. A. (2011). *Introduction to psychometric theory*. New York: Routledge.

Rim, S. Y., Trope, Y., Liberman, N., & Shapira, O. (2013). The highs and lows of mental representation: A construal level perspective on the structure of knowledge. In D. E. Carlston & D. E. Carlston (Eds.), *The Oxford handbook of social cognition* (pp. 194–219). New York: Oxford University Press.

Robinson, R. J., Hensel, E. C., Morabito, P. N., & Roundtree, K. A. (2015). Electronic cigarette topography in the natural environment. *PLoS One, 10*(6), e0129296. https://doi.org/10.1371/journal.pone.0129296

Robles, T. F., Shetty, V., Zigler, C. M., Glover, D. A., Elashoff, D., Murphy, D., & Yamaguchi, M. (2011). The feasibility of ambulatory biosensor measurement of salivary alpha amylase: Relationships with self-reported and naturalistic psychological stress. *Biological Psychology, 86*(1), 50–56. https://doi.org/10.1016/j.biopsycho.2010.10.006

Ross, L., Greene, D., & House, P. (1977). The "false consensus effect": An egocentric bias in social perception and attribution processes. *Journal of Experimental Social Psychology, 13*(3), 279–301. https://doi.org/10.1016/0022-1031(77)90049-X

Sakai, J. T., Mikulich-Gilbertson, S. K., Long, R. J., & Crowley, T. J. (2006). Validity of transdermal alcohol monitoring: Fixed and self-regulated dosing. *Alcoholism-Clinical and Experimental Research, 30*(1), 26–33. https://doi.org/10.1111/j.1530.0277.2006.00004.x

Schwarz, N. (2007). Cognitive aspects of survey methodology. *Applied Cognitive Psychology, 21*(2), 277–287. https://doi.org/10.1002/acp.1340

Selvam, A. P., Muthukumar, S., Kamakoti, V., & Prasad, S. (2016). A wearable biochemical sensor for monitoring alcohol consumption lifestyle through Ethyl glucuronide (EtG) detection in human sweat. *Scientific Reports, 6*, 23111. https://doi.org/10.1038/Srep23111

Sieving, R. E., Eisenberg, M. E., Pettingell, S., & Skay, C. (2006). Friends' influence on adolescents' first sexual intercourse. *Perspectives on Sexual and Reproductive Health, 38*(1), 13–19. https://doi.org/10.1363/psrh.38.013.06

Spearman, C. (1904). "General intelligence" objectively determined and measured. *American Journal of Psychology, 15*, 201–292. https://doi.org/10.2307/1412107

Spearman, C. (1910). Correlation calculation from faulty data. *British Journal of Psychology, 1904–1920, 3*(3), 271–295. https://doi.org/10.1111/j.2044-8295.1910.tb00206.x

Spearman, C. (1931). The general factor in Spearman's theory of intelligence. *Nature, 127*, 57–57. https://doi.org/10.1038/127057a0

Statistical Bureau of Wuhan (2012). *Wuhan statistical yearbook-2012*. Beijing: China Statistics Press.

Steenkamp, J.-B. E. M., De Jong, M. G., & Baumgartner, H. (2010). Socially desirable response tendencies in survey research. *Journal of Marketing Research, 47*(2), 199–214. https://doi.org/10.1509/jmkr.47.2.199

Tavakoli, H. R., Hull, M., & Okasinski, L. M. (2011). Review of current clinical biomarkers for the detection of alcohol dependence. *Innovations in Clinical Neuroscience, 8*(3), 26–33.

Tourangeau, A. E., Lance, J. R., & Raninski, K. (2000). *The psychology of survey response*. Cambridge: The University of Cambridge Press.

Tourangeau, R., & Yan, T. (2007). Sensitive questions in surveys. *Psychological Bulletin, 133*(5), 859–883.

Trope, Y., & Liberman, N. (2010). Construal-level theory of psychological distance. *Psychological Review, 117*(2), 440–463. https://doi.org/10.1037/a0018963

Trope, Y., & Liberman, N. (2012). Construal level theory. In P. A. M. Van Lange, A. W. Kruglanski, & E. T. Higgins (Eds.), *Handbook of theories of social psychology* (Vol. 1, pp. 118–134). Thousand Oaks: Sage Publications Ltd.

Verhelst, N. D., & Verstralen, H. H. F. M. (2008). Some considerations on the partial credit model. *Psicológica, 29*(2), 229–254.

Warner, L. (1965). Random response: A survey techniqe for eliminating evaise answer bias. *Journal of American Statistical Association, 60*, 63–69.

Willis, G. (2015). Pretesting of health survey questionnaires: Cognitive interviewing, usability testing and behavioral coding. In T. P. Johnson (Ed.), *Health survey methods* (pp. 217–242). New York: Wiley.

Wright, S. A. (2012). Using construal level theory to detect social desirable bias. In Z. Gürhan-Canli, C. Otnes, & R. Z. Duluth (Eds.), *Advances in consumer research* (Vol. 40, pp. 687–685). Cincinnati: University of Cincinnati.

Wu, S. S., Chen, S., Burr, D., & Zhang, L. (2016). A new data collection technique for preserving privacy. *Journal of Privacy and Confidentiality, 7*(3), 99–129. Retrieved from http://repository.cmu.edu/jpc_forthcoming/8/.

Yuen, H. K., Wang, E., Holthaus, K., Vogtle, L. K., Sword, D., Breland, H. L., & Kamen, D. L. (2013). Self-reported versus objectively assessed exercise adherence. *American Journal of Occupational Therapy, 67*(4), 484–489.

Chapter 5
Integrative Data Analysis and the Study of Global Health

Andrea M. Hussong, Veronica T. Cole, Patrick J. Curran, Daniel J. Bauer, and Nisha C. Gottfredson

Abstract In this chapter, we introduce Integrative Data Analysis (IDA) for use in the field of Global Health. IDA is *a novel framework for simultaneous analysis of individual-level data pooled from multiple studies.* This framework has been applied to address questions about substance use, cancer, HIV, and rare diseases from studies around the world. Advantages of this approach include efficiency (i.e., reuse of extant data), statistical power (i.e., large combined sample sizes), the potential to address questions not answerable by a single contributing study (e.g., combining studies with overlapping ethnicities to examine cross-cultural differences or age periods to examine longer periods of development), and the opportunity to test replicability of effects across studies in the pooled analysis. We describe the IDA methodological framework, emphasizing unique issues in measurement harmonization and hypothesis testing. We illustrate the application of the method using examples. We also describe emerging tools to handle specific harmonization challenges. Finally, we consider the potential utility of IDA in Global Health and epidemiological research.

Citation: Hussong, A. M., Cole, V. T., Curran, P. J., Bauer, D. J., & Gottfredson, N. C. (in preparation). Integrative data analysis and the study of global health. In X. Chen (Eds), *Statistics for global health and epidemiology: Principles, methods and application*. New York, NY: Springer.

A. M. Hussong (✉) · P. J. Curran · D. J. Bauer
Department of Psychology and Neuroscience, University of North Carolina at Chapel Hill, Chapel Hill, NC, USA
e-mail: hussong@unc.edu; curran@unc.edu; dbauer@email.unc.edu

V. T. Cole
Wake Forest University, Winston-Salem, NC, USA
e-mail: colev@wfu.edu

N. C. Gottfredson
Gillings School of Public Health, University of North Carolina at Chapel Hill, Chapel Hill, NC, USA
e-mail: gottfredson@unc.edu

X. Chen, (Din) D.-G. Chen (eds.), *Statistical Methods for Global Health and Epidemiology*, ICSA Book Series in Statistics,
https://doi.org/10.1007/978-3-030-35260-8_5

Keywords Data pooling · Integrative data analysis · Data harmonization · Meta-analysis

5.1 Pooled Data Analysis and Global Health Research

We are in a data rich era in our scientific history, offering opportunities to address unanswered questions in the field of Global Health. However, better understanding health on a global scale requires more than data. It also requires tools that can extract meaningful knowledge from data. In some cases, this extraction requires innovative approaches to data pooling or combining data from different data sources (Cooper, Hedges, & Valentine, 2009). This may include integration of disparate datasets or data streams derived from sources that assess similar predictors and outcomes with some variation in measurement, sampling, or methodology. Methods that allow us to pool or integrate data across different sources are expanding rapidly (e.g., Hofer & Piccinin, 2009; Hussong, Curran, & Bauer, 2013; Pigott, Williams, & Polanin, 2012).

In the United States, the call for pooled data analysis comes from policymakers, publishers, funders, and scientists. For example, the National Institutes on Health (NIH) has funded international collaborative data collection efforts focused on drug use and HIV (the STTR collaborative; Chandler et al., 2015), injection drug use (the PRIMER study; Werb et al., 2016), and adherence to antiretroviral therapy for HIV (the MACH14 Collaborative; Liu et al., 2013). Investigator-initiated data collaboratives are also increasingly common and have produced significant contributions to our understanding of environmental influences on children's physical development (Jelenkovic et al., 2016; Silventoinen et al., 2016), prostate cancer (Key et al., 2015), mammography density and aging (Burton et al., 2017), and rare diseases (like hereditary transthyretin amyloidosis with polyneuropathy; Serrano, Atzinger, & Botteman, 2018).

A fundamental issue in conducting pooled data analysis is data sharing. In line with ethical guidelines (e.g., American Psychological Association, 2016), the Open Science Movement (National Academies of Sciences, Engineering, and Medicine, 2018) encourages data sharing to monitor the quality and veracity of published findings. In addition, NIH-supported measurement archives such as the Patient Reported Outcomes Measurement Information System (PROMIS; Cella et al., 2007) and the PhenX toolkit (Conway et al., 2014) serve as resources for investigators as they initiate new data collection efforts and need to identify highly reliable, valid, flexible, precise, and responsive assessment tools that can be widely used in independent studies to create a potentially broad database for pooled analysis.

Over the years, researchers have introduced several methods for data pooling and analysis. One group of methods focuses on horizontal integration or harmonization (to adapt a term from the equating literature; Steinberg & Thissen, 2013). This approach combines data for the same participants with data in two or more independent datasets (e.g., arrest records and hospital records) but when no link exists for identifying records in each dataset that belong to the same person. Another group of data pooling techniques combines data for different participants collected in two or more different datasets (or vertical integration). Perhaps the best known of these data pooling techniques is meta-analysis. Meta-analysis is a set of techniques that traditionally focused on analyses of summary statistics from a group of study results testing the same hypothesis (Cooper et al., 2009). A more recent extension of meta-analysis is individual participant data Meta-Analysis (IPD Meta-Analysis; Pigott et al., 2012). This form of meta-analysis is more common in medical research and has been used to address the problem of data pooling for randomized control trials as well as observational data. IPD Meta-Analysis may incorporate primary data from each participant in the pooled studies or a mix of primary data and summary statistics from studies for which primary data are not available. This approach has similarities as well to Mega-Analysis (McArdle, Hamagami, Meredith, & Bradway, 2000; McArdle, Prescott, Hamagami, & Horn, 1998). Together, these techniques form a toolkit for researchers interested in analyzing pooled data. We offer to this toolkit an approach that we call *Integrative Data Analysis (IDA;* Hussong et al., 2013*)*.

5.2 Integrative Data Analysis

5.2.1 Defining Integrative Data Analysis

Integrative Data Analysis (IDA) is a framework for the simultaneous analysis of raw data pooled from multiple studies (Hussong et al., 2013). IDA is a vertical integration technique that differs from traditional meta-analysis by performing pooled analysis on the raw data from individual studies instead of on summary statistics. In this way, IDA has some similarities with IPD meta-analysis. However, IDA possesses a few unique features, most notably its ability to directly address between-study differences in measurement.

IDA has been applied in pooled data analyses that evaluate treatments for depression (e.g., Brown et al., 2016), map the epidemiology of rare diseases (e.g., Serrano et al., 2018), and describe the trajectories of symptomatology in high-risk youth (e.g., Hussong, Flora, Curran, Chassin, & Zucker, 2008). Advantages of IDA evident in these studies include increased efficiency (i.e., reuse of extant data), statistical power (i.e., large combined sample sizes), and robust modeling of rare events. Moreover, IDA has the potential to address new questions not answerable by a single contributing study (e.g., combining studies with overlapping ethnicities to examine cross-cultural differences) and the opportunity to test replicability of effects across studies in the pooled analysis. Importantly, IDA can pool data from multiple studies with some variations in measurement, sample characteristics and methodology (Curran, Cole, Bauer, Hussong, & Gottfredson, 2016).

5.2.2 Research Questions Suitable for IDA

Although IDA can be a potentially powerful methodological approach, it is not appropriate for every pooled data application. Based on our own research, answers to the following four questions can help researchers decide whether to pursue IDA as a method for a given research problem (see Table 5.1).

First, does your research involve pooling data from separate studies that do not contain the same individuals? To ensure independent sample distribution, IDA requires that the data to be pooled come from separate studies that have no overlap in study participants. Otherwise, IDA will not be an appropriate selection.

Second, does the research problem call for testing the effects of a variable (e.g., gender or ethnicity) that is fully confounded with study membership? IDA cannot control for or test for study differences in a pooled analysis if study membership is fully confounded with variation in measures of interest. For example, if study A is all boys and study B is all girls, IDA cannot test whether there are gender differences in some outcome by pooling participants in studies A and B. In this case, it will be impossible to determine whether observed differences are due to study membership or gender.

Third, do all the pooled studies have scales (or items) assessing central constructs? Although missing data approaches (e.g., full information maximum likelihood estimation) may sometimes bend this rule, IDA typically requires that all

Table 5.1 Is Integrative Data Analysis (IDA) is the right method for your research?

IDA may be used if you answer YES to all four questions	Comments
Q1: Do you have separate studies with different participants in each study?	IDA was developed to pool data from separate studies with non-overlapping participants. It was not developed to match the same participant in different datasets (e.g., to engage in vertical equating).
Q2: Are study differences not entirely confounded with variables of interest for hypothesis testing?	IDA cannot control for or test for study differences in a pooled analysis if study membership is confounded with variation in measures of interest. For example, if study A is all boys and study B is all girls, IDA cannot test whether there are gender differences in some outcome by pooling participants in studies A and B.
Q3: Do you have scales (or items) assessing central constructs in each study?	IDA typically includes measures of each construct in each study which allows testing of study differences or replication.
Q4: Are there shared anchor items within each cross-study scale?	IDA assumes that some items on a scale are invariant across studies, serving to anchor the meaning of the construct. Identifying anchor items is part of the IDA method. However, if there is no content overlap in the items that make up a scale (or in the single items that tap a construct), then IDA may not be fruitful. Making a cross-walk for your scale is a way to answer this question.

studies contribute measures of each construct that will be included in a given analysis to allow testing of study differences or replication of effects.

And, fourth, is there the potential to harmonize measures (i.e., equate scores) on the constructs across studies? If there is no content overlap in the items that constitute a scale (or in single items that tap a construct), then IDA may not be fruitful and will likely yield biased or misleading results. (We discuss measurement harmonization in detail below.)

For those interested in pursuing IDA to address a research problem, we outline the IDA methodology as a guide (and refer you to other key references such as Curran et al. (2017) and Hussong et al. (2013). Because IDA is more of a methodological approach than a specific analytic procedure, we offer guidelines for researchers in making decisions about two key challenges in pooled data analysis consistent with IDA; namely, measurement harmonization and hypothesis testing.

5.3 Measurement Harmonization

5.3.1 Need for Measurement Harmonization

A key set of challenges in pooled data analysis concern measurement. Although many efforts by government funders and research consortiums have targeted more consistent use of core measures within a given field to facilitate data pooling (e.g., NIH's PROMIS and PHEN-X), measures are often altered in various ways. Typical reasons for these alterations include to align response scales and timeframes on similar measures, to change outdated or culturally inappropriate language, or to modify wording for a given reporter (e.g., adolescent versus parent report). Although these alterations are well-intended and sometimes necessary, a long history of psychometric research cautions that changes to an instrument's directions, timeframe, item stems, response scale, and even placement within a battery can impact the validity and reliability of a scale and the comparability of the altered scale to the original (Wainer & Thissen, 2001). Such cautions are equally noteworthy when it comes to pooling data from measures that may have been altered across studies because of potential differences in measurement properties for individuals in different subsamples, for whom a single item on an instrument may have different meaning. The more that the composition of samples differs across datasets in a pooled analysis, the more pronounced the challenges of measurement harmonization become.

5.3.2 Logical Harmonization

Measurement harmonization describes a set of techniques designed to address the challenge of creating comparable measures across pooled studies (Granda,

Wolf, & Hadorn, 2010). The most common approach is logical harmonization. In this approach, item responses can be re-scored, if needed, to be comparable across studies (e.g., by collapsing a response scale or combining two items; Granda et al., 2010). Regardless of whether rescoring is needed, this approach assumes that items with similar wording or content (based on face validity or expert ratings) function similarly in different studies. After items from different studies have undergone logical harmonization, three types of measurement items for the same instrument will be generated in a pooled dataset: (a) identical items that were administered in exactly the same way across studies, (b) logically harmonized items, and (c) unique items that appear in some (or maybe even only one) of the pooled studies. In practice, we often refer to identical and logically harmonized items together as common items.

Logical harmonization is common practice, particularly for single-item scales. For example, variation across studies assessing alcohol use may include the use of different item stems. Although the stems appear equivalent, they may invoke a different cognitive frame for participants in responding to the questions. "In the past year, how often did you drink alcohol?" as an item stem may or may not be equivalent to a more detailed item stem (i.e., "In the past year, how often did you drink alcohol including beer, wine, hard liquor, mixed drinks, and wine coolers"), an item stem with a different timeframe (i.e., "In the past two weeks, how often did you drink alcohol?"), or an item stem that assesses alcohol use quantity rather than frequency (i.e., "In the past two weeks, how many drinks of alcohol have you consumed?"). Although each of these items provides information about alcohol use, they may not be equivalent. If the investigator is mostly interested in whether a participant has ever used alcohol or not (e.g., in an IDA study on drinking onset among youth in the world), then any response to these questions other than '0' or 'never' can be recoded as 'yes' and the rest as 'no'. This would result in a logically harmonized measure of alcohol use that attempts to equate item content (in stems, time frames and directions) and response scales. For single-item scales, there are few alternatives to logical harmonization so this becomes an endpoint in measurement harmonization.

This is unfortunate because logical harmonization makes an untestable assumption of invariant measurement. With multiple item scales, the investigator can go beyond logical harmonization to test this assumption. An example of multi-item logical harmonization is the scales for HIV-related stigma as used in a three-study IDA as depicted in Fig. 5.1. This illustrative pooled dataset contains 18 items, although each of the three studies contains 9 items. There are five shared items between Studies 1 and 2; two shared items between Study 1 and Study 3; and two shared items between Study 2 and Study 3.

In some approaches to data pooling, unique items may be discarded and traditional scoring (i.e., creating means or sum scores) applied to the remaining common items. The dangers of this approach are threefold. First, the smaller subset of items may not fully capture the construct of interest (i.e., HIV-related stigma) as well as the full set of items that include unique items, potentially reducing construct validity but also reliability. Second, the assumption that items in the

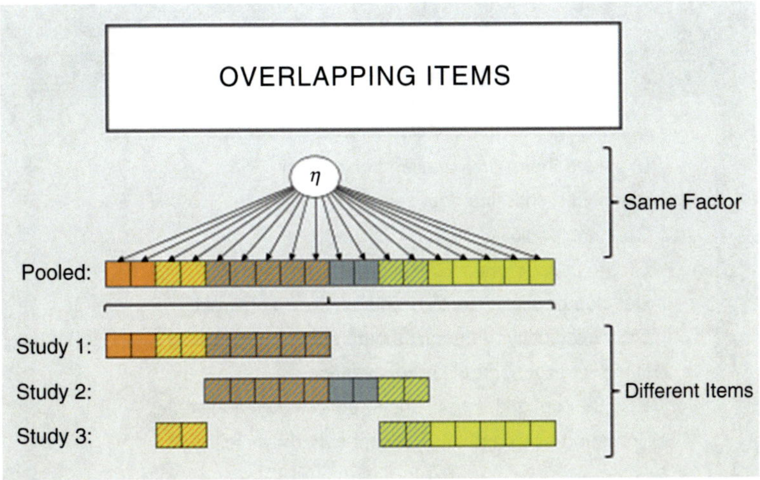

Fig. 5.1 Harmonizing overlapping items from different studies for IDA. Solid items in Study 1 only (orange), Study 2 only (blue), and Study 3 only (yellow). Shared items combine colors from multiple studies

pooled dataset are interchangeable (i.e., that logical harmonization was successful) is untested and violations of this assumption are not incorporated into the scoring model. And, third, even when items are identical across studies the potential for scales to function differently in one sample versus another is a well-documented psychometric challenge that may be compounded in pooled data analysis (Wainer & Thissen, 2001). Even an identical measure may perform differently in studies due to differences in sample composition (e.g., Study 1 has more men than Study 2), assessment protocol (e.g., study 1 primes the HIV-related stigma measure by first administering a discrimination measure in the battery whereas study 2 primes with a self-esteem measure), settings for data collection, and a host of methodological factors. For these reasons, the IDA framework requires that the assumptions of logical harmonization by evaluated with a second approach to measurement harmonization, namely psychometric harmonization.

5.4 Harmonization

5.4.1 Psychometric Harmonization and IDA

Our strategy for psychometric harmonization borrows heavily from measurement invariance testing in factor analysis (Meredith, 1993; Millsap, 2012; Millsap & Meredith, 2007) and on linking and equating test scores from educational assessment (Holland, 2007; Holland & Dorans, 2006). However, as shown in

TYPICAL STEPS IN IDA

1. Explicate theoretical question of interest
2. Identify contributing data sets
3. Conduct feasibility study
4. Create collaborative IDA research team
5. Develop pool of potential items for each construct
6. Create logically harmonized data set
7. Conduct psychometric hormonization
8. Estimate optimal scores anchored to a common scale
9. Transport scores to analyses for hypothesis testing

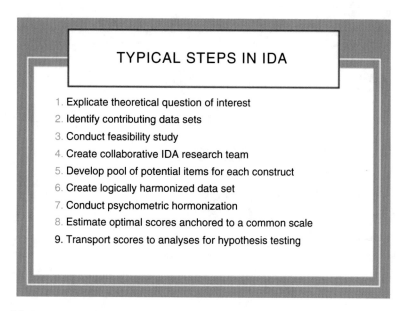

Fig. 5.2 Item selection for psychometric harmonization analysis

Fig. 5.2, our guidelines for conducting IDA do not begin with measurement but with identification of a strong hypothesis, identifying datasets, conducting a feasibility analysis and creating an IDA team. This framework is focused on variables of interest, drawn from studies that make theoretical sense for pooling and that include measures of all key constructs to produce a pool of common and unique items, and is supported by a clear set of guidelines for productive collaboration (see Hussong et al., 2013 for details about these steps).

A simple tool to guide item selection across studies and the creation of the integrated dataset is the measurement crosswalk (see Table 5.2 for an example). The crosswalk identifies the item pool for a given construct, documents variation in the measure or set of items across studies (e.g., in directions, item stems, reporters, time frames, response scales), and lays out the possibilities for logical harmonization.

This crosswalk is an important tool for IDA team communication and allows for expert evaluation of proposed item harmonization decisions. In addition, the crosswalk is an important guide for data management that identifies the naming convention for common items, re-scoring algorithms for different response scales across studies, and form of the integrated dataset. The crosswalk is also a tool for the analyst and study team that can provide a roadmap for expected and unexpected patterns of study differences in the pooled dataset.

Table 5.2 An example of measurement crosswalk

	Test form 1	Test form 2
Instructions	The next questions deal with alcohol, smoking and various other drugs. There is a lot of talk these days about this subject, but very little accurate information	
Response scale	0 occasions (0), 1–2 (1), 3–5 (2), 6–9 (3), 10–19 (4), 20–39 (5), 40 or more (6), Refuse to answer (.)	
Binge drinking	1. How many times have you had five or more drinks in a row in your lifetime?	How many times have you had five or more drinks in a row in your lifetime?
Tobacco	2. On how many occasions (if any) have you smoked cigarettes in your lifetime?	On how many occasions (if any) have you smoked cigarettes in your lifetime?
	3. On how many occasions (if any) have you taken or used smokeless tobacco (snuff, plug, dipping tobacco, chewing tobacco) in your lifetime?	In your lifetime, how often have you used chewing tobacco or snuff?
	4. On how many occasions (if any) have you smoked cigars or used pipe tobacco in your lifetime?	On how many occasions (if any) have you smoked cigars or used pipe tobacco in your lifetime?
	5. On how many occasions (if any) have you used electronic cigarettes in your lifetime?	In your lifetime, how often have you used e-cigs for tobacco?
Marijuana	6. On how many occasions (if any) have you used marijuana (weed, pot) or hashish (hash, hash oil) in your lifetime?	On how many occasions (if any) have you used marijuana (weed, pot) or hashish (hash, hash oil) in your lifetime?
Hallucinogens/MDMA	7. On how many occasions (if any) have you used LSD ("acid"), MDMA ("ecstasy") or other hallucinogens (like mescaline, peyote, "shrooms", or psilocybin, PCP) in your lifetime?	In your lifetime, how often have you used hallucinogens (like LSD, acid, mushrooms, PCP, special K, ecstasy)?
Cocaine	8. On how many occasions (if any) have you used cocaine (sometimes called "coke", "crack", "rock") in your lifetime?	On how many occasions (if any) have you used cocaine (sometimes called "coke", "crack", "rock") in your lifetime?

(continued)

Table 5.2 (continued)

	Test form 1	Test form 2
Amphetamines	9. Amphetamines are sometimes prescribed by doctors for people who have trouble paying attention, are hyperactive, have ADHD, or have trouble staying awake. They are sometimes called "uppers," "ups", or "pep pills", and include drugs like Adderall® and Ritalin®. Drugstores are not supposed to sell them without a prescription from a doctor. Amphetamines do NOT include any nonprescription drugs, such as over-the-counter diet pills or stay-awake pills. On how many occasions (if any) have you taken amphetamines on your own—that is, without a doctor telling you to take them—in your lifetime?	In your lifetime, how often have you used stimulants or amphetamines (such as Ritalin®, Adderall®, speed, uppers or ups)?
	10. On how many occasions (If any) have you taken Adderall® (without a doctor's orders) in your lifetime?	In your lifetime, how often have you taken Ritalin® or Adderall® in ways not prescribed for you by a doctor? (Do not include taking less than was prescribed for you.)
Opioids/ sedatives	11. Sedatives, including barbiturates and Quaaludes, are sometimes prescribed by doctors to help people relax or get to sleep. They are sometimes called "downs", "downers", "soapers", "quads", and "ludes" and include phenobarbital, Tuinal®, Nembutal®, and Seconal®. On how many occasions (if any) have you taken sedatives on your own— that is, without a doctor telling you to take them—in your lifetime?	In your lifetime, how often have you used barbiturates (prescription-type sleeping pills like Quaaludes, downs, yellow-jackets) or tranquilizers (prescription type drugs such as Valium®, Librium®, Xanax®, Klonopin®)?
	12. Tranquilizers are sometimes prescribed by doctors to calm people down, quiet their nerves, or relax their muscles. Librium®, Valium®, and Xanax® are all tranquilizers. On how many occasions (if any) have you taken tranquilizers on your own— that is without a doctor telling you to take them—in your lifetime?	*No matching item; harmonize by pooling item 11 and 12 from Test Form 1.*
	13. There are a number of types of narcotics, such as heroin. Some, like methadone, opium, morphine, codeine, Demerol®, Vicodin®, OxyContin®, and Percocet®, are sometimes prescribed by doctors. On how many occasions (if any) have you taken narcotics on your own—that is, without a doctor telling you to take them—in your lifetime?	There are a number of types of narcotics, such as heroin. Some, like methadone, opium, morphine, codeine, Demerol®, Vicodin®, OxyContin®, and Percocet®, are sometimes prescribed by doctors. On how many occasions (if any) have you taken narcotics on your own—that is, without a doctor telling you to take them—in your lifetime?

Source for Test Form 1: Monitoring the Future Survey: Johnston, O'Malley, Bachman, & Schulenberg, 2013

5.4.2 Psychometric Harmonization Model

After creating a pooled dataset based on the decisions embedded in a crosswalk, psychometric harmonization may begin. Although there are multiple approaches to psychometric harmonization, here we highlight the use of Moderated Non-Linear Factor Analysis (MNFLA; Bauer & Hussong, 2009; Curran et al., 2016; see Hussong, Flora, et al., 2008; Mun et al., 2015; Mun, Jiao, & Xie, 2016 for a discussion of other approaches). MNLFA is a highly flexible approach to analytic harmonization that blends the traditions of confirmatory factor analysis (CFA; Bollen & Hoyle, 2012) with item response theory (IRT; Steinberg & Thissen, 2013). The purpose of MNLFA is not to find interchangeable items across pooled studies but to create factor scores using both common and unique items from these studies to infer scores for an underlying factor representing the construct of interest thought to give rise to the item responses (see Fig. 5.1). Provided that enough (but not necessarily all) items measure the construct in the same way across studies – an empirically testable proposition—these scores can then be compared directly across studies. Importantly, this approach accounts for the presence of items that, despite being logically harmonized, do not in fact measure the construct equivalently.

In, MNFLA, we assume that all items used in the pooled studies assess a single construct (e.g., alcohol-related consequences) and can be measured by a single underlying factor. Items are referred to as y_{ij} and the latent factor is referred to as η_j, where i indexes items and j indexes people. For instance, for binary items, the relationship between the factor and the items can be expressed as

$$logit\left(\mu_{ij}\right) = \nu_{ij} + \lambda_{ij}\eta_j \tag{5.1}$$

where μ_{ij} represents the probability that item i will be endorsed by participant j, consistent with an item-level CFA. This probability is determined by a logistic relationship to the latent factor defined by an intercept ν_{ij} and a factor loading (slope) λ_{ij}. (Not that other item types can also be accommodated through the selection of appropriate link functions to relate expected values to latent factors, see Bauer & Hussong, 2009). Like a traditional CFA, these intercepts and slopes vary across items (the i subscript) but, unlike traditional CFA, they can also vary deterministically across persons (the j subscript).

The between-participant difference is determined by treating the parameters ν_{ij} and λ_{ij} as functions of person-specific covariates. Denoting the pth covariate for the jth subject x_{pj}, the measurement parameters are affected by covariates as follows:

$$\nu_{ij} = \nu_{0ij} + \sum_{p=1}^{P} + \kappa_{pi}x_{pj} \tag{5.2}$$

$$\lambda_{ij} = \lambda_{0ij} + \sum_{p=1}^{P} \omega_{pi}x_{pj}. \tag{5.3}$$

The parameters denoted by κ_{pi} and ω_{pi} reflect differential item functioning (DIF) for intercepts and loadings, respectively, indicating that these items do not measure the latent factor equivalently for people with different values on the background characteristic.

In typical IRT or CFA applications, these covariates are often individual demographic characteristics, such as gender or age. From the perspective of IDA, a key insight is that a subject's study membership can be treated as a covariate, allowing DIF based on study to be modeled. For instance, if the wording of an item differs across studies and this leads to an increase in endorsement of the item in one study versus another, this would result in (intercept) DIF for this item. If any items possess DIF, full measurement invariance is not present across studies. When a minority of items have DIF, this is referred to as partial invariance and is generally still considered to produce acceptable measurement comparability across studies at the level of the latent factor. When most or all items have DIF, then the validity of direct comparisons is dubious (Byrne, Shavelson, & Muthén, 1989).

Finally, in MNLFA, the latent factor mean (here denoted α_j) and variance (here denoted ψ_j) may also vary as a function of background characteristics allowing the mean level or variability of a construct to be higher for some participants than others. Between-participant differences in the mean or variance of a construct are known as impact and, as in the case of DIF, may occur based on study. For instance, if we were measuring alcohol consequences in a harmonized dataset comprised of a clinical sample and a community sample, we might expect mean and variance impact based on study. Mean and variance impact are conveyed through the following equations:

$$\alpha_j = \alpha_0 + \sum_{p=1}^{P} \gamma_p x_{pj} \tag{5.4}$$

$$\psi_j = \psi_0 \exp\left(\sum_{p=1}^{P} \delta_p x_{pj}\right) \tag{5.5}$$

where γ_p represents the impact of x_{pj} on the mean and δ_p represents impact of x_{pj} on the variance. To assign a scale for the latent factor, typically one sets α_0 to zero and ψ_0 to one, standardizing the scale of the factor when all background characteristics are scored zero. This again differs from a standard CFA or IRT analysis in which the mean and variance of the factor would typically each be assumed equal across persons. The effects of covariates on the factor mean, denoted by γ_p, and variance, denoted by δ_p, are collectively referred to as impact. A depiction of the full MNLFA model appears in Fig. 5.3.

The goal of MNFLA as an analytic harmonization approach in IDA is to test and account for study differences in pooled data analysis for latent constructs in terms of both study impact and DIF. This is of significance for global health and epidemiologic research, where between-study differences may relate to both the underlying construct of interest and the measurement process. For example, items

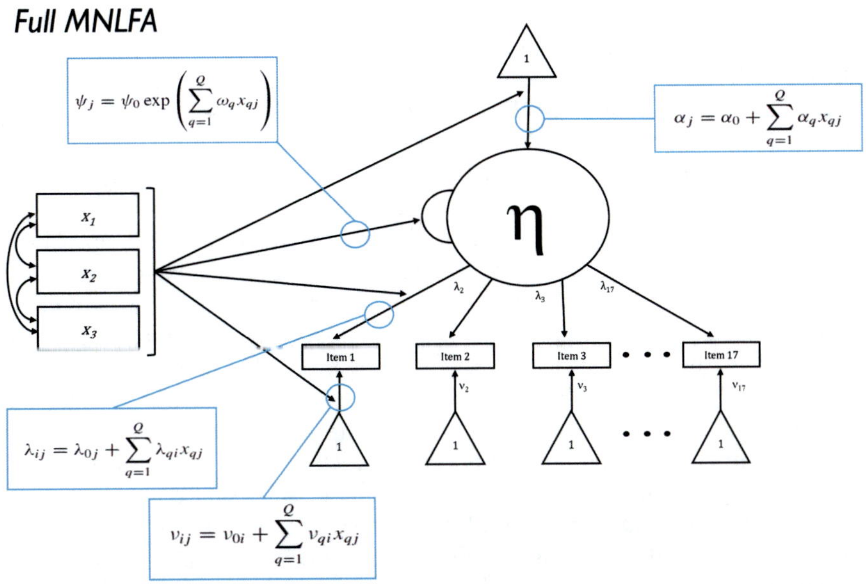

Fig. 5.3 Full moderated non-linear factor analysis

from a study that has administered a measure of alcohol-related consequences in its original form (e.g., the widely used Rutgers Alcohol Problems Inventory, RAPI, White & Labouvie, 1989) may relate differently to the underlying construct of alcohol-related consequences when compared to a second study in which some of these items have been altered, a response scale changed, or items dropped. These alterations to the scale may impact the performance of individual items or even lead individuals to respond to the original and altered items differently. Within the CFA tradition, such differences are said to result in non-invariant measurement. Within the IRT tradition, such differences are said to reflect differential item performance or DIF. Generalizing from these traditions, MNLFA provides a flexible framework for testing patterns of DIF in a set of items posited to underlie a given latent factor as a function of study membership. (Indeed, MNLFA provides even greater flexibility to test whether a set of categorical and/or continuous background characteristics uniquely as well as interactively account for DIF; see Bauer & Hussong, 2009 for a description).

MNLFA may be used to conduct IDA in harmonized datasets using a series of steps. We summarize these steps here and expand upon them in the empirical example, but readers are referred to the original formulation of these steps (Curran et al., 2014; Gottfredson et al., 2018) for further detail. The first step is to conduct descriptive and graphical analyses to understand the distributions of the items both within and across studies and the potential impact of covariates on these distributions. This may entail examining frequency tables and histograms to determine whether sparse response categories may be collapsed. The second step is to conduct factor analyses in order to determine the dimensionality of the construct. Though multidimensional MNLFA is certainly possible (see Bauer, 2017), we deal exclusively with the unidimensional case here. As with exploratory and confirmatory factor analyses, MNLFA assumes that observations are independent. When working with nested data (i.e., children in families, repeated measures), we therefore recommend fitting these models to a calibration sample, constructed by randomly sampling one observation from each cluster.

Third, MNLFA then models effects of study and covariate predictors on the mean and variance of the latent construct. Bringing these predictors into the model not only makes the specification of the model more accurate (by explicitly incorporating known sources of heterogeneity), but it also provides additional information with which to improve score estimates for the participants. We then move to testing models that incorporate DIF. A clear advantage of the MNLFA framework is that it allows DIF testing across studies as well as covariates (and even interactions among them) simultaneously. This is particularly useful when study membership is correlated with other potential sources of DIF (e.g., studies differ in proportion of men versus women, such that it may be important to account for and parse sex DIF from study DIF). DIF testing is accomplished by allowing variables indexing these potential sources of DIF to moderate the intercept and factor loading for an item. Again due to model complexity, we typically use an iterative process to estimate DIF on an item-by-item basis and trim non-significant predictors before incorporating all identified DIF in a summary model (Curran et al., 2014). Although this can be a tedious process, Gottfredson et al. (2018) offer an R program called aMNLFA (for automated MNLFA) that streamlines this analytic procedure[1].

Fourth, this final model is used to generate scores of the latent variable of interest. By incorporating DIF into the scoring model we can correct for bias in the scores that would result from differential measurement across study (i.e., failures of logical harmonization) and as a function of other covariates (e.g., age, sex, ethnicity). For instance, suppose that a harmonized item was constructed from two items measuring similar content but with slightly different item stems (e.g., an item assessing alcohol motives worded as "to get buzzed" in one study and "to get high" in another). If endorsement rates for these items differed in part due to wording differences in the item stems (i.e., buzzed versus high), and not just due to underlying differences in the construct of interest (i.e., stronger motives to use alcohol for such effects), then we would expect to detect study DIF for this item. Failing to account for study DIF would lead to artificially elevated scores for participants receiving the easier-to-endorse prompt. Generating scores from a model that incorporates DIF removes such potential sources of bias, ensuring that the scores are commensurate across studies (or other subpopulations).

There is, however, a question of how much DIF is too much DIF. If nearly all items display DIF, this would imply no commonality of measurement between subpopulations and a lack of comparability of scores. DIF among some items is

[1] http://nishagottfredson.web.unc.edu/amnlfa/

often expected and just how much DIF is tolerable is a matter of debate (Cheung & Rensvold, 1998; Reise, Widaman, & Pugh, 1993; Steenkamp & Baumgartner, 1998). Strictly speaking, only one invariant (non-DIF) item is required to put the measures on an equivalent scale across subpopulations, but the odds of correctly detecting which items are invariant versus not are reduced when many items display DIF (Yoon & Millsap, 2007). The less DIF, the more confidence one can have that the scale of measurement is truly invariant across persons.

In the final step of MNLFA, we examine the distribution and often the validity and reliability of scores. This includes both graphical analysis of the scores and assessments of the relationship between scores and predictors and outcomes of interest. These steps are expanded upon in the illustrative example below.

5.5 Illustrative Example

The goal of this analysis was to create an indicator for polysubstance use, a well-documented problem in Global Health (Hussong & Smith, 2018). Self-report instruments were used to assess the frequency with which participants used several common substances (e.g., alcohol, tobacco, amphetamines).

In this example we demonstrate an IDA combining data from two larger data collections. The first, the Real Experiences and Lives in the University (REAL-U) Study assessed substance use, psychopathology, academic functioning, and a variety of related constructs among college students. The second, the Millennial Friendship Study (MFS), assessed similar constructs. Additionally, MFS focused on relationships and contains dyads rather than individual respondents as in REAL-U; however, for the purposes of the current study, we only used one member of each dyad. In both REAL-U and MFS, two slightly different forms of the substance use measure were used for data collection (Table 5.2). The combination of data collections and test forms yields four studies: Study A (REAL-U, Test Form 1, $N = 225$); Study B (REAL-U, Test Form 2, $N = 301$); Study C (MFS, Test Form 1, $N = 236$); and Study D (MFS, Test Form 2, $N = 204$).

5.5.1 *Logical Harmonization of Individual Items*

Test Forms 1 and 2 are shown in Table 5.1. The polysubstance use measure (based on the Monitoring the Future Survey; Johnston et al., 2013) initially took the form of fourteen self-report items, each assessing a subject's lifetime frequency of using a given substance. Note that, while response options were identical between Test Forms 1 and 2, item stems were subtly different between the two forms. After a review of item content and endorsement rates, items were logically harmonized in two ways. First, we collapsed across some questions measuring similar substances. Specifically, one tobacco item was created using the maximum value a participant's responses to Questions 2–5; one amphetamine item was created using the maximum value a participant's responses to Questions 9 and 10; and one opiates/sedatives item was created using the maximum value a participant's responses to Questions 11–13.

Second, to deal with sparse response categories, we collapsed across response options for the bulk of items. For tobacco, we created a three-category item, which took a value of 0 if a subject had ever used tobacco, a value of 1 if the subject had used tobacco 1 to 5 times, and a value of 2 if the subject had used tobacco more than 5 times. For cocaine, hallucinogens/ecstasy, amphetamines, and opiates/sedatives, we created a binary item which took a value of 1 if a subject had ever used the substance and 0 otherwise. The original 7-point scale was retained for binge drinking and marijuana use, as higher categories were more frequently endorsed for these items. The result of these data management steps was the seven substance use items in the leftmost column of Table 5.2.

5.5.2 Steps 1 and 2: Descriptive Analysis

In order to include a covariate in an MNLFA model, configural invariance needs to be established on the basis of this covariate—that is, the same number and general configuration of factors should account for the covariance among the indicators across all levels of that covariate (Meredith, 1993). In preliminary analyses, it quickly became clear that there was not configural invariance based on gender. In particular, the relationship between all the substances and the latent construct was weaker, and the overall level of endorsement for all the substances considerably higher, among male participants. Due to well-documented differences between male and female young adults in terms of substance use (Chen & Jacobson, 2012), this is not surprising. But due to this lack of partial invariance, our example focused exclusively on female participants.

5.5.3 Step 3: Iterative MNLFA

After some preliminary analyses, including visual examination and exploratory factor analyses of these items in female respondents, we proceeded to conduct MNLFA using the aMNLFA package in R that utilizes Mplus (Curran et al., 2014; Gottfredson et al., 2018). We also tested the impact and DIF effects from two covariates on polysubstance use: sorority membership and the four different studies. Given the generally higher prevalence of substance use among students involved in Greek life (McCabe, Veliz, & Schulenberg, 2018), positive mean impact from sorority membership on substance use was predicted. Some DIF based on study was also predicted, given the differences in sampling and item wording across the four samples. Sample DIF was expected for the tobacco, opioid/sedatives, amphetamines, and hallucinogens/MDMA items, as the wording of these items differed between the different forms of the instrument.

A first set of models to test impact (i.e., differences in the latent variable mean or variance based on the covariates) was fit using the aMNLFA.initial() function. This initial set of models included: (1) a model testing the main effects of Greek life and study membership on the mean of substance use (mean impact) and (2) a model testing the main effects of Greek life and study membership on the variance of substance use (variance impact). The only impact effect was a positive effect of Greek life on the mean value of substance use, such that sorority members reported overall higher substance use than nonmembers. There were no mean-level differences between studies, and no variance impact for either variable.

A series of initial DIF models was then fit, also using the aMNLFA.initial() function. This step comprised seven item-wise models testing the effects of Greek life and study membership on the intercepts and loadings of each of the items (intercept and loading DIF). This step returned several intercept DIF effects, indicating differences in the overall levels of endorsement for certain substances based on study and/or sorority membership. There were intercept effects of sample membership on tobacco use and opiates, such that members of Studies C and D were less likely to endorse tobacco use, and members of Study D were more likely to endorse opioid and sedative use, than members of Study A. There was a positive effect of Greek life on binge drinking, as well as a negative effect of Greek life on the use of tobacco, marijuana, and amphetamines. Additionally, there were loading effects of sorority membership such that amphetamine use was more strongly related, and tobacco and marijuana use less strongly related, to overall substance use liability.

These impact and DIF effects were all tested simultaneously, using the aMNLFA.simultaneous() function, in the model shown in the left column of Table 5.3. Effects that were rendered non-significant were pruned from this model. The critical value for retaining a DIF effect, $\alpha = 0.05$, was sequentially adjusted using the Benjamini-Hochberg correction for multiple comparisons (Benjamini & Hochberg, 2000). The resultant model is shown in the right panel of Table 5.3. This model, which is denoted as the final model and fit using the aMNLFA.final() function, retained only three threshold DIF effects. There was a positive effect of study membership on the use of opioids and sedatives, such that members of Study D (who were in the MFS sample originally and answered Test Form 2) were more likely to endorse using these drugs than members of Study A (who were in the REAL-U sample originally and answered Test Form 1). Because the members of these samples differ both in terms of their original study membership and test form, it is difficult to determine whether this DIF reflects differences in measurement or sampling frame of the two studies. There was a positive effect of sorority membership on binge drinking, such that members of sororities were more likely to endorse binge drinking than their non-Greek counterparts, given the same overall level of substance use.

Table 5.3 aMNLFA results using the REAL-U IDA Analogue Study

Variable Coding		Simultaneous model			Final model		
		Estimate	SE	p value	Estimate	SE	p value
Substance Use							
Baseline parameters							
Intercept		0			0		
Variance		1			1		
Mean impact							
Sorority membership		0.428	0.104	<.001	0.338	0.083	<.001
Measurement							
Baseline parameters							
Loadings							
Tobacco		1.828	0.164	<.001	1.611	0.128	<.001
Binge Drinking		1.598	0.109	<.001	1.588	0.109	<.001
Amphetamines		1.491	0.188	<.001	1.489	0.188	<.001
Opioids/Sedatives		1.528	0.178	<.001	1.563	0.181	<.001
Marijuana		2.964	0.247	<.001	2.769	0.214	<.001
Hallucinogens/MDMA		3.350	0.414	<.001	3.441	0.432	<.001
Cocaine		3.735	0.536	<.001	3.625	0.505	<.001
Thresholds							
Tobacco	1	0.607	0.185	0.001	0.810	0.111	<.001
	2	2.612	0.216	<.001	2.776	0.159	<.001
Binge Drinking	1	−1.705	0.126	<.001	−1.706	0.126	<.001
	2	−0.485	0.107	<.001	−0.485	0.107	<.001
	3	0.342	0.106	0.001	0.341	0.106	0.001
	4	0.995	0.112	<.001	0.991	0.112	<.001
	5	1.879	0.128	<.001	1.870	0.127	<.001
	6	3.030	0.157	<.001	3.015	0.156	<.001
Amphetamines	1	2.428	0.191	<.001	2.434	0.193	<.001
Opioids/Sedatives	1	3.512	0.344	<.001	3.536	0.347	<.001
Marijuana	1	−0.445	0.160	0.005	−0.468	0.149	0.002
	2	0.534	0.163	0.001	0.509	0.151	0.001
	3	1.555	0.182	<.001	1.532	0.171	<.001
	4	2.269	0.203	<.001	2.249	0.193	<.001
	5	3.251	0.237	<.001	3.233	0.229	<.001
	6	4.225	0.277	<.001	4.202	0.269	<.001
Hallucinogens/MDMA	1	5.094	0.537	<.001	5.079	0.548	<.001
Cocaine	1	6.139	0.771	<.001	5.848	0.700	<.001
Differential Item Functioning							
Loadings							
Sorority membership							
Tobacco		−0.491	0.241	0.041			
Amphetamines		2.612	0.954	0.006	2.466	0.859	0.004
Marijuana		−0.566	0.266	0.033			

(continued)

Table 5.3 (continued)

Variable Coding		Simultaneous model			Final model		
		Estimate	SE	p value	Estimate	SE	p value
Thresholds							
Sorority membership							
Tobacco		−0.052	0.243	0.831			
Binge Drinking		0.446	0.181	0.014	0.587	0.150	<.001
Amphetamines		−1.790	1.014	0.077	−1.222	0.786	0.12
Marijuana		−0.097	0.289	0.737			
Sample membership							
Tobacco	B vs. A	0.080	0.221	0.718			
	C vs. A	−0.485	0.213	0.023			
	D vs. A	−0.460	0.234	0.049			
Opioids/sedatives	B vs. A	0.565	0.371	0.127	0.576	0.372	0.122
	C vs. A	0.177	0.358	0.621	0.252	0.359	0.482
	D vs. A	0.923	0.365	0.011	0.986	0.367	0.007

5.5.4 Step 4: Examine MNLFA Scores

Figure 5.4 shows item characteristic curves (ICC) reflecting DIF effects based on sorority membership. One particularly interesting finding is the strong positive effect of sorority membership on the loading for amphetamine use. Note that the corresponding intercept effect must be included, even though it is not significantly different from zero. Note also that this intercept effect is negative, which would initially suggest a lower probability of amphetamine use among sorority members, holding overall substance use constant. However, here the positive loading effect combines with this negative intercept effect to produce a different pattern of response probabilities entirely. Specifically, while neither sorority members nor non-members are very likely to endorse using amphetamines at all, the probability of amphetamine use increases sharply for sorority members who are one standard deviation above the mean in overall substance use. By contrast, the overall probability of amphetamine use increases much more gradually for non-members.

The final step of this analysis was to use the parameter estimates from this final model to generate model-implied substance use scores using the aMNLFA.final() function. These scores may then be used in subsequent analyses as measures of overall substance use, adjusting for differences in sorority membership and study membership.

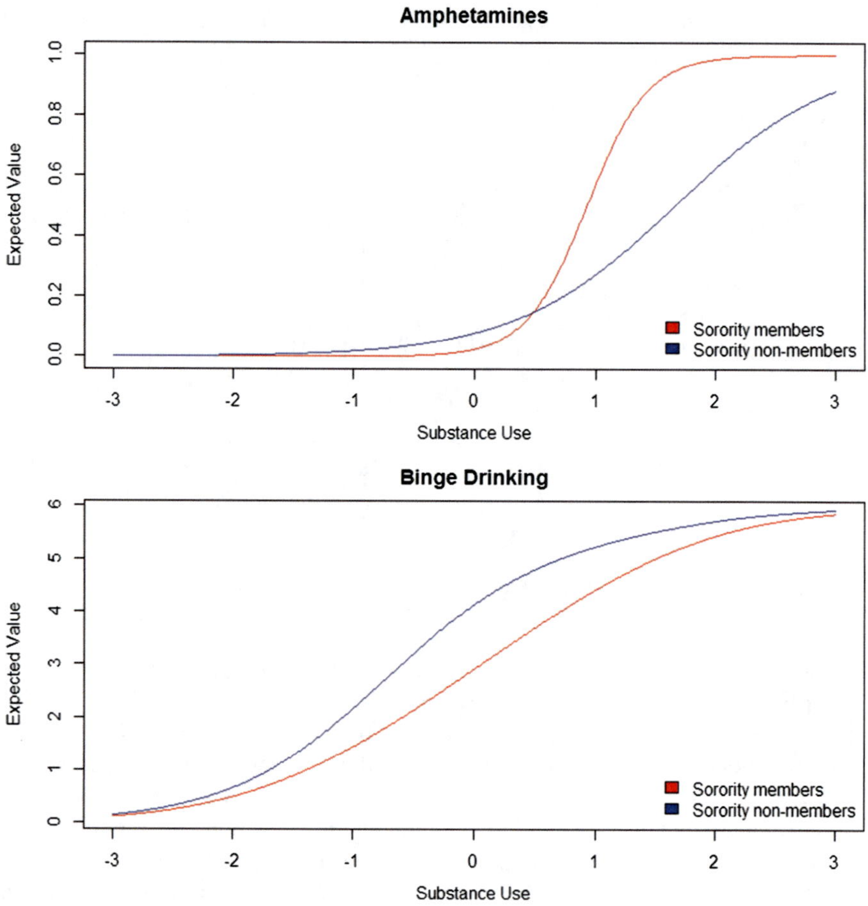

Fig. 5.4 Item characteristic curves for two items by group membership

5.6 Hypothesis Testing in IDA

5.6.1 Challenges to Hypothesis Testing

Common challenges and advantages of hypothesis test using IDA are highlighted here and outlined in Fig. 5.5 using published studies as examples. The first example integrates three longitudinal studies of children of alcoholic parents and matched controls. The first study was the Michigan Longitudinal Study (MLS; Zucker et al., 2000) with multi-wave data assessed from early childhood to early adulthood. The second study was the Adolescent and Family Developmental Project (AFDP; Chassin, Rogosch, & Barrera, 1991) with five waves of data from family-based interview x for adolescents aged 11–15 at baseline and continued to adulthood. The

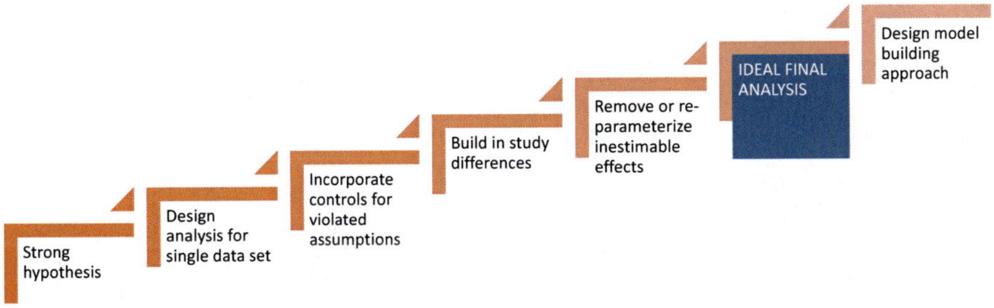

Fig. 5.5 Building an analysis for hypothesis testing in IDA

third study was the Alcohol, Health and Behavior Project (AHBP; Sher, Walitzer, Wood, & Brent, 1991) with 6 waves of data starting obtained from participants in the first year of college into their thirties.

Together, these three studies span the first four decades of life when early risk factors for later substance outcomes first emerge (childhood), when substance use initiation typically occurs (adolescence), when peak rates of substance use disorders are evident (young adulthood), and when deceleration in substance involvement is first apparent (adulthood). Table 5.4 presents a summary of the pooled sample as a function of study membership and chronological age. Each cell in the table identifies the number of individuals assessed in a given wave of a given study at a given age. The column totals identify the total number of individuals assessed at a given age pooling across study and wave.

There are multiple challenges presented in this three study IDA. For example, the three contributing studies varied substantially in design, including issues of participant recruitment, assessment strategies and instrumentation (see Hussong et al., 2007, 2008; Hussong, Flora, et al., 2008 for a summary of design characteristics). One purpose of IDA is to control for such between-study differences to examine our substantive questions of interest. The pursuit of this goal via IDA permitted us to study a longer developmental period than could be assessed by any one study, larger subsamples of families with specific forms of alcoholism, and trajectories of symptomatology in analyses with greater statistical power.

The first step for hypothesis testing using IDA is to develop a *strong hypothesis*. Being clear on the details of what is being examined, the measures that will be used to examine it, and the nature of the individual and pooled samples is essential. To gauge feasibility of the analysis, we recommend *designing a statistical model* to test the hypothesis by first treating the pooled sample as if it were a single study or for the single largest study in the pooled dataset. This approach encourages the researcher to identify the correct statistical model for a given hypothesis and to test whether standard assumptions for a model are met, can be met with data manipulation or transformation, or are not viable. This includes a careful examination of harmonized scores, including those derived from aMNLFA. *Incorporation of controls or corrections for violated assumptions* will increase internal validity in IDA models just as with any statistical model.

Table 5.4 Cross Study (three-study) Longitudinal IDA Design

MLSA1	168									19	147	2					
		Participant Age															
Study	N	2	3	4	5	6	7	8	9	10	11	12	13	14	15	16	17
MLS1	399	18	143	121	88	27	2										
MLS2	339				7	99	115	89	28	1							
MLS3	401							14	128	139	102	18					
MLS4	418										13	145	133	113	12	1	
MLS5	500													19	144	149	147
MLS6	482																17
MLS7	482																
MLSA2	158										17	132	9				
MLSA3	204											8	188	8			
MLSA4	247												17	214	16		
MLSA5	219													11	193	15	
MLSA6	202														11	179	12
MLSA7	203															14	182
AFDP1	454									32	78	85	107	102	46	4	
AFDP2	449										29	77	84	106	101	48	4
AFDP3	447											29	75	86	103	100	50
AFDP4	749																10
AFDP5	755																
AFDP6	735																
AHBP1	485																8
AHBP2	480																
AHBP3	468																
AHBP4	467																
AHBP5	454																
AHBP6	406																
AHBP7	383																
Total		18	143	121	95	126	117	103	156	191	386	496	613	657	625	509	429

For example, our first use of IDA tested the hypothesis that trajectories of internalizing symptomatology between 10 and 33 years of age were elevated among children of alcoholic parents relative to their peers throughout early development (Curran et al., 2008). The pooled sample consisted of a total of 1827 individual participants (512 drawn from the MLS, 830 from the AFDP, and 485 from the AHBP). Everyone provided between one and five repeated measures resulting in a total of 7377 person-by-time observations, however no individual provided data for all age periods. Indeed, MLS provided annual assessments between ages 11–17 with ongoing assessments lagged by 3 years. AFDP used a cohort sequential design, assessing 11–15 year olds at baseline followed by two annual assessments and then assessments lagged by 5 years. AHBP was a college cohort study and administered

Table 5.4 (continued)

18	19	20	21	22	23	24	25	26	27	28	29	30	31	32	33	34	35	36	37	38+
1																				
31	10																			
143	148	144	30																	
		17	143	148	144	30														
7																				
4																				
147	116	123	128	71	45	44	38	26	1											
				13	34	55	50	84	100	92	143	91	62	20	11					
									10	30	50	50	80	105	90	140	90	60	20	10
396	70	4	4	2	1															
8	394	68	4	4	1	1														
	8	362	88	4	4	1	1													
		6	340	110	6	3	2													
					3	283	154	8	4	0	2									
										112	225	59	7	1	2					
															31	221	113	12	5	1
736	743	724	737	352	238	417	245	118	115	234	420	200	149	126	134	361	203	72	25	11

Note: *MLS* Michigan Longitudinal Study, *MLSA* Michigan Longitudinal Study annual assessments (see Zucker et al., 2000); *AFDP* Adolescent and Family Development Project, *AHBP* Alcohol Health and Behavior Project. Each number appended to the study indicator indicates wave of assessment (e.g., AFDP3 is the third assessment wave in the AFDP project)

annual assessments for four years followed by assessment lags of 4–5 years. In many ways, the pooling of longitudinal data in this analysis raises similar challenges as any cohort sequential study in which assumptions about sample comparability (and negligent historical confounds) are tested by comparing individuals from different cohorts during overlapping periods of the trajectory. In this case, we needed to control for study differences not only in levels of internalizing symptoms at each time point but in the overall shape of trajectories (or rate of change in internalizing symptoms) over time.

Given the hypothesis and structure of the data, we chose to fit a series of multilevel piecewise growth models to examine the fixed and random effects characterizing the developmental trajectories of internalizing symptomatology between ages 10 and 33 and whether parent alcoholism significantly predicted elements of these trajectories. We included main effect predictors for study membership of both the intercepts and slopes of these trajectories. But we also accounted for differences in the nested structure of two of the contributing studies. For both MLS and AFDP, multiple children from the same family could participate in the study, violating the assumption that observations are independent in this modeling framework. To address this need, we adjusted for non-independence within the modeling framework.

This example also highlights the critical next step in IDA hypothesis testing of *building in study differences*. IDA scoring procedures and hypothesis testing work in tandem, and accounting for study differences in all parts of the model is a core tenant of this approach. We build in study differences into the hypothesis testing models in two ways. First, we code for main effects of study differences. As with any nominal variable, there are multiple ways to code for study differences. In this case, we coded AFDP as the comparison condition (using dummy codes comparing MLS to AFDP and AHBP to AFDP) because AFDP participants overlapped with both MLS and AHBP in age periods assessed. For other studies, we have used alternate approaches to coding study differences. In some cases, there was no clear comparison study and we used effect coding to test the extent to which study membership impacted outcomes in comparison to an overall average effect in the pooled sample (see STTR example to follow). The choice of how to code study differences is driven by whether testing study differences is of substantive interest and, if so, what codes capture posited study differences for interpretation; whether there is a primary control group or not; and how the coding scheme impacts interpretation of other effects in the model.

The second way we build study differences into these models is by testing for study differences in the effects of predictors on outcomes, typically via testing interactions. In our example, we included study membership as a predictor of internalizing trajectory intercepts but also as a moderator of the effect of age on internalizing symptoms to test for study differences in trajectory slopes. In these models, we controlled for child gender and parental education (as a proxy for socio-economic status) and include interactions between these control variables and study membership to control for study differences in the effects of these potential confounds (given study differences in sample composition and measurement). Although not directly a study effect, we also find that including other variables that serve as DIF indicators in MNLFA models as main effects in hypothesis testing reduces parameter bias. Computer simulation studies indicate that omitting covariates from scoring models but including them in hypothesis testing models can result in biased findings (Curran, Cole, Bauer, Rothenberg, & Hussong, 2018).

After building a complex model that tests stated hypotheses, incorporates controls and study differences, and is consistent with or addresses model assumptions, we *review the model for each study to identify potential inestimable effects*. We learned this lesson in analysis testing the time-varying effects of symptomatology on substance use across adolescents using the same data as in this example. In that analysis, we were interested in whether internalizing symptoms predicted substance use 1 year later, after controlling for co-occurring externalizing symptoms, across a 7-year developmental period (ages 11–18) using data from both MLS and AFDP. Using a time-varying covariate model, we found that models would not estimate when we relied on parent-reported symptomatology. In reviewing the original study designs, we realized that parents reported on youth symptomatology only every 3 years in MLS, though they did so every year in AFDP. Thus, one-year time lag data were only available in AFDP, meaning that data were unavailable to test interactions between a dummy variable indicating study membership and internalizing symptoms predicting next-year substance use. This is one example of the ways in which we have identified gaps in data coverage within the IDA framework for testing a given hypothesis because we were using the data to create a novel design, demonstrating again that knowledge of the details of contributing studies' designs is critical.

The result of these initial five steps in IDA hypothesis testing is an *ideal final analysis model* (referring to Fig. 5.5). Sometimes, this model may be too complex for reliable estimation. Although this may occur in any analytic model, those guided by IDA may be at particular risk for complexity that interferes with estimation because of the need to incorporate additional parameters to account for study differences. We address this challenge by *designing a model building approach* that allows for testing sets of parameters using a priori rationale paired with model trimming to reduce model complexity.

A typical model building approach is was used in our example in which we tested whether parent alcoholism predicting elevated trajectories of internalizing symptoms over the early life course. Our initial model included study membership as a predictor of internalizing trajectories, allowing us to establish the functional form of change in internalizing symptoms over the age period represented in our pooled data analysis. We then added control variables (gender and parent education) as well as interactions between control variables and study membership as predictors of trajectory elements (intercepts and slopes), then trimmed higher-order predictors that were non-significant to simply the model. Next, we included our variables of interest (parent alcoholism) indicators and their interactions with study membership to test our hypothesis. This approach allowed us to test our central hypothesis in a model that included only control variables that contributed to the prediction of outcomes, reducing model complexity and potential related problems such as multicollinearity. (For additional examples of how this method can be applied to different research problems, we refer the reader to Hussong, Cai, et al., 2008; Hussong, Flora, et al., 2008; Hussong et al., 2007).

In sum, hypothesis testing in IDA is heavily guided by hypothesis testing within whatever analytic method is deemed most appropriate for the hypothesis at hand. However, given the potential for model complexity and the need to consider study differences at multiple points in these models, a model building approach is often most useful. This approach as outlined here relies on incorporating study differences into the predictive model both as main effects (to control for study differences in the observed outcome) but also as potential moderators of other predictors in the model. These study moderators directly test the extent to which predictor-outcome relations replicate over studies included in the pooled analysis.

5.6.2 *Another Example of IDA in Global Health Research*

The study of Global Health engenders unique complexities in measurement, data linkage, and analysis. As an illustration, we summarize the Seek-Test-Treat-Retain (STTR) Research Harmonization Initiative to examine HIV treatment cascade studies conducted in many countries around the globe (Chandler et al., 2015, 2017). A core construct examined in this initiative is alcohol-related problems, primarily assessed by the AUDIT. Traditionally, research using the AUDIT relies on both cut-scores (Babor et al. 2001; Saunders, Aasland, Babor, De La Fuente, & Grant, 1993) and sum scores (Chen, Miller, Grube, & Waiters, 2006; Knibbe, Derickx, Kuntsche, Grittner, & Bloomfield, 2006). However, in the context of a multi-country study, these approaches may be limited. For this reason, Hussong et al. (2019) used MNLFA to create scores that psychometrically harmonized the AUDIT measures across all studies.

We analyzed baseline AUDIT data pooled from eight STTR study sites. Sample sizes of these studies ranged from 50 to 2405 and target populations also varied with regard to sampling frame, geographic location, and inclusion/exclusion criteria (see Hussong et al., 2019, Table 5.2). The pooled sample included 4667 participants and was 82% male, 52% Black, 24% White, 13% Hispanic, and 8% Asian or Pacific Islander, with a mean age of 38.86 (range 18–74). All studies took place across various criminal justice settings (e.g., jails, prisons, or community supervision programs) and included both persons living with HIV and HIV-uninfected individuals.

We first conducted logical harmonization with the AUDIT items. Although participants at all study sites completed the AUDIT to assess problem drinking, there were study-specific alterations to the measure. Alterations to the scale included changes in the length of the reporting window (up to 12 months), the wording of the binge item question (to capture sex differences in recommended cut-points), and the response scale. Across studies, we logically harmonized response scales to match traditional AUDIT response scales such that they ranged from 0 to 4 for items assessing frequency of alcohol use, quantity of alcohol consumed during drinking episodes, binge drinking, inability to stop drinking once started, failing to meet obligations due to drinking, needing a first drink to get started in the morning, feelings of guilt or remorse following drinking, and memory loss due to drinking; and response scales of 0 (no), 2 (yes), or 4 (not in the past year) for items 9–10 assessing whether the participant or another indivdual had been injured as a result of drinking and whether another individual has been concerned about the participant's drinking habits.

With the logically harmonized dataset, we applied traditional scoring algorithms to create cut-scores (i.e., sum scores of 8 or more (for men) or 4 or more (for women and those over 60 years of age) following Babor, Higgins-Biddle, Saunders, & Monteiro, 2001). We then examined item distributions within and across studies and conducted a series of exploratory factor analyses (EFA). Based on these analyses, we transformed all items to a binary response scale for MNLFA. In MNLFA models, sample membership was effect-coded to capture study differences. Sample membership was allowed to affect both the mean and variance of the latent factor (assessing differences in drinking severity, impact) as well as the intercepts and loadings of selected items (assessing differences in item performance across studies, DIF).

MNLFA results indicated that there were some differences in factor mean and variance (i.e., impact) by study samples as well as between-sample differences in item intercepts but not factor loadings. In other words, the assumption of invariance for logical harmonization was not supported. In comparisons across the three scoring approaches (i.e., cut-scores, sum scores, and MNLFA scores), the sum scores were more zero-inflated (i.e., piling up at zero) than MNLFA score, which had greater variation and were less likely to show floor effects. The correlation between sum scores and MNLFA scores was $r = 0.90$ but MNLFA scores captured greater individual variation than either sum scores or cut-scores. This property of MNLFA scores permits covariates to better differentiate (and predict) individuals' drinking severity.

In subsequent predictive validity analysis, we found that MNLFA scores predicted past 30 days binge drinking more strongly did cut- and sum-scores. Between-study differences in AUDIT scores associated with binge drinking were detected in analyses using sum and MNLFA scores but not in those using cut-scores. Our results suggest that relative to the other two scoring approaches, MNLFA scores captured more information or variation in problem drinking, better predicting binge drinking and more effectively detecting between-study differences in AUDIT-binge drinking associations.

5.7 Advances in IDA Methods

Although there are many new developments afoot in data pooling, here we highlight two recent tools for addressing specific challenges in measurement harmonization that can be applied in the context of IDA.

5.7.1 New Regularization Method to Identify DIF Items

Although the aMLNFA procedure represents a tremendous improvement over manually fitting all the models needed to identify DIF iteratively, we have recently explored the use of regularization techniques to optimize this process.

Regularization is a machine learning approach. It starts with a complex model containing many parameters and/or predictors, and then simplifies the model to reward sparsity, that is, to remove largely irrelevant parts of the model. When used to identify DIF, the initial model includes DIF everywhere. We then impose a penalty when fitting the model (the Least Absolute Shrinkage Selection Operator (LASSO) penalty) to shrink some of the DIF parameters to zero, allowing them to be removed from the model. The penalty is increased through a tuning parameter and as it increases more and more DIF parameters are removed until no DIF parameters remain.

The optimal value for the tuning parameter is determined by balancing model fit with model parsimony. One way to quantify this balance is by the Bayes' Information Criterion (BIC). The tuning parameter value generating the minimum BIC is then taken as optimal. Ideally, this best-BIC model should contain only those DIF parameters needed to reproduce the data well and not superfluous DIF parameters that over-fit the data. The advantages of this approach are twofold. First, it provides a fully automated method for MNFLA with multiple variables (i.e., study, age, sex, and other demographic and socioeconomic factors). Second, it avoids iterative hypothesis testing that may lead to inflated Type I errors. Preliminary results suggest that this method outperforms traditional DIF detection approaches in contexts that may frequently arise in IDA (i.e., when there is DIF for multiple items and the combined sample size is large; Bauer, Belzak, & Cole n.d.).

5.7.2 *Trifactor Modeling Method*

An additional challenge that can arise when combining multiple data sources is the need to incorporate assessments obtained from two or more independent reporters. Although this introduces an added layer of complexity to the analysis, using IDA to obtain multiple reporter assessments is a distinct advantage of this approach. It has long been known that the use of a single reporter inextricably confounds the assessment of the underlying trait with the perspective of the reporter (Achenbach, Krukowski, Dumenci, & Ivanova, 2005; Renk, 2005). For example, using the mother's report of her child's behavior by necessity limits the assessments as seen through the lens of the mother (e.g., Boyle & Pickles, 1997). Other perspectives that might provide additional insights into the child's behavior could include the father, a teacher, or a best friend. Although there is much consensus on the need for multiple reporter assessments, the analytic methods available to incorporate these separate sources of information in some principled fashion have been at best limited (Achenbach, 2011), and this is further complicated when considering multiple reporters within an IDA.

To address these limitations, Bauer et al. (2013) proposed a novel analytic approach that was explicitly designed to incorporate multiple reporter assessments within a single psychometric modeling framework. This could be applied to either traditional single-sample designs or to more complex IDA applications. They referred to this approach as the *trifactor model* (or TFM) because three levels of latent variables (or factors) are used to capture different sources of variability carried by a set of items. The first is a *common factor* that represents the pooled information shared by all three reporters. The second are a set of *perspective factors* that are uniquely defined for each reporter. Finally, the third are a set of *specific factors* that are uniquely defined for each item that is shared across the three reporters.

The TFM can be expanded in a variety of interesting ways. First, not all reporters need to respond to the same set of items. Thus, within an IDA application some reporters might respond to one set of items while other reporters respond to a subset of these items but respond to additional items that are unique to their own report. Second, complete-case data is not required such that some contributing samples might have three reporters available, some might have two, and some might have just one, yet these can all be combined within a single TFM. Third, the TFM allows for the incorporation of reporter-specific characteristics as covariates in the model that help in part determine the unique reporter perspective such as parental alcoholism diagnosis or teacher years of experience. Finally, the TFM can generate factor score estimates for the common factor that represent the optimal pooled combination of all available reporters net the potentially biasing effects of the perspective and specific factors, and these scores are then available for subsequent analysis. Complete details about these and other aspects of the TFM are available in Bauer et al. (2013).

5.7.3 Summary and Conclusions

With the accelerating accrual of high-quality datasets assessing Global Health, we anticipate that the demand for effective data pooling techniques will increase. Among these techniques, IDA offers a means of vertical harmonization across distinct datasets with overlapping measurement of core constructs. Two potentially unique aspects of the IDA framework include the heavy emphasis placed on analytic harmonization whenever possible and the testing of study differences (and not just controlling for study main effects) in hypothesis testing. As pooled data analyses become increasingly common, we anticipate that the strengths of various approaches will become more widely adopted across all approaches and lead to more powerful frameworks. Issues such as the appropriate ways to account for sampling and design frames (e.g., appropriately including sample weights, retaining the integrity of a randomized control design) remain unexplored areas in IDA. As necessity is the mother of invention, we believe that the most important advances in IDA, and data pooling more generally, will be driven by the need to address critical issues in fields such as Global Health.

Technical Appendix: Moderated Nonlinear Factor Analysis (MNLFA)

Below are the Mplus scripts used to conduct the analyses in the chapter. As described in the chapter, data come from two studies: the Millennial Friendship Study (MFS) and Real Experiences and Lives in the University (REAL-U) study. Based on all possible combinations of test battery and study, three groups were formed: Group A (REAL-U; test form 1); Group B (REAL-U; test form 2); Group C (MFS; test form 1); and Group D (MFS; test form 2). In the below syntax and data, the groups have been recoded here as G1 (corresponding to the original Group C), G2 (corresponding to the original Group B), and G3 (corresponding to the original Group D). With this caveat, the variables are as follows:

- Items
  - TBCO = Tobacco use; ordinal with 3 levels
  - BDRK = Binge drinking; ordinal with 7 levels
  - MNJA = Marijuana use; ordinal with 7 levels
  - AMPH = Amphetamine use; binary
  - HLCN = Hallucinogen use; binary
  - COCN = Cocaine use; binary
  - OPSD = Opioid or sedative use; binary
- Covariates
  - FRAT = Sorority membership; binary. Hypothesized to produce both impact and DIF.
  - G1, G2, G3 = Study grouping, coded as described above. Hypothesized to produce DIF only.

  There are three main sets of models which are run sequentially.

- The first is the ***initial models***. These encompass:
  - A model for mean impact (the first model shown below);
  - A model for variance impact (the second model shown below); and
  - Item-wise models testing the presence of DIF on all items (the third model shown below). Note that only the model for tobacco is shown; corresponding models were run for all of the other items.
- After running these initial models, a ***simultaneous model*** is produced. This model contains all effects that were found to be significantly different from zero in the initial models.
- Finally, after the simultaneous model, the ***final model*** is fit. This model prunes non-significant effects from the simultaneous model.

After running these models, a scoring model is produced, in which parameters are fixed at their estimated values from the final model. This step is not shown here, as it is not discussed in the chapter.

Initial Models

Mean and Variance impact models (this page); measurement invariance model for each item (next page)

```
TITLE:
    Mean Impact Model
DATA:
    FILE = "calibration.dat";
VARIABLE:
    NAMES = ID TBCO BDRK AMPH OPSD MJNA HLCN COCN FRAT G1 G2 G3;
    MISSING=.;
    USEVARIABLES= TBCO BDRK AMPH OPSD MJNA HLCN COCN FRAT ;
    AUXILIARY= ID ;
    CATEGORICAL= TBCO BDRK AMPH OPSD MJNA HLCN COCN ;
ANALYSIS:
    ESTIMATOR=ML;ALGORITHM=INTEGRATION;INTEGRATION=MONTECARLO;
    PROCESSORS=4;
MODEL:
    [ETA@0]; ETA@1;
    ETA BY TBCO*(l1);
    ETA BY BDRK*(l2);
    ETA BY AMPH*(l3);
    ETA BY OPSD*(l4);
    ETA BY MJNA*(l5);
    ETA BY HLCN*(l6);
    ETA BY COCN*(l7);
    ETA ON FRAT ;
OUTPUT:
tech1;

TITLE:
    Variance Impact Model
DATA:
    FILE = "calibration.dat";
VARIABLE:
    NAMES = ID TBCO BDRK AMPH OPSD MJNA HLCN COCN FRAT G1
     G2 G3;
    MISSING=.;
    USEVARIABLES= TBCO BDRK AMPH OPSD MJNA HLCN COCN FRAT ;
    AUXILIARY= ID ;
    CATEGORICAL= TBCO BDRK AMPH OPSD MJNA HLCN COCN ;
    CONSTRAINT= FRAT ;
ANALYSIS:
    ESTIMATOR=ML;ALGORITHM=INTEGRATION;INTEGRATION=MONTECARLO;
    PROCESSORS=4;
```

```
MODEL:
     ETA ON FRAT ;
     ETA*(veta);
     ETA BY TBCO*(l1);
     ETA BY BDRK*(l2);
     ETA BY AMPH*(l3);
     ETA BY OPSD*(l4);
     ETA BY MJNA*(l5);
     ETA BY HLCN*(l6);
     ETA BY COCN*(l7);
MODEL CONSTRAINT:
     new( v1*0 );
     veta=1*exp( v1*FRAT);
OUTPUT:
tech1;
```

```
TITLE:
    Measurement Invariance Model for TBCO
DATA:
    FILE = "calibration.dat";
VARIABLE:
    NAMES = ID TBCO BDRK AMPH OPSD MJNA HLCN COCN FRAT G1 G2 G3;
    MISSING=.;
    USEVARIABLES= TBCO BDRK AMPH OPSD MJNA HLCN COCN FRAT G1
     G2 G3 ;
    AUXILIARY= ID ;
    CATEGORICAL= TBCO BDRK AMPH OPSD MJNA HLCN COCN ;
    CONSTRAINT= FRAT G1 G2 G3 ;
ANALYSIS:
    ESTIMATOR=ML;ALGORITHM=INTEGRATION;INTEGRATION=MONTECARLO;
    PROCESSORS=4;
MODEL:
    [ETA@0]; ETA@1;
    ETA BY TBCO*(l1);
    ETA BY BDRK*(l2);
    ETA BY AMPH*(l3);
    ETA BY OPSD*(l4);
    ETA BY MJNA*(l5);
    ETA BY HLCN*(l6);
    ETA BY COCN*(l7);
    TBCO on FRAT G1 G2 G3;
MODEL CONSTRAINT:
    new(l1_00*1
    l1_1*0
    l1_2*0
    l1_3*0
    l1_4*0);
    l1=l1_00
    +l1_1*FRAT
    +l1_2*G1
    +l1_3*G2
    +l1_4*G3;
OUTPUT:
tech1;
```

Simultaneous Model

```
TITLE:
    Round 2 Calibration Model
DATA:
    FILE = "calibration.dat";
VARIABLE:
    NAMES = ID TBCO BDRK AMPH OPSD MJNA HLCN COCN FRAT G1 G2 G3;
    MISSING=.;
    USEVARIABLES= TBCO BDRK AMPH OPSD MJNA HLCN COCN FRAT G1
     G2 G3 ;
    AUXILIARY= ID ;
    CATEGORICAL= TBCO BDRK AMPH OPSD MJNA HLCN COCN ;
    CONSTRAINT= FRAT G1 G2 G3 ;
ANALYSIS:
    ESTIMATOR=ML;ALGORITHM=INTEGRATION;INTEGRATION=MONTECARLO;
    PROCESSORS=4;
MODEL:
    [ETA@0]; ETA@1;
    ETA BY TBCO*(l1);
    ETA BY BDRK*(l2);
    ETA BY AMPH*(l3);
    ETA BY OPSD*(l4);
    ETA BY MJNA*(l5);
    ETA BY HLCN*(l6);
    ETA BY COCN*(l7);
    TBCO on FRAT G1 G2 G3;
MODEL CONSTRAINT:
    new(l1_00*1
    l1_1*0
    l1_2*0
    l1_3*0
    l1_4*0);
    l1=l1_00
    +l1_1*FRAT
    +l1_2*G1
    +l1_3*G2
    +l1_4*G3;
OUTPUT:
techl;
```

Final Model

```
TITLE:
    Round 3 Calibration Model
DATA:
    FILE = "calibration.dat";
VARIABLE:
    NAMES = ID TBCO BDRK AMPH OPSD MJNA HLCN COCN FRAT G1 G2 G3;
    MISSING=.;
```

```
    USEVARIABLES= TBCO FRAT G1 G2 G3 BDRK AMPH OPSD MJNA
      HLCN COCN;
    AUXILIARY= ID ;
    CATEGORICAL= TBCO BDRK AMPH OPSD MJNA HLCN COCN ;
    CONSTRAINT= FRAT ;
ANALYSIS:
    ESTIMATOR=ML;ALGORITHM=INTEGRATION;INTEGRATION=MONTECARLO;
    PROCESSORS=4;
MODEL:
    [ETA@0]; ETA@1;
    ETA BY TBCO*(l1);
    ETA BY BDRK*(l2);
    ETA BY AMPH*(l3);
    ETA BY OPSD*(l4);
    ETA BY MJNA*(l5);
    ETA BY HLCN*(l6);
    ETA BY COCN*(l7);
    ETA ON FRAT;
    BDRK on FRAT;
    AMPH on FRAT;
    OPSD on G1 G2 G3;
MODEL CONSTRAINT:
     l3_00*1
     l3_1*0
     );
     l_3=l3_00+l3_1*FRAT;
OUTPUT:
tech1;
```

References

Achenbach, T. M. (2011). Commentary: Definitely more than measurement error: But how should we understand and deal with informant discrepancies? *Journal of Clinical Child & Adolescent Psychology, 40*, 80–86. https://doi.org/10.1080/15374416.2011.533416

Achenbach, T. M., Krukowski, R. A., Dumenci, L., & Ivanova, M. Y. (2005). Assessment of adult psychopathology: Meta-analyses and implications of cross-informant correlations. *Psychological Bulletin, 131*, 361–382. https://doi.org/10.1037/0033-2909.131.3.361

American Psychological Association. (2016). Ethical principles of psychologists and code of conduct. *American Psychologist, 71*, 900.

Babor, T. F., Higgins-Biddle, J. C., Saunders, J. B., & Monteiro, M. G. (2001). *The alcohol use disorders identification test: Guidelines for use in primary care*. Geneva: World Health Organization.

Bauer, D.J. (2017). A more general model for testing measurement invariance and differential item functioning. *Psychological methods, 22*, 507–526. https://doi.org/10.1037/met0000077. PMCID: PMC5140785.

Bauer, D.J., Belzak, W.C.M. & Cole, V.T. (in press). Simplifying the assessment of measurement invariance over multiple background variables: Using regularized moderated nonlinear factor analysis to detect differential item functioning. *Structural Equation Modeling: A Multidisciplinary Journal*. https://doi.org/10.1080/10705511.2019.1642754.

Bauer, D. J., Howard, A. L., Baldasaro, R. E., Curran, P. J., Hussong, A. M., Chassin, L., & Zucker, R. A. (2013). A trifactor model for integrating ratings across multiple informants. *Psychological Methods, 18*, 475–493.

Bauer, D. J., & Hussong, A. M. (2009). Psychometric approaches for developing commensurate measures across independent studies: Traditional and new models. *Psychological Methods, 14*(2), 101–125. https://doi.org/10.1037/a0015583

Benjamini, Y., & Hochberg, Y. (2000). On the adaptive control of the false discovery rate in multiple testing with independent statistics. *Journal of Educational and Behavioral Statistics, 25*(1), 60–83. https://doi.org/10.2307/1165312

Bollen, K. A., & Hoyle, R. H. (2012). Latent variables in structural equation modeling. In R. H. Hoyle (Ed.), *Handbook of structural equation modeling* (pp. 56–67). New York, NY: The Guilford Press.

Boyle, M. H., & Pickles, A. R. (1997). Influence of maternal depressive symptoms on ratings of childhood behavior. *Journal of Abnormal Child Psychology, 25*, 399–412. https://doi.org/10.1023/A:1025737124888

Brown, C. H., Brincks, A., Huang, S., Perrino, T., Cruden, G., Pantin, H., ... Sandler, I. (2016). Two-year impact of prevention programs on adolescent depression: An integrative data analysis approach. *Prevention Science, 19*, 74–94. https://doi.org/10.1007/s11121-016-0737-1

Burton, A., Maskarinec, G., Perez-Gomez, B., Vachon, C., Miao, H., Lajous, M., ... McCormack, V. (2017). Mammographic density and ageing: A collaborative pooled analysis of cross-sectional data from 22 countries worldwide. *PLoS Medicine, 14*(6), 1–21. https://doi.org/10.1371/journal.pmed.1002335

Byrne, B., Shavelson, R., & Muthén, B. (1989). Testing for the equivalence of factor covariance and mean structures: The issue of partial measurement invariance. *Psychological Bulletin, 105*, 456–466.

Cella, D., Yount, S., Rothrock, N., Gershon, R., Cook, K., Reeve, B., ... Rose, M. (2007). The Patient-Reported Outcomes Measurement Information System (PROMIS): Progress of an NIH roadmap cooperative group during its first two years. *Medical Care, 45*(5 Suppl 1), S3–S11. https://doi.org/10.1097/01.mlr.0000258615.42478.55

Chandler, R., Gordon, M. S., Kruszka, B., Strand, L. N., Altice, F. L., Beckwith, C. G., ... Crane, H. M. (2017). Cohort profile: Seek, test, treat and retain United States criminal justice cohort. *Substance Abuse Treatment, Prevention, and Policy, 12*, 24. https://doi.org/10.1186/s13011-017-0107-4

Chandler, R. K., Kahana, S. Y., Fletcher, B., Jones, D., Finger, M. S., Aklin, W. M., ... Webb, C. (2015). Data collection and harmonization in HIV research: The seek, test, treat, and retain initiative at the National Institute on Drug Abuse. *American Journal of Public Health, 105*(12), 2416–2422. https://doi.org/10.2105/AJPH.2015.302788

Chassin, L., Rogosch, F., & Barrera, M. (1991). Substance use and symptomatology among adolescent children of alcoholics. *Journal of Abnormal Psychology, 100*, 449–463.

Chen, M., Miller, B. A., Grube, J. W., & Waiters, E. D. (2006). Music, substance use and aggression. *Journal of Studies on Alcohol, 67*(3), 373–381. https://doi.org/10.1097/OGX.0000000000000256.Prenatal

Chen, P., & Jacobson, K. C. (2012). Developmental trajectories of substance use from early adolescence to young adulthood: Gender and racial/ethnic differences. *The Journal of Adolescent Health: Official Publication of the Society for Adolescent Medicine, 50*(2), 154–163. https://doi.org/10.1016/j.jadohealth.2011.05.013

Cheung, G., & Rensvold, R. (1998). Cross-cultural comparisons using non-invariant measurement items. *Applied Behavioral Science Review, 6*, 93–110.

Conway, K. P. K. P., Vullo, G. C. G. C., Kennedy, A. P. A. P., Finger, M. S. M. S., Agrawal, A., Bjork, J. M., ... Sher, K. J. K. J. (2014). Data compatibility in the addiction sciences: An examination of measure commonality. *Drug and Alcohol Dependence, 141*, 153–158. https://doi.org/10.1016/j.drugalcdep.2014.04.029

Cooper, H., Hedges, L., & Valentine, J. (2009). *The handbook of research synthesis and meta-analysis*. New York, NY: Russell Sage Foundation.

Curran, P. J., Cole, V., Bauer, D. J., Hussong, A. M., & Gottfredson, N. (2016). Improving factor score estimation through the use of observed background characteristics. *Structural Equation Modeling, 23*(6), 827–844. https://doi.org/10.1080/10705511.2016.1220839

Curran, P. J., Cole, V., Giordano, M., Georgeson, A. R., Hussong, A. M., & Bauer, D. J. (2017). Advancing the study of adolescent substance use through the use of integrative data analysis. *Evaluation & the Health Professions, 41*(2), 216–245. https://doi.org/10.1177/0163278717747947

Curran, P. J., Cole, V. T., Bauer, D. J., Rothenberg, W. A., & Hussong, A. M. (2018). Recovering predictor–criterion relations using covariate-informed factor score estimates. *Structural Equation Modeling: A Multidisciplinary Journal, 25*(6), 860–875.

Curran, P. J., Hussong, A. M., Cai, L., Huang, W., Chassin, L., Sher, K. J., & Zucker, R. A. (2008). Pooling data from multiple longitudinal studies: The role of item response theory in integrative data analysis. *Developmental Psychology, 44*(2), 365–380. https://doi.org/10.1037/0012-1649.44.2.365

Curran, P. J., McGinley, J. S., Bauer, D. J., Hussong, A. M., Burns, A., Chassin, L., . . . Zucker, R. (2014). A moderated nonlinear factor model for the development of commensurate measures in integrative data analysis. *Multivariate Behavioral Research, 49*(3), 214–231. https://doi.org/10.1080/00273171.2014.889594

Gottfredson, N. C., Cole, V. T., Giordano, M. L., Bauer, D. J., Hussong, A. M., & Ennett, S. T. (2018, online). Simplifying the implementation of modern scale scoring methods with an automated R package: Automated moderated nonlinear factor analysis (aMNLFA). *Addictive Behaviors*. 94:65–73. doi:https://doi.org/10.1016/j.addbeh.2018.10.031

Granda, P., Wolf, C., & Hadorn, R. (2010). Harmonizing survey data. In J. A. Harkness, M. Braun, B. Edwards, T. P. Johnson, L. Lyberg, P. P. Mohler, et al. (Eds.), *Survey methods in multinational, multiregional, and multicultural contexts* (pp. 315–332). Hoboken, NJ: Wiley. https://doi.org/10.1002/9780470609927.ch17

Hofer, S. M., & Piccinin, A. M. (2009). Integrative data analysis through coordination of measurement and analysis protocol across independent longitudinal studies. *Psychological Methods, 14*(2), 150–164. https://doi.org/10.1037/a0015566

Holland, P. (2007). A framework and history for score linking. In N. J. Dorans, M. Pommerich, & P. W. Holland (Eds.), *Linking and aligning scores and scales* (pp. 5–30). New York, NY: Springer.

Holland, P., & Dorans, N. (2006). Linking and equating. In R. L. Brennan (Ed.), *Educational measurement* (4th ed., pp. 187–220). Westport, CT: American Council on Education/Prager.

Hussong, A., & Smith, R. K. (2018). Parent-based interventions for adolescent substance use. In J. E. Lansford (Ed.), *Handbook of adolescent development research and its impact on global policy* (pp. 280–298). New York, NY: Oxford University Press.

Hussong, A. M., Cai, L., Curran, P. J., Flora, D. B., Chassin, L. A., & Zucker, R. A. (2008). Disaggregating the distal, proximal, and time-varying effects of parent alcoholism on children's internalizing symptoms. *Journal of Abnormal Child Psychology, 36*(3), 335–346. https://doi.org/10.1007/s10802-007-9181-9

Hussong, A. M., Curran, P. J., & Bauer, D. J. (2013). Integrative data analysis in clinical psychology research. *Annual Review of Clinical Psychology, 9*, 61–89. https://doi.org/10.1146/annurev-clinpsy-050212-185522

Hussong, A. M., Flora, D. B., Curran, P. J., Chassin, L. A., & Zucker, R. A. (2008). Defining risk heterogeneity for internalizing symptoms among children of alcoholic parents. *Development and Psychopathology, 20*(1), 165–193. https://doi.org/10.1017/S0954579408000084

Hussong, A. M., Gottfredson, N. C., Bauer, D. J., Curran, P. J., Haroon, M., Chandler, R., . . . Springer, S. A. (2019). Approaches for creating comparable measures of alcohol use symptoms: Harmonization with eight studies of criminal justice populations. *Drug and Alcohol Dependence, 194*(September 2018), 59–68. doi:https://doi.org/10.1016/j.drugalcdep.2018.10.003

Hussong, A. M., Wirth, R. J., Edwards, M. C., Curran, P. J., Chassin, L. A., & Zucker, R. A. (2007). Externalizing symptoms among children of alcoholic parents: Entry points for an antisocial pathway to alcoholism. *Journal of Abnormal Psychology, 116*(3), 529–542. https://doi.org/10.1037/0021-843X.116.3.529

Jelenkovic, A., Sund, R., Hur, Y. M., Yokoyama, Y., Hjelmborg, J. V. B., Möller, S., ... Silventoinen, K. (2016). Genetic and environmental influences on height from infancy to early adulthood: An individual-based pooled analysis of 45 twin cohorts. *Scientific Reports, 6*, 1–14. https://doi.org/10.1038/srep28496

Johnston, L. D., O'Malley, P. M., Bachman, J. G., & Schulenberg, J. E. (2013). *Monitoring the future national survey results on drug use, 1975-2012. Volume II: College students and adults ages 19-50*. Ann Arbor, MI: Institute for Social Research.

Key, T. J., Appleby, P. N., Travis, R. C., Albanes, D., Alberg, A. J., Barricarte, A., ... Allen, N. E. (2015). Carotenoids, retinol, tocopherols, and prostate cancer risk: Pooled analysis of 15 studies. *American Journal of Clinical Nutrition, 102*(5), 1142–1157. https://doi.org/10.3945/ajcn.115.114306

Knibbe, R. A., Derickx, M., Kuntsche, S., Grittner, U., & Bloomfield, K. (2006). A comparison of the alcohol use disorder identification test (Audit) in general population surveys in nine european countries. *Alcohol and Alcoholism, 41*(SUPPL. 1), 29–25. https://doi.org/10.1093/alcalc/agl072

Liu, H., Wilson, I. B., Goggin, K., Reynolds, N., Simoni, J. M., Golin, C. E., ... Bangsberg, D. R. (2013). MACH14: A multi-site collaboration on ART adherence among 14 institutions. *AIDS and Behavior, 17*(1), 127–141. https://doi.org/10.1007/s10461-012-0272-4

McArdle, J., Hamagami, F., Meredith, W., & Bradway, K. (2000). Modeling the dynamic hypotheses of Gf-Gc theory using longitudinal life-span data. *Learning and Individual Differences, 12*, 53–79.

McArdle, J., Prescott, C., Hamagami, F., & Horn, J. (1998). A contemporary method for developmental-genetic analyses of age changes in intellectual abilities. *Developmental Neuropsychology, 14*, 69–114.

McCabe, S. E., Veliz, P., & Schulenberg, J. E. (2018). How collegiate fraternity and sorority involvement relates to substance use during young adulthood and substance use disorders in early midlife: A national longitudinal study. *Journal of Adolescent Health, 62*(3, Suppl), S35–S43. https://doi.org/10.1016/j.jadohealth.2017.09.029

Meredith, W. (1993). Measurement invariance, factor analysis and factorial invariance. *Psychometrika, 58*(4), 525–543.

Millsap, R., & Meredith, W. (2007). Factorial invariance: Historical perspectives and new problems. In R. Cudeck & R. C. MacCallum (Eds.), *Factor analysis at 100: Historical developments and future directions* (pp. 131–152). Mahwah, NJ: Erlbaum.

Millsap, R. E. (2012). *Statistical approaches to measurement invariance*. London: Routledge.

Mun, E.-Y., de la Torre, J., Atkins, D. C., White, H. R., Ray, A. E., Kim, S.-Y., ... Huh, D. (2015). Project INTEGRATE: An integrative study of brief alcohol interventions for college students. *Psychology of Addictive Behaviors, 29*(1), 34–48. https://doi.org/10.1037/adb0000047

Mun, E.-Y., Jiao, Y., & Xie, M. (2016). Integrative data analysis for research in developmental psychopathology. In D. Cicchetti & D. Cicchetti (Eds.), *Developmental psychopathology: Theory and method* (pp. 1042–1087). Hoboken, NJ: Wiley.

National Academies of Sciences, Engineering, and Medicine. (2018). *Open science by design: Realizing a vision for 21st century research*. Washington, DC: National Academies Press.

Pigott, T., Williams, R., & Polanin, J. (2012). Combining individual participant and aggregated data in a meta-analysis with correlational studies. *Research Synthesis Methods, 3*(4), 257–268. https://doi.org/10.1002/jrsm.1051

Reise, S., Widaman, K., & Pugh, R. (1993). Confirmatory factor analysis and item response theory: Two approaches for exploring measurement invariance. *Psychological Bulletin, 114*, 552–566.

Renk, K. (2005). Cross-informant ratings of the behavior of children and adolescents: The "gold standard". *Journal of Child and Family Studies, 14*, 457–468. https://doi.org/10.1007/s10826-005-7182-2

Saunders, J. B., Aasland, O. G., Babor, T. F., De La Fuente, J. R., & Grant, M. (1993). Development of the alcohol use disorders identification test (AUDIT): WHO collaborative project on early detection of persons with harmful alcohol consumption-II. *Addiction, 88*(6), 791–804. https://doi.org/10.1111/j.1360-0443.1993.tb02093.x

Serrano, D., Atzinger, C. B., & Botteman, M. F. (2018). Understanding the disease course and therapeutic benefit of tafamidis across real-world studies of hereditary transthyretin amyloidosis with polyneuropathy: A proof of concept for integrative data analytic approaches. *Neurology and Therapy, 7*(1), 141–154. https://doi.org/10.1007/s40120-018-0096-x

Sher, K., Walitzer, K., Wood, P., & Brent, E. (1991). Characteristics of children of alcoholics: Putative risk factors, substance use and abuse, and psychopathology. *Journal of Abnormal Psychology, 100*, 427–448.

Silventoinen, K., Jelenkovic, A., Sund, R., Hur, Y. M., Yokoyama, Y., Honda, C., … Ji, F. (2016). Genetic and environmental effects on body mass index from infancy to the onset of adulthood: An individual-based pooled analysis of 45 twin cohorts participating in the COllaborative project of Development of Anthropometrical measures in Twins (CODATwins). *American Journal of Clinical Nutrition, 104*(2), 371–379. https://doi.org/10.3945/ajcn.116.130252

Steenkamp, J., & Baumgartner, H. (1998). Assessing measurement invariance in cross national consumer research. *Journal of Consumer Research, 25*, 78–90.

Steinberg, L., & Thissen, D. (2013). Item response theory. In J. S. Comer & P. C. Kendall (Eds.), *The Oxford handbook of research strategies for clinical psychology* (pp. 336–373). New York, NY: Oxford University Press.

Wainer, H., & Thissen, D. (2001). True score theory: The traditional method. In H. Thissen & W. David (Eds.), *Test scoring* (pp. 23–72). Mahwah, NJ: Lawrence Erlbaum.

Werb, D., Garfein, R., Kerr, T., Davidson, P., Roux, P., Jauffret-Roustide, M., … Strathdee, S. A. (2016). A socio-structural approach to preventing injection drug use initiation: Rationale for the PRIMER study. *Harm Reduction Journal, 13*(1), 1–11. https://doi.org/10.1186/s12954-016-0114-1

White, H. R., & Labouvie, E. W. (1989). Towards the assessment of adolescent problem drinking. *Journal of Studies on Alcohol, 50*(1), 30–37.

Yoon, M., & Millsap, R. (2007). Detecting violations of factorial invariance using data-based specification searches: A Monte Carlo study. *Structural Equation Modeling: A Multidisciplinary Journal, 14*, 435–463.

Zucker, R., Fitzgerald, H., Refior, S., Puttler, L., Pallas, D., & Ellis, D. (2000). The clinical and social ecology of childhood for children of alcoholics: Description of a study and implications for a differentiated social policy. In H. Fitzgerald, B. Lester, & B. Zuckerman (Eds.), *Children of addiction: Research, health, and policy issues* (pp. 109–141). New York, NY: Routledge Falmer.

Chapter 6
Introduction to Privacy-Preserving Data Collection and Sharing Methods for Global Health Research

Guanhong Miao, Hanzhi Gao, Yan Wang, and Samuel S. Wu

Abstract In global health and epidemiological research, collecting and sharing data for sensitive topics, such as income, age, sex partners, drug use, HIV infection, stigma, and religion, has been a long-standing challenge. In this chapter, we introduce a range of methods for privacy-preserving data collection and sharing. After a comprehensive review of the classic randomized response techniques and related extensions, we present a new privacy-preserving data collection method capitalizing on the matrix masking theory. In addition to an introduction to the theory and principles, examples are used to illustrate the procedures in applying the method in practice.

Keywords Privacy · Randomized response technique · Random matrix masking · Data sharing

6.1 Introduction

In the big data era, with the explosion of data from various sources, we are facing unprecedented challenges of how to properly protect privacy while maximizing the opportunity to collaborate and exchange data from multiple data providers. While Europe's new General Data Protection Regulations (GDPR) is currently reshaping the cyber world, the Health Insurance Portability and Accountability Act (HIPAA) of 1996 and subsequent rulings have imposed legal requirements on privacy protection in the data collection and handling in medical research in both the developed and developing countries till today.

G. Miao · H. Gao · S. S. Wu (✉)
Department of Biostatistics, University of Florida, Gainesville, FL, USA
e-mail: gmiao@ufl.edu; gaohanzhi@ufl.edu; samwu@biostat.ufl.edu

Y. Wang
Department of Epidemiology, University of Florida, Gainesville, FL, USA
e-mail: ywang48@ufl.edu

X. Chen, (Din) D.-G. Chen (eds.), *Statistical Methods for Global Health and Epidemiology*, ICSA Book Series in Statistics,
https://doi.org/10.1007/978-3-030-35260-8_6

To meet the requirement of HIPAA, a number of traditional and new privacy protection methods have been routinely used, such as anonymity, de-identification, encryption, access control, and personnel training. However, application of these methods requires at least one authorized institution to store the data at a designated server or a trustful curators to respond to queries in a limited time. That suggest that these methods are vulnerable to internal attacks by "insiders"—system administrators, principal investigators, data analysts who have full access to the raw data. Security breaks of this type have become more and more common as shown by the well-publicized hacking incidences at major retailers, credit bureaus and banks (Huffington Post, 2011; Reuters, 2015, 2017). Thus, these methods cannot ensure high levels of confidentiality. When used in data collection they may also result in low response rate.

To avoid privacy and confidentiality breach by a third party while minimizing the risk of being hacked, new methods with stronger privacy-preserving data collection, storage and sharing are needed. The ultimate goal of these methods is that with such methods, an obfuscated dataset can be collected and transported directly between the collaborators; there is no need for a third party in mediating data transitions who also gain full access to the data to be shared; and it may also enhance survey response because of the high levels of privacy and confidentiality.

Among various methods devised to collect obfuscated data, the oldest randomized response technique (RRT) (Warner, 1965) provides an illustrative example. In RRT, response to a survey question is altered according to some randomization schemes in which a survey respondent answers the question, mitigate concerns about privacy. This method and many derivatives have been used in research.

Among various methods for data transportation and sharing, triple matrix-masking (TM^2) technique provides a powerful tool (Wu, Chen, Burr, & Zhang, 2017). After data are masked, they can be transported and shared through any communication channels with no concerns of privacy and confidentiality. Since RRT and TM^2 serve the same purpose of privacy-preserving data collection and both are based on randomized mechanisms, before describing TM2, we give a brief introduction to RRT.

6.2 Randomized Response Technique and Its Extensions

Global health and epidemiology may deal with research questions that are sensitive, invasive, or stigmatizing. In responding to a survey involving these type of questions, survey participant may want to skip or provided edited answers. The following are some typical questions. How old are you? What is your monthly income? Do you have a legal visa to work in the United States? Have you ever used heroin? Do you have any kind of communicable disease? Have you ever had a sexual relationship with a person of the same sex? The list of such questions goes on forever.

In responding to any of these questions, a participant may perceive it as a threat to provide a true answer because of potential social paneity or cost (Lee, 1993). The threat can be intrinsic if certain responses have a negative impact on personal image, or questions are too personal or stressful to respondents; the threat can also be extrinsic if a true response can lead to risk of social sanctions. In these settings, participants can either skip the questions, leading to missing data; or intentionally give socially desirable answers; resulting biased data.

To overcome this limitation for better quality data, several *indirect questioning techniques* have been devised. Typical examples include RRT, Item Count Technique, Nominative Technique, the Three Card Method, Non-randomized Response Models, and Negative Survey. The purposes of these methods are to mitigate or fully eliminate qualms or misperception of self-incrimination for high response rates and unbiased data.

In this chapter, we will focus on RRT and its extensions which usually lead to the lowest response distortion (Locander, Sudman, & Bradburn, 1976). Interested readers can refer to Chaudhuri and Christofides (2013) for more detailed quantitative characteristics of RRT, ICT and other indirect questioning methods.

6.3 Warner's Method

The Mirrored Question Design developed by Warner (1965) is one of the classic RRT. In this method, randomized responses are used to increase survey respondents' cooperation and to estimate the proportion of true "yes" to a sensitive question many respondents may not respond truthfully otherwise (Lensvelt-Mulders, Hox, Van der Heijden, & Maas, 2005). Because of its simplicity and innovation, this method has been studied extensively and subsequently further developed by many other researchers (Boruch, 1971; Fox & Tracy, 1986; Greenberg, Abul-Ela, Simmons, & Horvitz, 1969; Kuk, 1990; Mangat, 1994; Mangat & Singh, 1990).

6.3.1 Principles and Method

The basic idea of Warner's method is that during the survey, an respondent is offered a randomization device to determine whether to answer the question in its original or reverse format. Commonly used randomization devices include spinner, dices, coins, date of birth or any other random generators that has a known probability. By introducing the random noise with known distribution, respondents conceal their responses and therefore protect the privacy by their own; while researchers can still learn the population-level prevalence. The procedure of Warnerr's method is illustrated in Fig. 6.1.

For example, a researcher wanted to investigate the prevalence of a range of risky sexual behavior (e.g., involvement in unprotected sex) in under-graduate

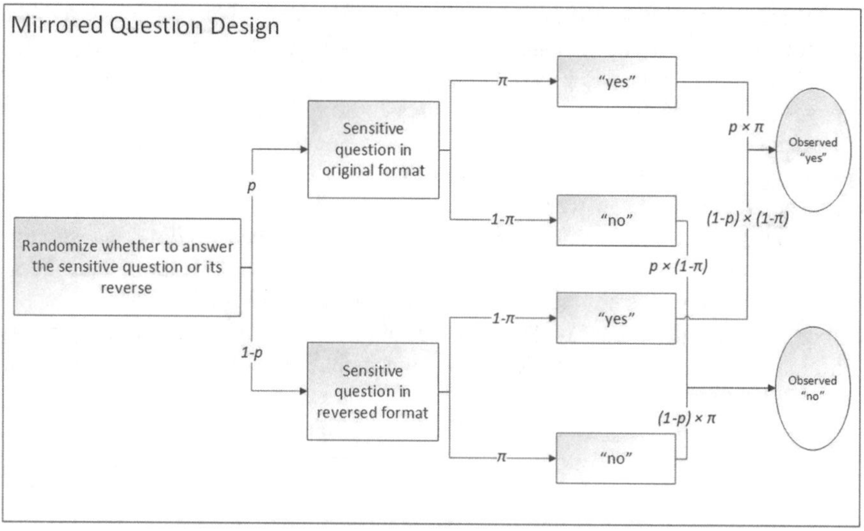

Fig. 6.1 Probability tree for the mirrored question design (Warner's RRT)

students. Due to the highly intrusive and sensitive nature of this topic and related survey questions, direct questioning may end up with large amount of missing and misreports, jeopodizing any effort to obtain an accurate estimates of the prevalence of these behaviors.

6.3.2 *Application of Warner's Method in Study Risky Behaviors Among College Students*

To verify Warner's method, Arnab and Mothupi (2015) conducted a study to investigate sexual risky behaviors among students in a university in Botswana. In this study, results from Warner's method was compared to those of other methods without the option of validation of the results against a known criterion. In the study, 200 students were interviewed. Each respondent was provided a pack of well shuffled cards. The pack consists of two types of cards with known proportions and all the cards were identical in appearance.

If a student drew the type 1 card, he/she was instructed to give "yes" or "no" answer truthfully to the following question printed on the card.

A. I have been involved in unprotected sex with a partner.

If the student drew the type 2 card, he/she was instructed to give "yes" or "no" answer truthfully to a reversed stated question printed on the ard.

$\overline{A}$. I have never been involved in unprotected sex with a partner.

Respondent performed the card draw in the absence of the interviewer, so the interviewer was blind to which card the respondent picked. The privacy of the respondent was guaranteed, since nobody else except the students who knew which of the two questions they answered. However, data collected through this method can be used to obtain accurate estimate of the prevalence of unprotected sex given a relatively large sample and the pre-determined proportions of card type 1 and type 2 in the pack and observed proportion with a "yes" answers.

The proportion of card type 1 is the key parameter, p, which can be used to quantify the burden of cooperation (Warner, 1965) or the privacy spent. The respondent being interviewed is asked for less information if p is closer to 0.5. The two extreme cases are when p equals 0.5, the interviewee would be furnishing no information at all; and when p equals 1, the whole procedure would reduce to direct questioning. The ideas in Warner's original paper were formalized by researchers 40 years later that privacy spent in the entire procedure of this method could be analytically quantified using the idea of differential privacy (Dwork, 2008; Dwork, McSherry, Nissim, & Smith, 2006).

Suppose the underlying true proportion ("yes" to the original sensitive question, i.e., proportion of the students who have been involved in unprotected sex in our example) is π, the proportion of observed "yes" is *P(YES)*, and the number of answers in total is n. Then the unbiased estimator of the true proportion π can be obtained using the following formula,

$$\hat{\pi} = \frac{P(YES) + p - 1}{2p - 1} \tag{6.1}$$

And the sampling variance of this estimator is,

$$\mathrm{var}\left(\hat{\pi}\right) = \frac{\pi\,(1-\pi)}{n} + \frac{p\,(1-p)}{n(2p-1)^2} \tag{6.2}$$

In this comparative study, the estimated proportion is 47.4% under Warner's method and 13.1% under "closed box" method (respondents were asked to fill the questionnaire and put in a locked box), which means that Warner's method provides a more valid estimate under what Tourangeau and Yan (2007) called the "more-is-better" assumption. Note that "more-is-better" assumption is not always warranted, and blind reliance on it is dangerous (Höglinger, 2016).

More real-world applications of *mirrored question design* include but not limited to a study of corruption among public bureaucrats in Bolivia (Gingerich, 2010), a multi-item design on legalizing marijuana use (Himmelfarb, 2008), and a study of whether respondents are in favor of capital punishment (Lensvelt-Mulders, Hox, & Van Der Heijden, 2005).

6.3.3 *Limitations of Warner's Method*

Compared to direct questioning, Warner's method may not be too superior in terms of improvement in response rate, since the two alternative questions—the original and its reversed form—are sensitive in nature. Survey respondents may think the existence of some mathematical tricks for the investigators to sort out their real status (John, Loewenstein, Acquisti, & Vosgerau, 2018; Umesh & Peterson, 1991). In terms of efficiency, the second term on the right side of equation (6.2) represents the variance added by the Warner's method. It can be seen clearly that Warner's method is less efficient than face-to-face direct questioning if everyone answers truthfully. Despite these disadvantages, it is no doubt that Warner has opened new avenues to address the issue of sensitive data collection and inspired numerous applications and extensions of research in this area (Blair et al. 2015; Christophides, 2016).

6.3.3.1 Other Extensions of Warner's Method

Following Warner's invention in 1965, new theoretical and practical contributions to the RRT methodology have been reported. Typical examples include the *forced response design*, the *disguised response design,* and the *unrelated question design*. These newly established methods are now widely accepted and implemented in epidemiology and global health research.

Forced response design, introduced by Boruch (1971) has been further developed and simplified by Fox and Tracy (1986). In this method, respondents are instructed to use a randomization device to determine whether to answer truthfully to a sensitive question or simply reply with a forced answer of "yes" or "no" with a probability p_1 or p_0, respectively. It is easier for respondents to understand this method and therefore better follow the instruction. A study by Moriarty and Wiseman (1976) showed that participants actually did believe that their privacy was protected. However, other studies also showed that not all respondents felt comfortable providing a forced response (Edgell, Himmelfarb, & Duchan, 1982).

The forced question design are often used in research, such as the study of vote choices regarding a Mississippi abortion referendum conducted by Rosenfeld, Imai, and Shapiro (2016), the study of crowdsourcing technology of Google (Erlingsson, Pihur, & Korolova, 2014), the xenophobia and anti-Semitism study in Germany (Krumpal, 2012), the study of consumer use of adult entertainment (De Jong, Pieters, & Fox, 2010), the study of fabrication in job applications (Donovan, Dwight, & Hurtz, 2003), and the study of social security fraud (Van der Heijden & van Gils, 1996).

Disguised response design was proposed by Kuk (1990). This method was developed to overcome the limitation of the use of sensitive questions in the two methods described above. In Kuk's design, the "yes" or "no" answer is replaced with more innocuous words or other objects so that a respondent will feel hard to give false "Yes" response (Van der Heijden & van Gils, 1996). Specifically, in

Disguised response design, the randomization device used is not dice or coin but two stacks of cards. Respondents are not forced to answer a specific question or to give a false answer. Instead, respondents draw cards from each stack and name the color of card from the right (or left) stack according to their underlying true answer to the sensitive question. An example of *disguised question design* is the study on non-compliance to rules in the area of social benefits in Dutch (Frank, Van den Hout, & Van der Heijden, 2009; Van Der Heijden, Van Gils, Bouts, & Hox, 2000).

Unrelated question design or unrelated question model (UQM) is suggested by Horvitz, Shah, and Simmons (1967), and further developed by Greenberg et al. (1969), to address the same problem of *mirrored question design* and *forced question design* and to improve the acceptance to sensitive questions. Under this design, a respondent uses randomization devices to determine whether to answer a sensitive or an unrelated insensitive question. The basic procedure of this method is similar to Warner' method. However, Question $\overline{A}$ from Warner's method is replaced with a neutral question, such as "I was born in Florida". This design has been used in the area of doping and illicit drug use in athletes, including studies by Ulrich et al. (2018), Striegel, Ulrich, and Simon (2010), Dietz et al. (2013), and Schröter et al. (2016). Also, the design has been implemented in abortion studies in Taiwan (Chow & Rider, 1972), North Carolina (Abernathy, Greenberg, & Horvitz, 1970), Turkey (Tezcan & Omran, 1981), and Mexico (Lara, García, Ellertson, Camlin, & Suárez, 2006; Lara, Strickler, Olavarrieta, & Ellertson, 2004).

6.4 More Sophisticated Randomized Response Techniques: RAPPOR

Researchers at Google create a technology called Randomized Aggregatable Privacy-Preserving Ordinal Response (RAPPOR) (Erlingsson et al., 2014). In this method, randomized response techniques are used to analyze large amount of its users' data without compromising the privacy of any individual users in both one-time and longitudinal fashion. The RAPPOR algorithm is specifically designed for collecting statistics on values or strings over large number of clients and executed locally on the client's machine with privacy protection. For example, with this method, data can be obtained about the distribution of a characteristic of all users of an app (e.g., homepage URL domain of Chrome browsers, Windows processes, and search engine queries).

The procedure of local report generating is illustrated in Fig. 6.2, which can be found in the original paper (Erlingsson et al., 2014).

The first step: the client app hashes the true value v ("The number 68", which needs to be protected but is also of interest) onto a bloom filter, creating a bit vector B.

Hash function maps data of arbitrary size to a bit vector of a fixed size. Bloom filter is a data structure designed to tell you whether an element is definitely not

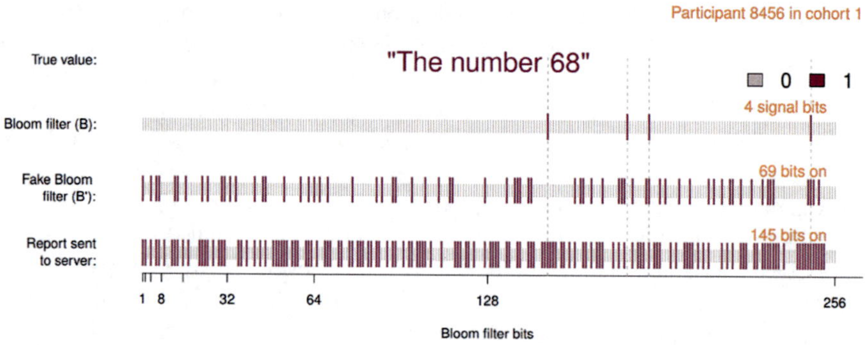

Fig. 6.2 Life of a RAPPOR report

in the set. (A nice illustration of hash function and bloom filter can be found at https://llimllib.github.io/bloomfilter-tutorial/). If the set of strings being collected is relatively small and well-defined, there would be no need to use a Bloom filter.

The second step is the permanent randomized response. Similar to forced response design, we apply a coin flip randomization mechanism at each bit. A new bit vector B' is then created and memorized by the client.

This step essentially serves as a "safe vault" of B. Since only B' is memorized, meaning that even the most powerful attacker have limited ability to learn the true value of B. In practice, learning the true value in its original format, v, is even harder. In sum, the second step provides a long-term privacy guarantees.

The last step is the instantaneous randomized response. A new one-time bit vector, S, is created using coin flip mechanism similar to Kuk's disguised response design based on B' and then sent to the server.

This step provides a short-term privacy guarantee, which can be tuned to balance short-term and long-term risks through the pre-determined parameters in the design. The next time the server asks for the same value, the client server will repeat the last step, create another randomized version S of B' and then send that over.

Note that, the only thing stored in the client app is the permanent randomized response B', and the only thing that ever leaves the client app is another randomized version S of B', meaning that individual's raw data v and raw bit vector B can then be well protected. However, population-level inference on v can still be made, which is illustrated by the following example.

Example The Chrome web browser has deployed RAPPOR to collect data among Chrome users who have opted in to send usage information to Google (http://www.chromium.org/developers/design-documents/rappor). Because homepage URL domains are often targeted and hijacked by malicious software, knowing which URL is commonly used can be very helpful for Google to find out who the main players are. Meanwhile, with daily collection from approximately 14 million respondents, Google can decode RAPPOR reports to accurately detect URLs used with high frequency.

Specifically, each user would first hash his or her homepage URL domain v (e.g., "www.google.com") onto a bit vector B, then randomizes the bit vector B twice and sends out the randomized bit vector S to Google.

Google then summarizes and recovers the frequencies of each bit in the "true" bit vectors (B's), using the formula similar to what we used in previous RRTs section.

Next, regression methods can be implemented based on the design matrix of bit vectors of 8616 candidate URLs (not necessarily cover all possible users' hompage URLs), to find out which URLs are present and their frequencies with statistical confidence.

As a result, even though less than 0.5% of 8616 candidate URLs are found present with enough statistical confidence, they collectively account for approximately 85% of the total probability mass. Excluding those expected domains (e.g., www.google.com), more than 30 unexpected URLs are discovered by RAPPOR analysis. At the same time, Google cannot know each user's homepage URL domain with absolute certainty even with randomized data from approximately 14 million respondents each day.

The reason why RAPPOR is routinely used in Google is that (1) RAPPOR successfully adapted RRTs from data collection over relatively small sample to crowdsourcing over large number of clients. (2) The large number of clients mitigates the efficiency loss of the RRTs. (3) RAPPOR provides privacy protection in both short-term and long-term fashion (4) RAPPOR provides rigorous mathematical proofs of the differential privacy it achieves. (5) RAPPOR algorithm is executed locally on the client's machine, and does not require a trusted third party. (6) The use of hash functions and Bloom filter enables RAPPOR to collect data in more complicated and even messy formats.

In the next part of this chapter, we will focus on another method called triple matrix-masking (TM^2), which is also closely related to randomized response techniques. It shares certain desirable features with RAPPOR, that is, it is also performed locally and can be applied to collect data over large number of users. Moreover, it does not suffer from efficiency loss, which is a common disadvantage of previous methods we introduced.

6.5 Random Orthogonal Matrix Masking (ROMM) for Data Sharing

Random Orthogonal Matrix Masking (ROMM) (Ting, Fienberg, & Trottini, 2008) is a disclosure restriction method with preservation of significant statistical quantities. Statistical results of linear model are invariant after raw data are masked using ROMM. Some categorical data analyses, such as chi-squared test and estimation of odds ratio and relative risk, also have identical results after orthogonal transformation. These properties enable multiple medical entities to share health research data using ROMM without disclosing any raw data at all.

For example, suppose k international and global health research entities have collected data on a common set medical conditions and outcomes (i.e., common variables). Each of them can orthogonally transform its own data and share the masked data with each other. Because the combination of orthogonally transformed data is an orthogonal transformation of combination of raw data, important statistical analysis (including linear regression and contingency table analysis) of the shared data will yield exactly the same results as if the raw data are shared.

6.5.1 Basic Principles and Methodology

Linear Model Suppose $Y_{n \times 1}$ is the vector for the response and $X_{n \times p}$ is the model matrix. The linear model can be written as

$$Y = X\beta + \epsilon,$$

where β is a $p \times 1$ dimensional vector of parameters and ϵ is a $n \times 1$ dimensional vector of zero-mean random error terms following normal distribution. The least square estimate $\hat{\beta}$ can be written as $\hat{\beta} = \left(X^T X\right)^{-1} X^T Y$ where X^T denotes transpose of matrix X.

An orthogonal matrix A is a square matrix which satisfies $A^T A = AA^T = I$ where I is the identity matrix. Now left-multiply Y and X by orthogonal matrix A and refit linear model. That is $AY = AX\beta_{new} + A\epsilon$. According to the property of orthogonal matrix, the new estimator $\hat{\beta}_{new} = \left((AX)^T AX\right)^{-1}(AX)^T AY = \left(X^T A^T AX\right)^{-1} X^T A^T AY = \left(X^T X\right)^{-1} X^T Y$ which is the same as the original linear regression estimator. In other words, applying orthogonal matrix transformation not only protects data, but also keeps estimators invariant.

Contingency Table Analysis Next consider analyzing data in 2×2 tables. Suppose raw data are two $n\times$ 1 vectors Z_1 and Z_2 where n is the number of observations. The elements in Z_1 and Z_2 are 0 or 1. Usually the data are summarized as counts in a 2×2 table. Let a denote the number of observations that are 0's in both Z_1 and Z_2, b denote the number of observations that are 0's in Z_1 and 1's in Z_2, c denote the number of observations with 1 in Z_1 and 0 in Z_2 and d with 1's in both Z_1 and Z_2. The contingency table can also be expressed using vectors: $Z_1^T Z_2 = d$, $Z_1^T Z_1 = c + d$ and $Z_2^T Z_2 = b + d$. It is easy to compute a, b, c and d given these three vector multiplication values and sample size n.

Researchers can multiply Z_1 and Z_2 with an orthogonal matrix A before release if they want to hide values of Z_1 and Z_2. The values in the contingency table are invariant as $(AZ_1)^T AZ_1 = {Z_1}^T Z_1$, $(AZ_2)^T AZ_2 = {Z_2}^T Z_2$ and $(AZ_1)^T AZ_2 = {Z_1}^T Z_2$. Therefore, orthogonal transformation will not influence the analysis of contingency table. The common analysis, such as chi-squared test and estimation of odds ratio and relative risk, will have identical results after an orthogonal transformation.

6.5.2 *Examples of Random Transformation*

The following example shows orthogonal transformation doesn't change linear regression estimators. A random subset of 10 observations from the LEAPS study (Duncan et al., 2011) is used to build the linear model. Eight variables of the original data are explained below.

Variable	Description
Response	Improved functional level of walking 1 year after the stroke (Yes = 1/No = 0)
Δ	Change in walking speed from 2-month to 12-month post-stroke (m/s)
Group	Treatment group, 1 = Locomotor Training Program; 0 = Home Exercise Program
Age	Age at stroke onset (years)
BBS	Berg Balance Scale in sitting, standing, reaching, shifting weight, and turning
IH	Inpatient Hospitalization post randomization (Yes = 1/No = 0)
MIF	Multiple or Injurious Falls post randomization (Yes = 1/No = 0)
ADL/iADL	Activities of daily living (ADL's) and instrumental activities of daily life (iADL's)

Table 6.1 lists 10 randomly selected observations from the LEAPS study.

Consider a linear model with intercept. The first column of the design matrix will be a column of ones. As orthogonal transformation is for the whole design matrix, we add a column of ones with column name "Intercept" to the dataset in Table 6.1 before transformation. A linear model is built with change of walking speed as response and age and Berg balance score as predictors. The design matrix would be a 10×3 matrix with a column of ones. Table 6.2 below gives the transformed

Table 6.1 Random subset of 10 observations from LEAPS study

ID	Response	Group	Δ	Age	BBS	IH	MIF	ADL/iADL
1	1	0	0.67	57	40	0	1	62.5
2	1	1	0.52	38	39	1	1	80
3	1	0	0.34	54	29	0	0	80
4	1	1	0.34	68	48	0	0	72.5
5	1	0	0.48	65	39	0	1	47.5
6	1	0	0.12	81	40	0	0	67.5
7	1	1	0.15	84	29	0	0	42.5
8	0	1	0.20	65	33	0	0	42.5
9	1	1	0.15	66	24	0	1	55
10	1	1	0.22	90	44	0	0	100

Table 6.2 Transformed subset of 10 observations from LEAPS study

Obs no	Delta	Age	BBS	Intercept
1	−0.07	19.12	17.62	0.24
2	−0.25	−99.09	−49.33	−1.37
3	−0.17	−49.74	−22.02	−0.76
4	0.25	43.27	29.62	0.74
5	0.45	67.79	44.01	0.77
6	0.51	105.81	59.33	1.56
7	0.52	102.41	52.5	1.56
8	−0.6	4.33	−20.69	−0.52
9	−0.22	−19.32	−19.72	−0.47
10	0.19	74.52	26.3	0.99

Table 6.3 Correspondence between two forms of counts in 2 × 2 table

		Original data			Orthogonal transformed data		
		Multiple or injurious falls			Multiple or injurious falls		
		No	Yes	Totals	No	Yes	Totals
Group	HEP	5	3	8	–	–	–
	LTP	6	6	12	–	$(AZ_1)^T AZ_2 = 6$	$(AZ_1)^T AZ_1 = 12$
	Totals	11	9	20	–	$(AZ_2)^T AZ_2 = 9$	20

dataset for linear model when using a key of 123 as the random seed to generate orthogonal matrices.

It is easy to check that linear regression results based on the original data in Table 6.1 are exactly the same as those using the orthogonally transformed data in Table 6.2.

Using the same dataset of LEAPS study, we illustrate the invariant property of the orthogonal transformation for contingency table analysis. The contingency table is for group variable (Z_1) and Multiple or Injurious Falls (Z_2). There are two treatment groups: locomotor training program (LTP) and home exercise program (HEP). As shown in Table 6.3, values in the contingency table remain invariant after orthogonal transformation. So odds ratio, relative risk estimation and chi-squared test remain the same before and after orthogonal transformation.

6.6 Triple Matrix-Masking (TM^2) Methods

Triple Matrix-Masking (TM^2) method (Wu, Chen, Burr, & Zhang, 2017) is designed for data collection based on orthogonal transformation and it keeps linear regression estimators invariant after matrix masking. TM^2 method not only prevents privacy leakage, but also maximizes data utility.

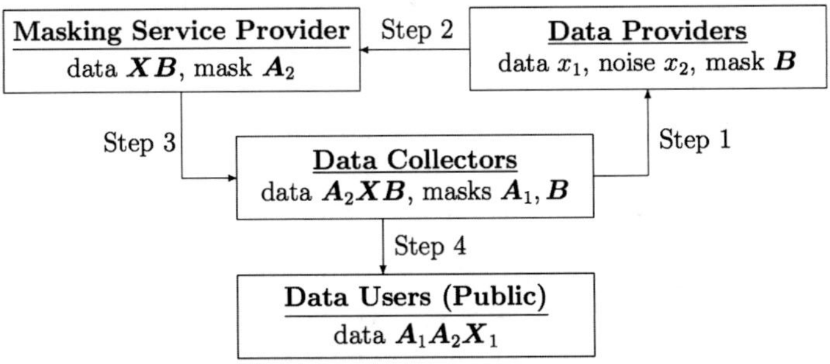

Fig. 6.3 This diagram shows each agency's knowledge of the dataset. Nobody knows the original data X_1 with each data provider (participant) only knows his/her row x_1

6.6.1 Principles and Methodology

There are three agencies in TM^2 method: data collector, data providers (participants) and masking service provider. The procedure (Fig. 6.3, an enhanced version of the one presented in Wu, Chen, Burr, & Zhang, 2017) can be described as follows:

Step 1. Data collector randomly generates a $p \times p$ orthogonal matrix B and saves it in every participant's data collection device.

Step 2. Each data collection device collects each participant's data x_1 (a p_1 dimensional vector) and merge with Gaussian noise x_2 (a p_2 dimensional vector) into a $p = p_1 + p_2$ dimensional vector $x = (x_1, x_2)$. Then x is right multiplied by B on the participant's device. Finally the device sends xB to the masking service provider.

Step 3. The masking service provider combines individual data xB into a $n \times p$ matrix XB after receiving data from all participants. $p_1 < n \leq p = p_1 + p_2$. Then generates another $n \times n$ random orthogonal matrix A_2. XB is left multiplied by A_2 and A_2XB is sent to the data collectors.

Step 4. Data collector multiplies A_2XB by B^{-1} to get A_2X. Take the first p_1 columns to get A_2X_1. Another $n \times n$ random orthogonal matrix A_1 is generated by data collector and left multiply it to A_2X_1. Dataset AX_1 (where $A = A_1A_2$) is publicly published.

Masking service provider has access to the right-masked data XB and the public left-masked data AX_1. Theoretical analysis shows that the original data X cannot be derived given XB and AX_1.

We apply TM^2 method to the dataset of 10 observations from LEAPS study. In the dataset, Inpatient Hospitalization (IH) and Multiple or Injurious Falls (MIF) are sensitive medical information that patients may not want to release publicly as it could adversely affect their opportunities of employment or insurance policies. The proposed TM^2 method protects participant's information by collecting and publishing only masked data through the following steps. In this example, $p_1 = 9$ (8 columns of variables and one column of intercept) and $p_2 = 11$.

Data collector generates a 20×20 ($p = p_1 + p_2 = 20$) random orthogonal matrix B and sends it to every data collection device. Each participant merges his/her own 9-dimensional data with a 11-dimensional Gaussian noise vector. After getting 20-dimensional vector x, it is immediately transformed by B and only masked data xB are sent to the masking service provider. The masking service provider aggregates data from 10 participants to get XB. A 10×10 random orthogonal matrix A_2 is generated and right multiplied by XB. A_2XB is sent to the data collectors. Since B is generated by data collector, data collector can get A_2X using B^{-1}. Take the first p_1 columns to get A_2X_1. Data collector then generate another orthogonal matrix A_1 and left multiply it to A_2X_1 to get published dataset $A_1A_2X_1$. Linear regression model using masked dataset $A_1A_2X_1$ has the same result as in Sect. 6.5.2.

6.6.2 *Extensions of TM² Methods*

Partial Masking TM^2 method can be designed to do partial masking which allows researchers to access part of the data while keeping sensitive information masked. Suppose response, group, change in walking speed and age are not sensitive information in previous LEAPS data. In order to achieve partial masking, we use orthogonal matrix $B = \begin{pmatrix} I_{4\times 4} & O_{4\times 16} \\ O_{16\times 4} & B^*_{16\times 16} \end{pmatrix}$ where $B^*_{16\times 16}$ is an orthogonal matrix. Then generate orthogonal matrices A_1 and A_2 that can keep the first 4 columns of X invariant. After applying TM^2 procedures using these three chosen matrices B, A_1 and A_2, dataset X is masked except the first 4 columns which information is not sensitive.

Collusion Resistant Multi-Matrix Masking Since orthogonal matrix B is known to the data collector and all individual data providers, privacy protection is not safe if one of them shares matrix B with masking service provider who knows XB and AX_1. Collusion resistant multi-matrix masking was introduced in (Wu, Chen, Bhattacharjee, & He, 2017) which solves this problem. There are k masking service providers in order to avoid privacy leakage.

Step 1. A participant's data vector x (a combination of a p_1-dimensional original vector and a p_2-dimensional Gaussian noise vector) is randomly decomposed into k parts: $x = v_1 + v_2 + \cdots + v_k$.

Step 2. v_i ($i = 1, \cdots, k$) is first sent to i-th masking service provider and right multiplied by B_i. Then masked data is sent to all other masking service providers to be right multiplied by their orthogonal matrix. After going through all masking service providers, we get v_iB ($B = \prod_{i=1}^k B_i$ where B_i, $i = 1, \cdots, k$ are commuting in product) and send it to data collector.

Step 3. Data collector adds up all the k parts of masked data v_iB ($1 \le i \le k$) and get xB. Aggregate all participants' data into XB. Send XB back to masking service providers to remove right multiplied orthogonal matrix B (each masking service provider i removes its corresponding matrix B_i) and add left multiplied orthogonal matrix A (each masking service provider i adds its corresponding matrix A_i and $A = \prod_{i=1}^{k} A_i$ where A_i, $i = 1, \cdots, k$ are commuting in product). AX is sent to data collector.

Step 4. Take the first p_1 columns to get AX_1. Data collector releases AX_1 and XB.

For collusion resistant multi-matrix masking, two orthogonal matrices A and B are enough to protect the data as each masking service provider provides parts of information for the generation of A and B. Unlike TM^2 method discussed before, it is hard to know matrix B in multi-matrix masking as the generation procedure is the cooperation of k masking service providers.

6.7 Conclusion Remarks

Useful data are available from different sources elsewhere but not accessible due to laws and regulations for privacy protection. The methods introduced in this chapter will enable epidemiologists and global health researchers to collect and share data overcoming these legal barriers.

The classic randomized response technique (RRT) is reviewed along with its new extensions. In addition, the efficiency loss of the RRT method will no longer be an issue if data from large samples are available. The method is appealing because it has rigorous quantification of privacy spent, does not need of a trusted third party, is flexible to collect data with various format. We also strongly believe that the new method of RAPPOR will be of particular significance for global health research capitalizing on large scale of data collection with privacy challenges

In addition to RRT and its extensions, we also present a privacy-preserving data collection method using random matrix masking. Matrix masked data can be published and freely transferred with little concern of data leaking. This method has several advantages. First, the masked data can by analyzed directly using statistical methods and software commonly used in research. Second, there is theoretical formulation and proofs that no party in the data collection process is capable of gaining insight into the data at the individual participant level.

We anticipate the need for further research in the area of privacy-preserving data collection and sharing. While linear regression and contingency table analysis can be directly applied to masked data with the same results, we need to develop masking technologies that allow for other statistical analysis tools such as longitudinal data analysis, missing data imputation, and machine learning. Also, new technologies are needed for "vertical data" sharing, where each entity contribute a subset of characteristics (variables) for the same cohort of research subjects. Currently available "vertical data" sharing method that keep statistical utility are not privacy-preserving—an entity can maliciously contribute fake data to obtain other entities' original data.

References

Abernathy, J. R., Greenberg, B. G., & Horvitz, D. G. (1970). Estimates of induced abortion in urban North Carolina. *Demography, 7*(1), 19–29.

Arnab, R., & Mothupi, T. (2015). Randomized response techniques: A case study of the risky behaviors' of students of a certain University. *Model Assisted Statistics and Applications, 10*(4), 421–430.

Blair, G., Imai, K., & Zhou, Y. Y. (2015). Design and analysis of the randomized response technique. *Journal of the American Statistical Association, 110*(511), 1304–1319.

Boruch, R. F. (1971). Assuring confidentiality of responses in social research: A note on strategies. *The American Sociologist, 6*, 308–311.

Chaudhuri, A., & Christofides, T. C. (2013). *Indirect questioning in sample surveys*. New York, NY: Springer Science & Business Media.

Chow, L. P., & Rider, R. V. (1972). The randomized response technique as used in the Taiwan outcome of pregnancy study. *Studies in Family Planning, 3*(11), 265–269.

Christophides, T. (2016). The classical randomized response techniques: Reading Warner (1965) and Greenberg et al. (1969). 50 years later. *Data Gathering, Analysis and Protection of Privacy through Randomized Response Techniques: Qualitative and Quantitative Human Traits, Handbook of Statistics, 34*, 29–41.

De Jong, M. G., Pieters, R., & Fox, J. P. (2010). Reducing social desirability bias through item randomized response: An application to measure underreported desires. *Journal of Marketing Research, 47*(1), 14–27.

Dietz, P., Ulrich, R., Dalaker, R., Striegel, H., Franke, A. G., Lieb, K., & Simon, P. (2013). Associations between physical and cognitive doping—a cross-sectional study in 2.997 triathletes. *PLoS One, 8*(11), e78702.

Donovan, J. J., Dwight, S. A., & Hurtz, G. M. (2003). An assessment of the prevalence, severity, and verifiability of entry-level applicant faking using the randomized response technique. *Human Performance, 16*(1), 81–106.

Duncan, P. W., Sullivan, K. J., Behrman, A. L., Azen, S. P., Wu, S. S., Nadeau, S. E., . . . Hayden, S. K. (2011). Body-weight–supported treadmill rehabilitation after stroke. *The New England Journal of Medicine, 364*(21), 2026-2036.

Dwork, C. (2008, April). Differential privacy: A survey of results. In *International conference on theory and applications of models of computation* (pp. 1–19). Berlin: Springer.

Dwork, C., McSherry, F., Nissim, K., & Smith, A. (2006, March). Calibrating noise to sensitivity in private data analysis. In *Theory of cryptography conference* (pp. 265–284). Berlin: Springer.

Edgell, S. E., Himmelfarb, S., & Duchan, K. L. (1982). Validity of forced responses in a randomized response model. *Sociological Methods & Research, 11*(1), 89–100.

Erlingsson, Ú., Pihur, V., & Korolova, A. (2014, November). Rappor: Randomized aggregatable privacy-preserving ordinal response. In *Proceedings of the 2014 ACM SIGSAC conference on computer and communications security* (pp. 1054–1067). New York, NY: ACM.

Fox, J. A., & Tracy, P. E. (1986). Randomized response: A method for sensitive surveys.

Frank, L. E., Van den Hout, A., & Van der Heijden, P. G. M. (2009). Repeated cross-sectional randomized response data: Taking design change and self-protective responses into account. *Methodology: European Journal of Research Methods for the Behavioral and Social Sciences, 5*(4), 145.

Gingerich, D. W. (2010). Understanding off-the-books politics: Conducting inference on the determinants of sensitive behavior with randomized response surveys. *Political Analysis, 18*(3), 349–380.

Greenberg, B. G., Abul-Ela, A. L. A., Simmons, W. R., & Horvitz, D. G. (1969). The unrelated question randomized response model: Theoretical framework. *Journal of the American Statistical Association, 64*(326), 520–539.

Himmelfarb, S. (2008). The multi-item randomized response technique. *Sociological Methods & Research, 36*(4), 495–514.

Höglinger, M. (2016). *Revealing the truth? Validating the randomized response technique for surveying sensitive topics.* Doctoral dissertation, ETH Zurich.
Horvitz, D.G., Shah, B. V., & Simmons, W. R. (1967). The unrelated randomized response model. In *Proceedings of the Social Statistics Section of the American Statistical Association* (pp. 65–72).
Huffinton Post. (2011). *Citigroup: $2.7 million stolen from customers as result of hacking.* Retrieved from http://www.huffingtonpost.com/2011/06/27/citigroup-hack_n_885045.html.
John, L. K., Loewenstein, G., Acquisti, A., & Vosgerau, J. (2018). When and why randomized response techniques (fail to) elicit the truth. *Organizational Behavior and Human Decision Processes, 148*, 101–123.
Krumpal, I. (2012). Estimating the prevalence of xenophobia and anti-Semitism in Germany: A comparison of randomized response and direct questioning. *Social Science Research, 41*(6), 1387–1403.
Kuk, A. Y. (1990). Asking sensitive questions indirectly. *Biometrika, 77*(2), 436–438.
Lara, D., García, S. G., Ellertson, C., Camlin, C., & Suárez, J. (2006). The measure of induced abortion levels in Mexico using random response technique. *Sociological Methods & Research, 35*(2), 279–301.
Lara, D., Strickler, J., Olavarrieta, C. D., & Ellertson, C. (2004). Measuring induced abortion in Mexico: A comparison of four methodologies. *Sociological Methods & Research, 32*(4), 529–558.
Lee, R. M. (1993). *Doing research on sensitive topics*. Thousand Oaks, CA: Sage.
Lensvelt-Mulders, G. J., Hox, J. J., & Van Der Heijden, P. G. (2005). How to improve the efficiency of randomised response designs. *Quality and Quantity, 39*(3), 253–265.
Lensvelt-Mulders, G. J., Hox, J. J., Van der Heijden, P. G., & Maas, C. J. (2005). Meta-analysis of randomized response research: Thirty-five years of validation. *Sociological Methods & Research, 33*(3), 319–348.
Locander, W., Sudman, S., & Bradburn, N. (1976). An investigation of interview method, threat and response distortion. *Journal of the American Statistical Association, 71*(354), 269–275.
Mangat, N. S. (1994). An improved randomized response strategy. *Journal of the Royal Statistical Society. Series B (Methodological), 56*, 93–95.
Mangat, N. S., & Singh, R. (1990). An alternative randomized response procedure. *Biometrika, 77*(2), 439–442.
Moriarty, M., & Wiseman, F. (1976). On the choice of a randomization technique with the randomized response model. In *Proceedings of the Social Statistics Section, American Statistical Association* (pp. 624–626).
Reuters. (2015). *Target to pay $10 million to settle lawsuit from massive data breach.* Retrieved from http://www.huffingtonpost.com/2015/03/18/target-hack-settlement_n_6899290.html.
Reuters. (2017). *Equifax says hack potentially exposed details of 143 million consumers.* Retrieved from http://www.huffingtonpost.com/entry/quifax-says-hack-potentially-exposed-details-of-143-million-consumers_us_59b1bc2de4b0354e4410b33e.
Rosenfeld, B., Imai, K., & Shapiro, J. N. (2016). An empirical validation study of popular survey methodologies for sensitive questions. *American Journal of Political Science, 60*(3), 783–802.
Schröter, H., Studzinski, B., Dietz, P., Ulrich, R., Striegel, H., & Simon, P. (2016). A comparison of the Cheater detection and the unrelated question models: A randomized response survey on physical and cognitive doping in recreational triathletes. *PloS One, 11*(5), e0155765.
Striegel, H., Ulrich, R., & Simon, P. (2010). Randomized response estimates for doping and illicit drug use in elite athletes. *Drug and Alcohol Dependence, 106*(2-3), 230–232.
Tezcan, S., & Omran, A. R. (1981). Prevalence and reporting of induced abortion in Turkey: two survey techniques. *Studies in Family Planning, 12*, 262–271.
Ting, D., Fienberg, S. E., & Trottini, M. (2008). Random orthogonal matrix masking methodology for microdata release. *International Journal of Information and Computer Security, 2*(1), 86–105.
Tourangeau, R., & Yan, T. (2007). Sensitive questions in surveys. *Psychological Bulletin, 133*(5), 859.

Ulrich, R., Pope, H. G., Cléret, L., Petróczi, A., Nepusz, T., Schaffer, J., ... Simon, P. (2018). Doping in two elite athletics competitions assessed by randomized-response surveys. *Sports Medicine, 48*(1), 211–219.

Umesh, U. N., & Peterson, R. A. (1991). A critical evaluation of the randomized response method: Applications, validation, and research agenda. *Sociological Methods & Research, 20*(1), 104–138.

Van der Heijden, P. G., & van Gils, G. (1996). Some logistic regression models for randomized response data.

Van Der Heijden, P. G., Van Gils, G., Bouts, J. A. N., & Hox, J. J. (2000). A comparison of randomized response, computer-assisted self-interview, and face-to-face direct questioning: Eliciting sensitive information in the context of welfare and unemployment benefit. *Sociological Methods & Research, 28*(4), 505–537.

Warner, S. L. (1965). Randomized response: A survey technique for eliminating evasive answer bias. *Journal of the American Statistical Association, 60*(309), 63–69.

Wu, S. S., Chen, S., Bhattacharjee, A., & He, Y. (2017). Collusion resistant multi-matrix masking for privacy-preserving data collection. In *2017 IEEE 3rd international conference on big data security on cloud (bigdatasecurity), IEEE international conference on high performance and smart computing (HPSC), and IEEE international conference on intelligent data and security (ids)* (pp. 1–7). Beijing: IEEE.

Wu, S. S., Chen, S., Burr, D. L., & Zhang, L. (2017). A new data collection technique for preserving privacy. *Journal of Privacy and Confidentiality, 7*(3), 99–129.

Part II
Essential Statistical Methods

Chapter 7
Geographic Mapping for Global Health Research

Bin Yu

Abstract Geographic mapping represents one of the most efficient approaches for students and researchers to establish a global perspective on a specific medical, health and behavioral issues. In this chapter, we introduce the application of the free software R program packages available in geographic mapping. We demonstrate various mapping methods and R program codes using country-specific data for population and population density as examples.

Keywords Global mapping · Population distribution · Global health · R software

An essential part of global health and epidemiology is to gain a comprehensive understanding of a disease or a health behavior in order to further investigate the causes and risk factors and to develop strategies for treatment, control and prevention. Traditional medical and health research focuses on individual persons who suffer from a disease, such as high blood pressure, heart disease, and cancer; or engaged in an unhealthy behavior, such as smoking cigarettes, drinking alcohol, using illegal drugs, and committing suicide. Establishment of public health in general and epidemiology in particularly expands our vision from focusing on individuals to including the population. Such an expansion in our vision results in new developments in research methodologies, and greatly increases our capabilities to grasp the causes and risk factors of many diseases and health risk behaviors. With new development in technologies and increased availability of public domain data, researchers in public health and medicine started stretching from the community-, country-, international-based approach to globe. Supported with achievements in international health research and development during the history of public health and medicine, more and more medical and health researchers are now

B. Yu (✉)
Department of Epidemiology, University of Florida, Gainesville, FL, USA
e-mail: byu@ufl.edu

X. Chen, (Din) D.-G. Chen (eds.), *Statistical Methods for Global Health and Epidemiology*, ICSA Book Series in Statistics,
https://doi.org/10.1007/978-3-030-35260-8_7

tackling challenging questions with a cross-cultural, multidisciplinary and global perspective. Such advancement requires new tools and methods, and global mapping provides one of such tools for researchers to further advance their research agenda.

7.1 Importance of Global Mapping

With the massive economic globalization, rapid developments in transportation and communication backed by accelerated advancement in information technologies, many countries over the world have completed the State I to Stage IV epidemiological transition (Omran, 1971). Along with the declines in infectious diseases, we are facing more and more new health challenges, such as cultural shock, depression, migration stress, cross-country or cross-board transmission of HIV/AIDS, autism, global epidemic of obesity, substance use, depression, and internet addiction (Elsabbagh et al., 2012; Griffiths, Kuss, Billieux, & Pontes, 2016; Morgen & Sørensen, 2014; Murray et al., 2014; Whiteford, Ferrari, Degenhardt, Feigin, & Vos, 2015). Furthermore, we know very little about the causes of many chronic diseases that are common, such as cancer and cardiovascular diseases (Harris, 2013). Integration of a global approach into our current research endeavor will be a promising approach to improve our understanding of both new and traditional medical and health challenges in the new era of economic and technological globalization (Chen, Elliott, & Wang, 2018; Chen & Wang, 2017; Chen, 2014; Cochi & Dowdle, 2011; DeLaet, 2015).

"One picture is worth a thousand words." This English saying is particularly relevant for public health researchers and decision-makers to establish a global picture of a medical, public health and a behavior issue. Putting data on a world map provides a simple but most efficient way for a person to establish a global perspective and to understand any medical, health or behavioral problems with a global significance. For example, we know that the total number of people in a country differs dramatically. When we put this number into a world map, a clear picture of global population distribution appears (see Fig. 7.7 later in this chapter). Many people may believe that HIV infection is most prevalent in Africa, based on scattered information from different sources. Is that true? The best way to grasp the global epidemic of HIV is to map the distribution by countries using different indicators (see examples in Chap. 8 in this book).

It is appealing to researchers, decision-makers and public health practitioners to see the global pictures of a disease, a health problem, or a health risk behavior; however, it is challenging for many people on how to map a problem on computer because of the lack of specialized training in computer sciences and efficient application of complex software such as the Arc-GIS (ESRI, Redlands, California, USA) (Olson et al., 2001). It is costly to purchase these software packages and it takes time to master the use of such software. Technical, financial and practical barriers prevent many of us from using the global mapping approach in investigating global medical and health issues. In this chapter, we introduce the methods and skills for global mapping using (1) software R that is free of charge (The R Foundation, 2018) and (2) data from sources that are freely available (see Chaps. 1 and 2 for details regarding existing data).

This chapter is divided into two sections. In the first section, we provide some fundamental knowledge about the free software R and preparations for geographic mapping. In the second section, we introduce the method to draw world map with data from individual countries as example.

7.2 Preparation for Geographic Mapping

7.2.1 Brief Introduction to R and R Studio

R is an open-source software as well as a language and environment for statistical computing. It is available free of charge to anyone who wants to use it for research and other practices (R Core Team, 2013). The software can do more statistical analysis than any other commercial software alone that may cost up to thousands of dollars. Another advantage of R is that it can produce graphics, figures and maps with publishable quality.

R consists of two parts, a base R, plus numerous programs, or packages for use to solve complex and/or more specific problems. For example, to draw maps using R, in addition to the base R, a number of R packages must be installed. We will introduce R packages in Sect. 7.3.1 when talking about mapping. Researchers keep developing new functions, tools and packages in R, making this software a very powerful source to solve new and challenging questions.

There are at least two ways for people to use R: (1) programming and executing a project directly through R, and (2) using the R Studio as an interface to program and execute a project. The former approach is more relevant for people who are specialized in data analysis and mapping while the latter is more efficient for non-specialized individuals. We introduce the second approach in this chapter.

7.2.2 Download and Install R

To do geographic mapping, the first thing is to download and install R on your computer. Please start the internet, open a browser, search for "R software", you may see a screen like the following:

The R Project for Statistical Computing
https://www.r-project.org/ ▾
R is a free **software** environment for statistical computing and graphics. It compiles and runs on a wide variety of UNIX platforms, Windows and MacOS.

Click on the green colored website address, the following page appears:

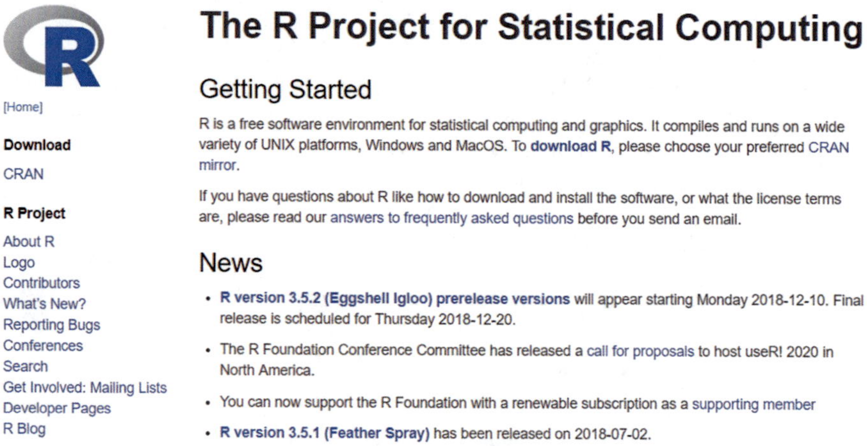
The R Project for Statistical Computing
[Home]
Download
CRAN
R Project
About R
Logo
Contributors
What's New?
Reporting Bugs
Conferences
Search
Get Involved: Mailing Lists
Developer Pages
R Blog
Getting Started
R is a free software environment for statistical computing and graphics. It compiles and runs on a wide variety of UNIX platforms, Windows and MacOS. To download R, please choose your preferred CRAN mirror.
If you have questions about R like how to download and install the software, or what the license terms are, please read our answers to frequently asked questions before you send an email.
News
R version 3.5.2 (Eggshell Igloo) prerelease versions will appear starting Monday 2018-12-10. Final release is scheduled for Thursday 2018-12-20.
The R Foundation Conference Committee has released a call for proposals to host useR! 2020 in North America.
You can now support the R Foundation with a renewable subscription as a supporting member
R version 3.5.1 (Feather Spray) has been released on 2018-07-02.

You can also direct come to this page by typing in the website URL address: https://www.r-project.org/

Click "Download R" highlighted in the first paragraph, and you will see a list of CRAN mirrors—the location where you can download R. Then scroll down to a place close to you and click on one of the links provided. Use the USA as an example. When scrolling down you will see the following:

USA

https://cran.cnr.berkeley.edu/	University of California, Berkeley, CA
http://cran.cnr.berkeley.edu/	University of California, Berkeley, CA
http://cran.stat.ucla.edu/	University of California, Los Angeles, CA
https://mirror.las.iastate.edu/CRAN/	Iowa State University, Ames, IA
http://mirror.las.iastate.edu/CRAN/	Iowa State University, Ames, IA
https://ftp.ussg.iu.edu/CRAN/	Indiana University
http://ftp.ussg.iu.edu/CRAN/	Indiana University
https://rweb.crmda.ku.edu/cran/	University of Kansas, Lawrence, KS
http://rweb.crmda.ku.edu/cran/	University of Kansas, Lawrence, KS
https://cran.mtu.edu/	Michigan Technological University, Houghton, MI
http://cran.mtu.edu/	Michigan Technological University, Houghton, MI
http://cran.wustl.edu/	Washington University, St. Louis, MO
http://archive.linux.duke.edu/cran/	Duke University, Durham, NC
https://mirrors.sorengard.com/cran/	Sorengard, Bronx NY
https://cran.case.edu/	Case Western Reserve University, Cleveland, OH
http://cran.case.edu/	Case Western Reserve University, Cleveland, OH
https://ftp.osuosl.org/pub/cran/	Oregon State University
http://ftp.osuosl.org/pub/cran/	Oregon State University
http://lib.stat.cmu.edu/R/CRAN/	Statlib, Carnegie Mellon University, Pittsburgh, PA
http://cran.mirrors.hoobly.com/	Hoobly Classifieds, Pittsburgh, PA
https://mirrors.nics.utk.edu/cran/	National Institute for Computational Sciences, Oak Ridge, TN

From the list, we note that the National Institute for Computational Sciences, Oak Ridge, TN is closer to the University of Florida where we located. By clicking on the link, three download options are available for different computer systems you are using:

- Download R for Linux
- Download R for (Mac) OS X
- Download R for Windows

Choose the one that matches with your computer and click on it. Follow the instructions to install R on your computer.

7.2.3 Download and Install R Studio

After completion of installing R in the previous step, you can move to install R Studio. You can do this by directly going to the R Studio website: (https://www.rstudio.com/products/rstudio/download/). Click on the link, you will see five versions of R Studio. For geographic mapping, the first one licensed by AGPL, free of charge is adequate.

To install, click the button "DOWNLOAD". From the drop down manual "Installers for Supported Platforms", select the version that matches your computer. For example, if you use Windows Vista/7/8/10, click on the link, then follow the instruction to install the R Studio.

7.2.4 Work Around R Studio

After completing the installation of the software R and the corresponding R Studio, you can start running R through the R studio. After starting R Studio, you will see the work interface as showing in the computer (Fig. 7.1).

The top line is the menu for programming and executing R, including files, edit, code, view, plots, and other common functions.

There are four windows under the manual. The first box located on the top left is the R script area. This box is also known as the syntax-highlighting editor where you can put your R program codes and execute the program codes. This is the most frequently used working space.

The box located on the top right is named as the work environment and history. Particularly, it includes the datasets you use for analyzing and mapping.

The box located at the bottom left is called the Console for R. This box is for showing the R codes that are executed and analytical results.

The box located at the bottom right is for display of maps, chart, and plots for review. It also shows the installed packages, helps and viewers.

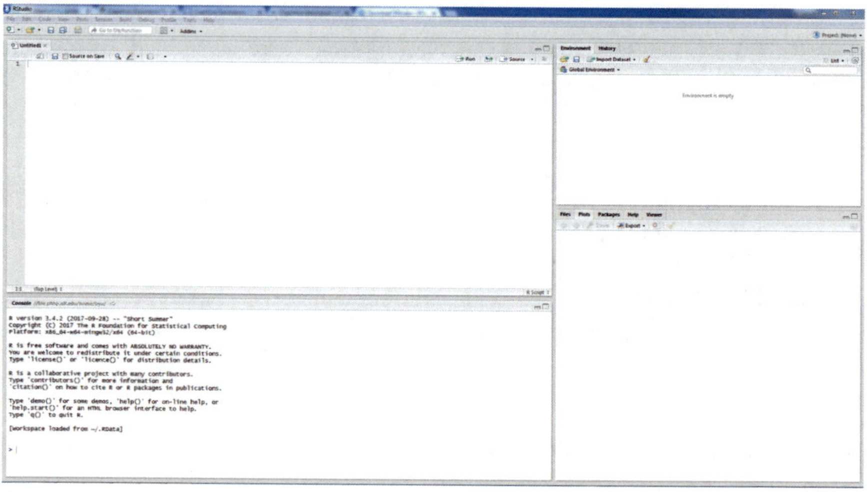

Fig. 7.1 The work interface of R studio

7.3 R Packages for Geographic Mapping

To conduct geographic mapping, in addition to the R base described in the previous sections, several R packages are needed. You need to know these packages, download and install them on your computer.

7.3.1 R Packages Needed

To conduct geographic mapping, different R packages are available. In this chapter, five R packages will be installed and used after you installed R base and the R Studio:

1. Package "dplyr": This package is needed for data management (Wickham, François, Henry, & Müller, 2019). The chapter will use this package to manage the data used for mapping.
2. Package "maps": This package is used for display of maps (Becker & Wilks, 2018). One function of this package is that it contains geographic information (longitude and latitude) to describe the shape of the whole world as well as the boundaries for specific countries in the world.
3. Package "mapproj": This package is used to convert latitude/longitude into projected coordinates (McIlroy, 2018). It contains the data to adjust a map for mapping analysis, including projection methods (e.g. mercator, sinusoidal,

cylequalarea, cylindrical, rectangular, etc.), and orientation (latitude, longitude, rotation).
4. Package "RColorBrewer": This package provides color schemes for graphics and maps (Neuwirth, 2014). An R color cheatsheet can be found in the following website (https://www.nceas.ucsb.edu/~frazier/RSpatialGuides/colorPaletteCheatsheet.pdf).
5. Package "ggplot2": This package is used to make various graphics, figures and maps in R (Wickham, Chang, et al., 2019).

7.3.2 Download and Install the Related R Packages

It is easy to install an R package after the R Base and the R Studio are installed. To install an R package through the R Studio, you first start R Studio. In the top left R script box, you simply type in:

```
install.packages("package name")
```

Put the name of the packages you want to install in the place "*package name*". Check if you spell the package name correctly. Remember that the package name is case-sensitive, small letters and capital letters indicate different packages.

After checking the package name, you can install it now by either pressing the key combination of "Ctrl + Enter" on your computer keyboard, or click on the "Run" button on the top right banner of the Script Box of the R Studio.

For example, you can install "ggplot2" by typing "install.packages ("ggplot2")" in the Script Box, and then press "Ctrl + Enter" to start installing. For each package that has been successfully installed, the result should appear in the R Console box located at the bottom left of the R Studio.

To facilitate your installation, you can type or copy of the following R codes to the Script Box on the top left of your R Studio to install all five required R packages.

```
install.packages("dplyr")
install.packages("maps")
install.packages("mapproj")
install.packages("RColorBrewer")
install.packages("ggplot2")
```

After all required packages are installed, the function "library" will be used to load the installed packages before actual mapping. For example, "library (ggplot2)" is used to load the package "ggplot2", thus this package is activated to use in the following steps.

```
library(ggplot2)
```

More details about loading R packages are provided in the following sections for different mapping purposes.

7.4 Mapping the World Using R

7.4.1 Creating a Base World Map

After completion of installing Base R, R Studio and the five R packages for mapping, we are ready to draw maps. A world map is a foundation for modeling diseases, health risk behaviors, and any other related health issues. In this section, we demonstrate the steps to draw a blank world map.

Packages and activation. We need two packages to create a blank world map, and they are: "maps", and "ggplot2". To activate or load a package into the computer so that they can be used for drawing map, we used the command "library ()". Copy the following lines of command to load the two packages:

```
library(maps)
```

This package contains the geographic information of the world for mapping. Specifically, there is a database called "world" in this package which provides information regarding names of individual countries, longitudes, and latitudes of the boundaries between countries.

```
library(ggplot2)
```

This package functions as a drawer to produce a world map.

Data preparation for mapping. In the Script box of the R Studio, type in the following R code to create a data set:

```
world_data <- map_data("world")
```

In the code, the "world_data" is the dataset name newly created, the rest of the code ask the computer to read data from the package "maps" about the world map and input the data, and the code "map_data" from package "ggplot2" asks the computer to derive the data from the package "maps" for mapping.

You can check the data in the dataset "world_data" by simply typing "world_data" in the script window, and you will see the contents of output as shown in Fig. 7.2.

	long	lat	group	order	region	subregion
1	-6.989912e+01	1.245200e+01	1	1	Aruba	<NA>
2	-6.989571e+01	1.242300e+01	1	2	Aruba	<NA>
3	-6.994219e+01	1.243853e+01	1	3	Aruba	<NA>
4	-7.000415e+01	1.250049e+01	1	4	Aruba	<NA>
5	-7.006612e+01	1.254697e+01	1	5	Aruba	<NA>
6	-7.005088e+01	1.259707e+01	1	6	Aruba	<NA>
7	-7.003511e+01	1.261411e+01	1	7	Aruba	<NA>
8	-6.997314e+01	1.256763e+01	1	8	Aruba	<NA>
9	-6.991181e+01	1.248047e+01	1	9	Aruba	<NA>
10	-6.989912e+01	1.245200e+01	1	10	Aruba	<NA>
12	7.489131e+01	3.723164e+01	2	12	Afghanistan	<NA>
13	7.484023e+01	3.722505e+01	2	13	Afghanistan	<NA>
14	7.476738e+01	3.724917e+01	2	14	Afghanistan	<NA>
15	7.473896e+01	3.728564e+01	2	15	Afghanistan	<NA>
16	7.472666e+01	3.729072e+01	2	16	Afghanistan	<NA>
17	7.466895e+01	3.726670e+01	2	17	Afghanistan	<NA>
18	7.455899e+01	3.723662e+01	2	18	Afghanistan	<NA>
19	7.437217e+01	3.715771e+01	2	19	Afghanistan	<NA>

Fig. 7.2 Display of "world" data containing geographic information

Information in this output file is described below:

The top row is the variable name, including long, lat, group, order, region and subregion. The variable "long" means longitude, it contains both positive and negative values, depending on the location of the country relative to the prime median. The values are negative if located on the left of the meridian and positive if located on the right. The variable "lat" indicates latitude. The variable "order" indicates the order that guides the package "ggplot2" to connect the dots defined by both the variable "long" and the variable "lat" to draw individual countries in the world map. The variable "group" is very important! It provides information guiding the package "ggplot2" to draw maps by selecting the right segments to connect by lines. If they are in the same group, then they can get connected, but if they are in different groups then they don't. The variables "region" and "subregion" tell package "ggplot2" to put region (country) or subregion defined by a set of points using "long' and "lat".

Drawing World Map. After reading data and data checking, now you can draw a blank work map using the following R codes:

```
mapbase<-ggplot(data=world_data,mapping=aes(x=long,y=lat,group
=group)) +
     coord_fixed(1.5) +
     geom_polygon(color="black", fill="grey") +
     labs(x="Longitude") +
     labs(y="Latitude")
```

The object mapbase is created to store the world map created using R. Function "ggplot()" is used to draw the map with the newly created dataset: world_data. The function "aes" for mapping is to construct aesthetic mapping, x is longitude, and y is latitude, group for drawing is the same as the original data.

The function "coord_fixed()" is used to define the ratio of x axis and y axis. It fixes the relationship between one unit in the y direction and one unit in the x direction. The function "geom_polygon()" directs "ggplot()" to draw polygons by linking the last point back to the first point with a line. The attributes of "geom_polygon()" help define the color of the map. "color="black"" asks to draw the board line black, and "fill="grey"" asks to fill in the area of individual countries with grey. The function "labs()" is used to define the axis labels.

To view the map just created, simply type "mapbase" in the script window. If doing correctly you will see a world map as shown in Fig. 7.3.

7.4.2 *Change Map Projections for Best View*

Steps for Projection. R mapping contains a function for us to alter the projection mode of the world map to fit our need. Several projections are available. In this section, we introduce mapping with the rectangular projection, one of the commonly used projections in world map presentation.

To alter map project, we first activate or load the package "mapproj" using the following R code.

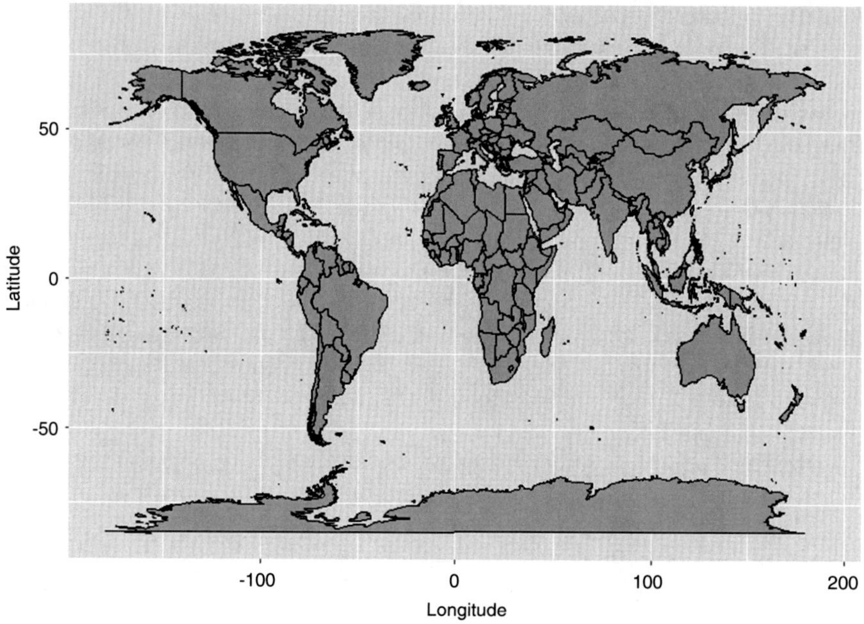

Fig. 7.3 World map created using R

```
library(mapproj)
```

This package contains the information to convert a world map into different views with a projection function.

After the package "mapproj" is loaded, you can convert the world map just created using the rectangular projection by typing in the following R codes.

```
mapbase_p<-ggplot(data=world_data,mapping=aes(x=long,y=lat,
group=group))+
     coord_fixed(1.5) +
     coord_map(projection="rectangular", parameters=c(lat0=40),
     xlim=c(-180, 180)) +
     geom_polygon(color="black", fill="grey") +
     labs(x="Longitude") +
     labs(y="Latitude")
```

The R codes above are an extension of the codes to draw the base world map in Fig. 7.3 by adding the following:

```
coord_map(projection="rectangular", parameters=c(lat0=40),
xlim=c(-180, 180)
```

The function "coord_map()" asks "ggplot2" to adjust the map using projection="rectangular" taking from the package "mapproj", which indicates equally spaced parallels and equally spaced straight meridians in the map and set the parameters for mapping to the values defined by "c(lat0=40)" which indicates

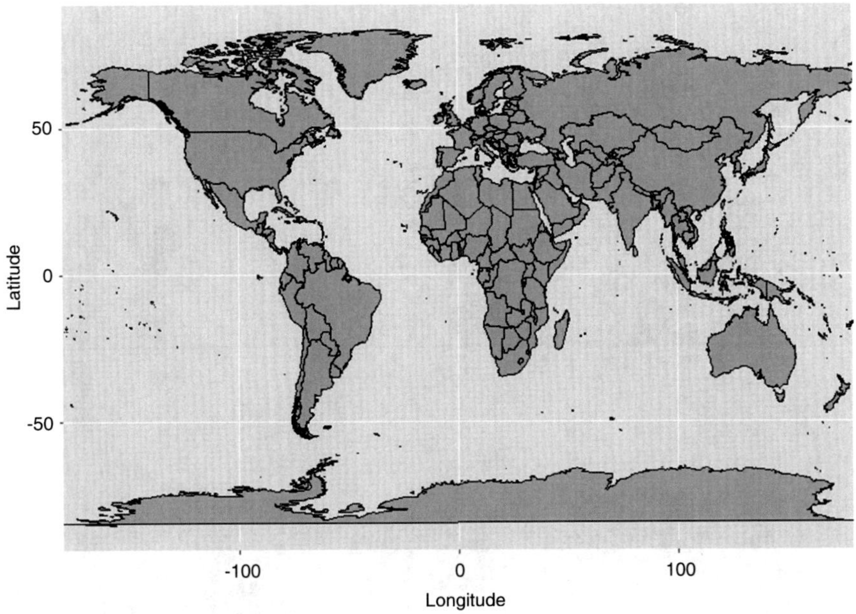

Fig. 7.4 Re-projected world map using R

the true scale used in the map. "xlim=c(-180, 180)" defines the map begins from the longitude −180 to +180.

View Results. With this projection, a curved area on the earth surface will be converted into a 2D flat plane like a rectangle. To see the projected map, simply type "mapbase_p" in the script window and run. If the R codes are entered correctly, you will see a map like the one in Fig. 7.4.

By comparing the project map in Fig. 7.4 with the original base map in Fig. 7.3, you may not see much difference. However, a careful comparison you may find that the areas toward both the North and South Pole are becoming larger in the projected map than in the base map.

Although the rectangular project has been used most commonly in research, more projection methods are available from the package "mapproj". You can consult the instructions for using this package for details.

7.4.3 *Map Rotation for a Different Central View*

Steps for Rotation. In mapping analysis, we often need to rotate the map to put the country of interest in the center of the map. The two maps in the base map and the projected base map, west Europe and Africa are located as the central view. If we

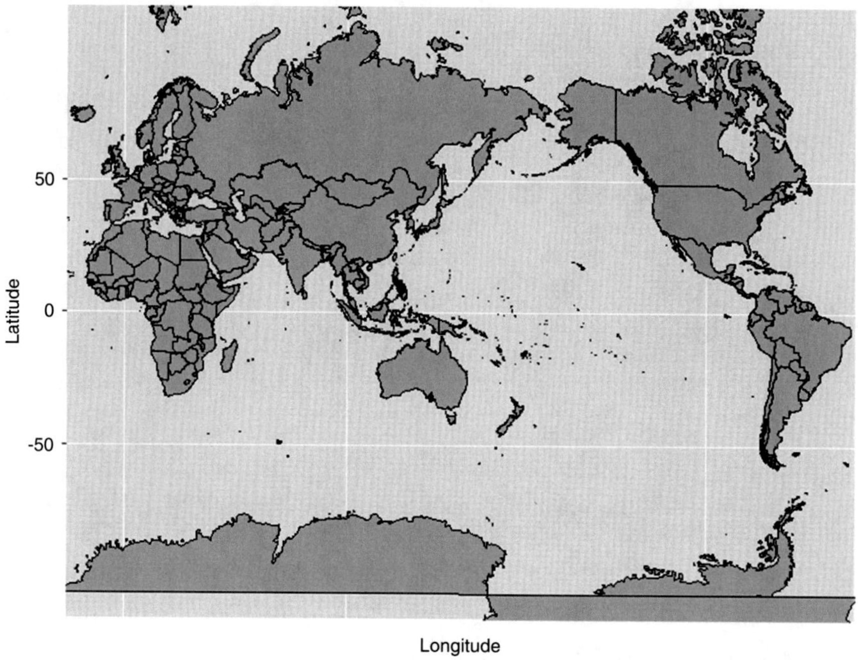

Fig. 7.5 Rotated world map using R. Note: To better visualize the rotated map, the region of Greenland was excluded

want to move China to the center, for example, we can rotate the map using the R code: orientation=c(90,150,0).

```
mapbase_o<-
ggplot(data=world_data,mapping=aes(x=long,y=lat, group=group))+
      coord_fixed(1.5) +
      coord_map(orientation=c(90, 150, 0), xlim=c(-180, 180)) +
      geom_polygon(color="black", fill="grey")+
      labs(x="Longitude") +
      labs(y="Latitude")
```

"orientation=c(90,150,0)" in "coord_map" is used to adjust the map center. This statement is describing where the "North Pole" should be when computing the projection. "90" is the latitude, "150" is the longitude, indicating the centered longitude, and "0" is the degree of clockwise rotation, and we keep it "0" here. "xlim=c(-180, 180)" sets the longitude on the map beginning from −180 to +180.

View Results. With this rotation, China will be presented roughly at the center of the world map. To see the rotated world map, simply type "mapbase_o" in the script window and run. If the R codes are entered correctly, you will see a map like the one in Fig. 7.5.

Comparing to the base map in Fig. 7.3, this rotated figure put China and the West Pacific in the central view, better-showing patterns in this region.

The same approach can be used to rotate the world map to meet your need for research and presentation by altering the parameters in the function "orientation=c(latitude, longitude, rotation)".

7.4.4 An Example with Both Projection and Rotation

After learning how to draw the base map, to project the map with different projection methods and to rotate the map for different research needs, in this section, we present an example on how to do both projection and rotation together. The R codes to perform this function are a combination of the R codes for the three world maps we have learned in the previous sections. The following are a set of R codes to create a map with a rectangular project and a rotation with China being centered in the view:

```
mapbase_op<-
ggplot(data=world_data,mapping=aes(x=long,y=lat, group=group)) +
     coord_fixed(1.5) +
     coord_map(projection="rectangular", parameters=c(lat0=40),
     orientation=c(90,150,0), xlim=c(-180,180),
     ylim=c(-60,90)) +
     geom_polygon(color="black", fill="grey")+
     labs(x="Longitude") +
     labs(y="Latitude") mapbase
```

As in the previous two figures, the R code "projection="rectangular"" was used to specify the project and the "orientation=c(90, 150, 0)" was used to specify the rotation with the same parameter values.

If you do everything correctly, you should see a map as displayed in Fig. 7.6 by typing "mapbase_op" in the script Window and run it.

7.5 Geographic Mapping of the World Population: A Practical Example

In this section, we demonstrate the application of R for geographic mapping using world population and population density data. We start with the mapping of the world population, then move to population density. The purpose is to let you exercise your skills for mapping. After gaining familiarity with this example, you can easily extend the approach to mapping other data you may have.

Data for population and geographic area are from World Bank (World Bank, 2018a, 2018b). The population density was calculated by dividing the total population with the total area for individual countries. Data for a total of 148 countries were included.

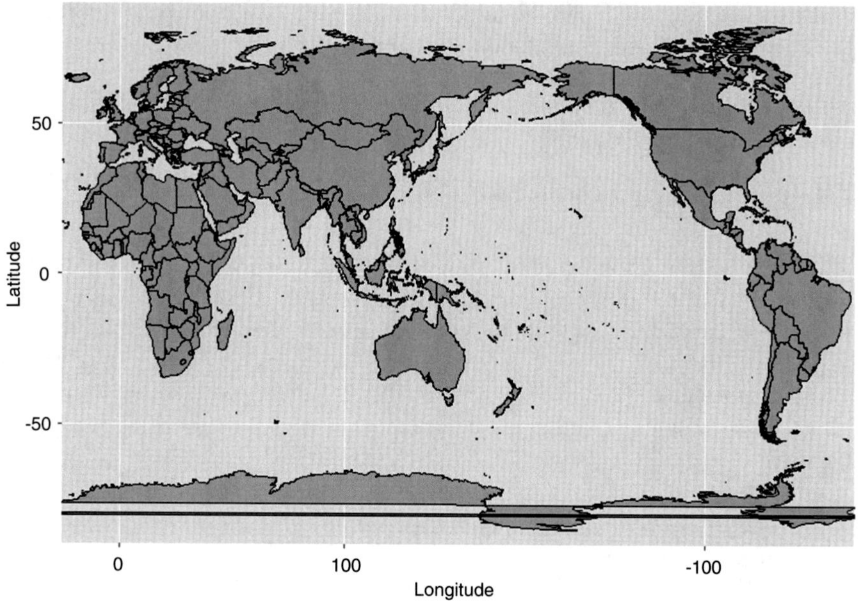

Fig. 7.6 World map with projection and rotation. Note: To better visualize the rotated map, the region of Greenland was excluded

7.5.1 Steps to Map a Subject Matter

With the basic skills described in the previous sections, we are now ready to map contents of interest to address global health issues. From our previous work, we recommend the Eight-Step approach for global mapping:

Step 1: Read data you want to map, such as population, diseases, birth, and death.
Step 2: Read the world map data as described in the previous sections.
Step 3: Merge the two datasets from the previous two steps.
Step 4: Create a base map.
Step 5: Define and select color schemes for mapping.
Step 6: Define the categories (or levels) of the data you want to be mapped.
Step 7: Add the data layer to the base map with the selected color scheme and the categories of the data.
Step 8: View and output of the map.

7.5.2 Data Preparation

To put data into a world map, in addition to the data for the world map previously described, you must prepare and add your data to the dataset for mapping.

Prepare and read in the world population data. Table 7.1 lists part of the data needed for global mapping. You can find these data from the World Bank websites (World Bank, 2018a, 2018b). Put the data in excel format and save it as popdata.csv (the file type csv is one of the most frequently used data types for R, although other data types are possible).

After the dataset is saved on the computer, you can read the data into R for mapping using the following R codes:

```
pop = read.csv("C:/Users/Data/popdata.csv", header = T)
```

This line of R codes tells the computer to read the data file "popdata.csv" saved in the specified location and put the data into "pop", a dataset R can use for mapping. The code "header=T" means the first row of the csv dataset of yours contains the name of all variables.

Please be advised, you must prepare your data by country so that your data can be linked to the countries carried in the dataset for world mapping. You also need to use exact the same name (or standardized codes) for individual countries. You can find such information in https://www.nationsonline.org/oneworld/country_code_list.htm.

You need name the characteristic variable as "region" for countries since this is the variable used in the world map data to identify individual countries.

Read data for the world map. We have already learned this in the previous sections. This is achieved using the following R codes:

```
worldmap <- map_data("world")
```

With this line of codes, it puts all the data for the world map into the dataset "worldmap" for mapping.

Merge the population data with world map data. After completion of the previous two steps and reading in "worldmap" and "pop" data into R, we will create a new dataset named as "worldpop" by merging these two datasets. R is powerful for

Table 7.1 Example dataset used in R in Chap. 8

Region	Population (1000)	Geographic size (km^2)	Population density (No. of people per km^2)
Afghanistan	32,527	652,860	49.82
Algeria	39,667	2,381,741	16.65
Angola	25,022	1,246,700	20.07
Argentina	43,417	2,736,690	15.86
Armenia	3018	28,470	106.01
...	...	...	...
Zimbabwe	15,603	386,850	40.33

merging two datasets. In our example here, you can merge the two datasets using the following R codes:

```
worldpop <- inner_join(worldmap, pop, by = "region")
```

With this line of the R codes, the merged data are stored in the dataset "worldpop". The key R function for data merging is "inner_join()". It asks R to combine the dataset "worldmap" with dataset "pop" by the variable "region". The variable for country names are presented in both the "worldpop" and the "pop" dataset.

7.5.3 Mapping Your Data

It will take several steps to map your data just prepared and merged with the world map data. This is achieved by first creating a base map of the world, then processing your data, creating a data map as a map layer and over laying it on to the base map.

Create the base map. To map your data, you create a blank world map as the base using the R codes described in Sect. 7.4.1. You can change the projection with the R codes described in Sect. 7.4.2; rotate the map using the R codes described in Sect. 7.4.3. In this example, we used rectangular projected map in the Sect. 7.4.2 as the base map.

Select and define color scheme for data mapping. To select and define a color scheme for mapping, we must load the previously installed package "RColor-Brewer" using the following R command:

```
library(RcolorBrewer)
```

This R package contains many color schemes for use. After the package is loaded, you can select the color scheme you like for your map. At the beginning, you may not know which one to use. The best way to find it out is to try by yourself. As an example, we used the following R codes to define a 5-level color scheme:

```
mapcolor <- brewer.pal(5, "YlorRd")
```

The function "brewer.pal()" from the package "RcolorBrewer" tells the computer to select the color scheme for mapping, the parameter 5 asks the computer to use five different colors and the code "YlorRd" asks the computer to draw the colors in five levels from yellow to red.

Define the categories of your data matching with the 5-level color scheme. There are different ways to categorize a variable. In this example, we manually categorize the "pop", population size by country in the dataset. We do this by calling the R function "cut()" to define a new variable "popcat" and add this variable to the merged dataset "worldpop". This is done by reading the population data using the point "worldpop$pop", and use R function "breaks=c()" to divide all countries in the dataset by population size into 5 groups using the specified cutoff values of "c(0, 10000, 35000 . . .)". After a categorical variable is created, label the variable using the function "lables=c()", which will be used later as map legend.

```
worldpop$popcat <- cut(worldpop$pop,
               breaks=c(0,10000,35000,55000,150000,1400000)),
               lables=c("0-10000","10000-35000","35000-55000",
               "55000-150000",">150000"))
```

Create a layer of map for the population data and overlay on to the base map. With the categorized population data described above, we now can create a map of the population size by category and add it to the base map. This can be achieved using the following R codes:

```
world_pop <- mapbase_p +
  geom_polygon(data=worldpop, aes(fill=popcat),color="black") +
  geom_polygon(color="black", fill=NA) +
  scale_fill_manual(values=mapcolor, guide_legend
  (title="Population (1000)", label=TRUE)) +
  theme_bw()+
  theme(legend.key.size=unit(0.5,"cm"),
       legend.text=element_text(size=8),
       legend.title=element_text(size=10),
       legend.position=c(0.04,0.25))+
     ditch_the_axes
```

From the codes above, we can see that we store the map of world population with the file name: world_pop. The map is created by adding (+) the mapbase with the population map to be created using the function "geom_polygon()" and the worldpop data specified by the R codes "data=worldpop". The R codes "aes(fill=popcat)" asks the computer to fill data for individual countries by category using the newly created variable popcat; "color="black"" tells the computer to draw the borders of all countries with black; "scale_fill_manual()" defines the colors and legend for mapping, and the first argument "values=mapcolor" asks the computer to draw the map with the color scheme previously defined in another step.

Lastly, the function "theme_bw()" is used to specify the classic dark-on-light ggplot2 theme. The next function "theme()" is for specifying the legends presented on the map, including the font, size, and position. The map code end with the command "ditch_the_axes" to remove the axes from the map, which is not needed.

Display the mapping result—World population map. Since the created map of the world population is stored in the file "world_pop", it is easy to display the map by simply typing the following R code in the script window, and then run the program.

```
world_pop
```

If you correctly do all the steps following the instruction in the previous sections, you will see a map showing the total population by country in the world as in Fig. 7.7. If cannot obtain a map or the map you get differs from Fig. 7.7, please go back and check your R codes. We recommend that you practice more times with the eight-step approach to gain efficiency.

From the newly created world map, it clearly shows the global pattern of the world population by countries. The world most populous countries are China, India, United States, and Brazil, and the least populous countries include those in West and

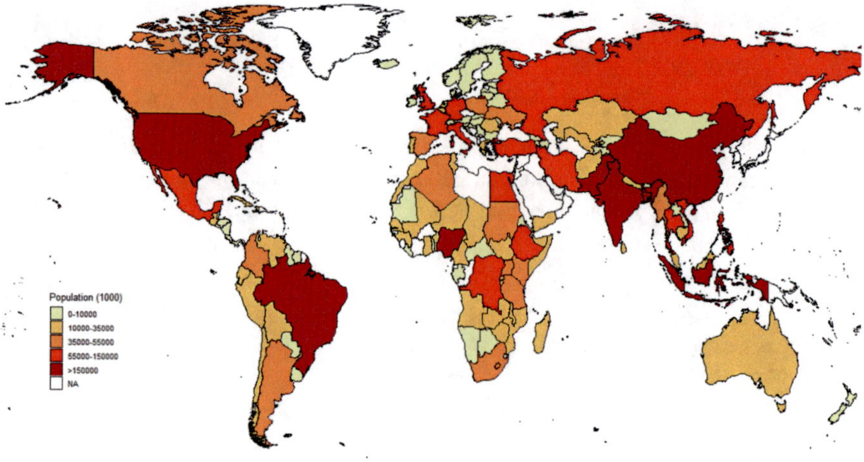

Fig. 7.7 Distribution of the world population by country

South Europe, Mongolia in Asian, a number of small countries scattered in Africa, West Pacific and South America.

7.6 Mapping the Density of World Population by Country

After knowing how to map world population by country, it will be very simple to model population density. What need to be done is to create a new variable for population density and categorize the variable for mapping. The following R codes present an example to create a categorized population density variable:

```
Worldpop$popdstcat <- cut(worldpop$popdensity,
                    breaks=c(0,6,20,50,130,7720)),
                    lables=c("0-6","6-20","20-50","50-130",">130"))
```

The cutoff points are determined based on data. You can determine this using frequency distribution, or use equal-length interval, or exponential intervals.

With the newly created population density variable "popdstcat", the following R codes can be used to generate the map of the density of world population by country as shown in Fig. 7.8.

```
map_popdensity <- mapbase_p +
   geom_polygon(data=worldpop, aes(fill=popdstcat),color
   ="black") +
   geom_polygon(color="black", fill=NA) +
   scale_fill_manual(values=mapcolor, guide_legend
   (title="Population density (per km2)", label=TRUE)) +
   theme_bw()+
   theme(legend.key.size=unit(0.5,"cm"),
```

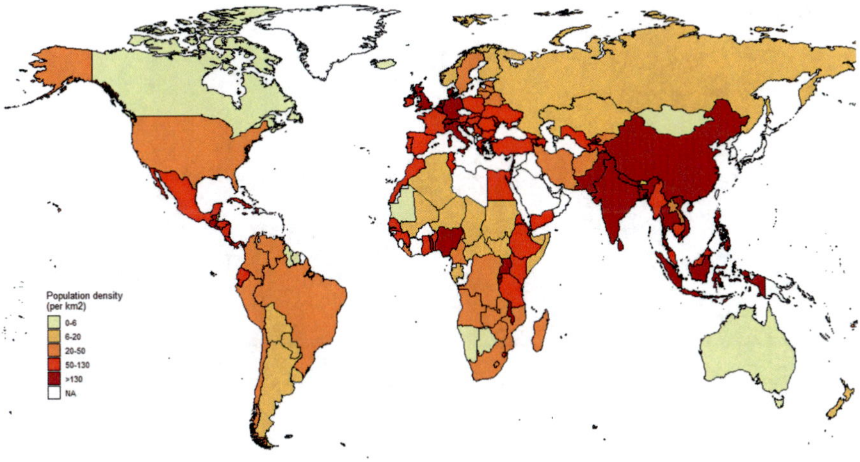

Fig. 7.8 Global pattern of population density by country

```
        legend.text=element_text(size=8),
        legend.title=element_text(size=10),
        legend.position=c(0.04,0.25))+
    ditch_the_axes
map_popdensity
```

Compared to the global pattern of world population by country in Fig. 7.7, population density by countries shows a very different pattern. Countries with high population density appear to form a band stretching from Europe to Asia and South Pacific; while countries with the lowest density are scattered around, including Canada, Australia. Mongolia and several countries in Africa and South America.

7.7 Conclusion Remarks

In this chapter, we focus on introducing the method to map data across the globe. The purpose is to assist researchers with limited training and resources to investigate medical, health and behavior issues with great global significance. By using this mapping technique, you will see the value of global mapping in assisting you to understand and grab global health issues and to establish and use a global perspective in your effort to examine local medical and health issues with global significance, and in decision-making and collective action to deal with global health challenges.

Appendix

```
R version 3.5.3 (2019-03-11)
Platform: x86_64-w64-mingw32/x64 (64-bit)
Running under: Windows >= 8 x64 (build 9200)

Matrix products: default

locale:
[1] LC_COLLATE=English_United States.1252  LC_CTYPE=English_United States.1252    LC_MONETARY=English_United States.1252
[4] LC_NUMERIC=C                           LC_TIME=English_United States.1252

attached base packages:
[1] stats     graphics  grDevices utils     datasets  methods   base

other attached packages:
[1] sqldf_0.4-11       RSQLite_2.1.1      gsubfn_0.7         proto_1.0.0        RColorBrewer_1.1-2 dplyr_0.8.0.1
[7] mapproj_1.2.6      maps_3.3.0         ggplot2_3.1.1

loaded via a namespace (and not attached):
 [1] Rcpp_1.0.1        pillar_1.3.1      compiler_3.5.3    plyr_1.8.4        tools_3.5.3       digest_0.6.18
 [7] bit_1.1-14        memoise_1.1.0     tibble_2.1.1      gtable_0.3.0      pkgconfig_2.0.2   rlang_0.3.4
[13] DBI_1.0.0         rstudioapi_0.10   yaml_2.2.0        withr_2.1.2       bit64_0.9-7       grid_3.5.3
[19] tidyselect_0.2.5  glue_1.3.1        R6_2.4.0          tcltk_3.5.3       purrr_0.3.2       blob_1.1.1
[25] magrittr_1.5      scales_1.0.0      assertthat_0.2.1  colorspace_1.4-1  labeling_0.3      lazyeval_0.2.2
[31] munsell_0.5.0     chron_2.3-53      crayon_1.3.4
```

References

Becker, R. A., & Wilks, A. R. (2018). Package ‘maps’. Retrieved April 18, 2019, from https://cran.r-project.org/web/packages/maps/maps.pdf

Chen, X. (2014). Understanding the development and perception of global health for more effective student education. *The Yale Journal of Biology and Medicine, 87*(3), 231–240.

Chen, X., Elliott, A. L., & Wang, S. (2018). Cross-country Association of Press Freedom and LGBT freedom with prevalence of persons living with HIV: Implication for global strategy against HIV/AIDS. *Global Health Research and Policy, 3*(1), 6. https://doi.org/10.1186/s41256-018-0061-3

Chen, X., & Wang, K. (2017). Geographic area-based rate as a novel indicator to enhance research and precision intervention for more effective HIV/AIDS control. *Preventive Medicine Reports, 5*, 301–307. https://doi.org/10.1016/j.pmedr.2017.01.009

Cochi, S. L., & Dowdle, W. R. (Eds.). (2011). *Disease eradication in the 21st century: Implications for global health*. The MIT Press. https://doi.org/10.7551/mitpress/9780262016735.001.0001

DeLaet, D. L. (2015). *Global health in the 21st century: The globalization of disease and wellness*. Routledge. https://doi.org/10.4324/9781315634425

Elsabbagh, M., Divan, G., Koh, Y.-J., Kim, Y. S., Kauchali, S., Marcín, C., … Fombonne, E. (2012). Global prevalence of autism and other pervasive developmental disorders. *Autism Research: Official Journal of the International Society for Autism Research, 5*(3), 160–179. https://doi.org/10.1002/aur.239

Griffiths, M. D., Kuss, D. J., Billieux, J., & Pontes, H. M. (2016). The evolution of Internet addiction: A global perspective. *Addictive Behaviors, 53*, 193–195. https://doi.org/10.1016/j.addbeh.2015.11.001

Harris, R. E. (Ed.). (2013). *Epidemiology of chronic disease: Global perspectives*. Burlington, MA: Jones & Bartlett Learning.

McIlroy, D. (2018). CRAN—Package mapproj. Retrieved April 18, 2019, from https://cran.r-project.org/web/packages/mapproj/index.html

Morgen, C. S., & Sørensen, T. I. A. (2014). Obesity: Global trends in the prevalence of overweight and obesity. *Nature Reviews Endocrinology, 10*(9), 513–514. https://doi.org/10.1038/nrendo.2014.124

Murray, C. J. L., Ortblad, K. F., Guinovart, C., Lim, S. S., Wolock, T. M., Roberts, D. A., … Brown, J. C. (2014). Global, regional, and national incidence and mortality for HIV, tuberculosis, and malaria during 1990-2013: A systematic analysis for the Global Burden of Disease Study 2013. *The Lancet, 384*(9947), 1005–1070. https://doi.org/10.1016/S0140-6736(14)60844-8

Neuwirth, E. (2014). ColorBrewer Palettes [R package RColorBrewer version 1.1-2]. Retrieved April 18, 2019, from https://cran.r-project.org/web/packages/RColorBrewer/index.html

Olson, D. M., Dinerstein, E., Wikramanayake, E. D., Burgess, N. D., Powell, G. V. N., Underwood, E. C., ... Kassem, K. R. (2001). Terrestrial ecoregions of the world: A new map of life on earth. *Bioscience, 51*(11), 933. https://doi.org/10.1641/0006-3568(2001)051[0933:TEOTWA]2.0.CO;2

Omran, A. R. (1971). The epidemiologic transition: A theory of the epidemiology of population change. *The Milbank Memorial Fund Quarterly, 49*(4), 509. https://doi.org/10.2307/3349375

R Core Team. (2013). *R: A language and environment for statistical computing*. Vienna, Austria: R Foundation for Statistical Computing.

The R Foundation. (2018). R: The R project for statistical computing. Retrieved December 25, 2018, from https://www.r-project.org/

Whiteford, H. A., Ferrari, A. J., Degenhardt, L., Feigin, V., & Vos, T. (2015). The global burden of mental, neurological and substance use disorders: An analysis from the Global Burden of Disease Study 2010. *PLoS One, 10*(2), e0116820. https://doi.org/10.1371/journal.pone.0116820

Wickham, H., Chang, W., Henry, L., Pedersen, T. L., Takahashi, K., Wilke, C., ... RStudio. (2019). ggplots: Create elegant data visualisations using the grammar of graphics [R package ggplot2 version 3.1.1]. Retrieved April 18, 2019, from https://cran.r-project.org/web/packages/ggplot2/index.html

Wickham, H., François, R., Henry, L., & Müller, K. (2019). Package "dplyr". Retrieved April 18, 2019, from https://cran.r-project.org/web/packages/dplyr/dplyr.pdf

World Bank. (2018a). *Land area (sq. km)*. Retrieved December 26, 2018, from https://data.worldbank.org/indicator/AG.LND.TOTL.K2

World Bank. (2018b). *Population, total*. Retrieved December 25, 2018, from https://data.worldbank.org/indicator/SP.POP.TOTL

Chapter 8
A 4D Indicator System of Count, P Rate, G Rate and PG Rate for Epidemiology and Global Health

Xinguang Chen, Bin Yu, and (Din) Ding-Geng Chen

Abstract How to end the HIV/AIDS epidemic is a typical global health question since the impact of HIV/AIDS is global and it cannot be ended without collaborative global effort. In this chapter, a new measurement system is introduced to inform HIV/AIDS control cross the globe. All countries with data available on area size, total population and total number of persons living with HIV (PLWH) were included, yielding a sample of 148 countries. Four indicators, including the *total count*, population-based *p rate*, geographic area-based *g rate* and population and geographic area-based *pg rate* were used as a 4D system to describe the global HIV epidemic. The total PLWH count provided data informing resource allocation for individual countries to improve HIV/AIDS care; and the top five countries with highest PLWH count were South Africa, Nigeria, India, Kenya, and Mozambique. Information from the remaining three indicators provided a global risk profile of the HIV epidemic, supporting HIV/AIDS prevention programming strategies. Five countries with highest p rates were Swaziland, Botswana, Lesotho, South Africa, and Zimbabwe; five countries with highest g rates were Swaziland, Malawi, Lesotho, Rwanda, and Uganda; and five countries with highest pg rates were

The original version of this chapter was revised: An appendix has been added at the end of this chapter and page numbers in the subsequent chapters were corrected. The correction to this chapter is available at https://doi.org/10.1007/978-3-030-35260-8_17

X. Chen
Department of Epidemiology, College of Public Health and Health Professions, College of Medicine, University of Florida, Gainesville, FL, USA

Global Health Institute, Wuhan University, Wuhan, China
e-mail: jimax.chen@ufl.edu

B. Yu
Department of Epidemiology, University of Florida, Gainesville, FL, USA
e-mail: byu@ufl.edu

(Din) D.-G. Chen
School of Social Work, University of North Carolina, Chapel Hill, NC, USA
e-mail: dinchen@email.unc.edu

X. Chen, (Din) D.-G. Chen (eds.), *Statistical Methods for Global Health and Epidemiology*, ICSA Book Series in Statistics,
https://doi.org/10.1007/978-3-030-35260-8_8

Barbados, Swaziland, Lesotho, Malta, and Mauritius. According to pg rates, two HIV hotspots (south and middle Africa and Caribbean region) and one HIV belt across Euro-Asian were identified. In addition to HIV/AIDS, the 4D measurement system can be used to describe morbidity and mortality for many diseases across the globe. We recommend the use of this measurement system in research to address significant global health and epidemiologic issues.

Keywords Global health research · HIV/AIDS epidemic · Geographic area-based g rate · Geographic and population-based pg rate · Global mapping

8.1 Introduction

One fundamental task for epidemiology, particularly global health epidemiology is to provide good tools to extract information from data for accurate understanding of the level, risk factors of a disease and its impact on population health (Rothman, Greenland, & Lash, 2008; Szklo & Nieto, 2018). In addition to the disease epidemiology, such information is essential for public health planning and strategic decision-making, prevention intervention programming and program evaluation (Bayer & Galea, 2015; Chen & Wang, 2017; Khoury, Iademarco, & Riley, 2016). Since the beginning of epidemiology and public health, two indicators most commonly used in research have been (1) the total count that informs us about the total number of persons who suffer from or died of a disease; and (2) rate that reflects the risk of a person suffering from or being died of a disease.

During early stages when a disease has just started to appear, the number of new cases is counted periodical (i.e., daily, weekly, or monthly); the counts are then accumulated to show the progress of the disease epidemic in a population, such as SARS (Wikipedia, 2019), Ebola (Meltzer et al., 2014), and bird flu (Ferguson, Fraser, Donnelly, Ghani, & Anderson, 2004) as being commonly practiced today. When a disease becomes an epidemic and lasts for long time to affect more and more people in a population, annual count of persons who suffered from or died of the disease is used to monitor the epidemic, such as the number of persons living with HIV/AIDS or died from AIDS each years (WHO, 2018). In vital statistics, the number of persons suffered from or died of different causes of diseases is documented on an annual or biannual basis as shown in many statistical yearbooks.

The headcount of a disease as an epidemiologic measure provides information very useful for decision-making at the population level. It is the basic data used in planning and decision-making to allocate resource for disease treatment and prevention (Bautista-Arredondo, Gadsden, Harris, & Bertozzi, 2008). For example, if a total of 1200 persons are diagnosed with cancer. Assuming that the government expenditure for treating one cancer patient per year on average is \$15,000, a total of \$18 million ($\$15{,}000 _* 1200$) every year must be allocated in the country's budget for treating all the cancer patients. In the United States, the Centers for Disease Control and Prevention uses this method to plan its Healthy People 2030 for resource allocation for all public health programs, and more details can be found at the URL: https://www.healthypeople.gov/.

Despite the usefulness, information provided by headcount is inadequate for measuring and comparing risks of a disease across regions and jurisdictions with a country and across countries in the world. This is because given the same level of likelihood for a disease to spread, the head count of a disease will differ for countries and regions with different population sizes. A country or region with a larger population will have more people at risk of suffering from a disease than a country or region with a smaller population given the same risk level. Epidemiologists have overcome the limitation of headcount data by using the indicator rate. Methodologically, a rate is a measure that adjusts the impact of population size in assessing disease risk (Chen, 2017; Chen & Wang, 2017). Disease rates therefore provide a measure more informative than disease count for comparison across regions within a country, and across countries in the world.

The two epidemiologic indicators, headcount and disease rate described above have been used almost everywhere from research to practice, including the World Health Organization, governmental and nongovernmental agencies; researchers and students in institutes and universities; and public health workers in communities and neighborhoods. While appreciating the value and utility of the two epidemiologic indicators, we cannot overlook their limitations. Although measures of disease rate are more informative than measures of headcount with regard to informing levels of risk of a disease at the population level, both headcount and disease rate cannot address another key factor–the size of geographic areas people reside (Chen, 2017; Chen & Wang, 2017). To fill in this methodology gap, in this chapter, we will introduce a new measurement system by incorporating geographic area size into measurement. We illustrate the new measurement system using the global HIV epidemic as an example.

8.2 Ending the HIV/AIDS Epidemic by 2030

The epidemic of the human immunodeficiency virus (HIV) and the acquired immunodeficiency syndrome (AIDS) is a typical global health problem (Chen, 2014; Merson, Black, & Mills, 2012). Worldwide, the number of persons living with HIV (PLWH) has totaled 36.9 million (WHO, 2018). The impact of HIV/AIDS on human health is global; therefore, effective HIV/AIDS control and prevention requires collaborative and global efforts (Deeks et al., 2016; International Aids Society Scientific Working Group on H I V Cure et al., 2012). No one individual country is immune to HIV infection and no one individual country alone can get rid of the HIV epidemic without involving other countries and agencies in the world.

In fighting the HIV/AIDS epidemic, two strategies are widely used: (1) Antiretroviral therapy (ART) and (2) prevention intervention programs. The first strategy is designated for treating persons living with HIV (PLWH) whose viral load has not been suppressed and this strategies has been widely implemented across the globe (Tanser, Barnighausen, Grapsa, Zaidi, & Newell, 2013; UNAIDS, 2017a). In addition to treading the infected, appropriate implementation of ART, such as treatment as prevention (TasP) can help PLWH to achieve viral suppression, reducing the number of infected persons who can infect others (Cohen, 2011; Granich et al., 2010).

The second strategy of prevention is for all persons who are at risk for HIV infection, including the PLWH who can be re-infected (Lyles et al., 2007). These programs include school- or community-based interventions for general population and venue-based high-risk population intervention (e.g., drug users, men who have sex with men, sex workers). To develop and implant either an ART program or a prevention intervention strategy, adequate data are always needed for strategic planning, evidence-based decision-making, and objective program evaluation (Courtenay-Quirk, Spindler, Leidich, & Bachanas, 2016; H. I. V. Modelling Consortium Treatment as Prevention Editorial Writing Group, 2012; Marsh & Farrell, 2015).

Based on the epidemic of HIV/AIDS and success in treatment and prevention, the Jointed United Nations Program on HIV/AIDS sets the goal to End the AIDS Epidemic by 2030 (UNAIDS, 2014b). To achieve the goal, the UNAIDS further asked that by 2020, 90% of PLWH know their HIV status, 90% of diagnosed PLWH receive sustained ART and 90% who receive ART have their blood viral load suppressed (90-90-90 strategy) (UNAIDS, 2017a). Pursuing these goals requires collaborative efforts to plan and deliver patient-centered ART and population-centered (both the general and at-risk population) prevention programs to reduce the risk of HIV transmission by all possible venues, including sexual contact, needle sharing and vertical maternal-child transition (AVERT, 2017; CDC, 2018b; National Health and Family Planning Commission of PRC, 2015; WHO, 2017).

8.3 Four-Dimensional Measurement System

8.3.1 Two Conventional Measure of Headcount and P Rate

From a precision public health perspective (Chen & Wang, 2017; Khoury et al., 2016), relevant and sufficient information is essential to plan and implement HIV/AIDS treatment and prevention strategies to achieve the goal of ending the HIV/AIDS epidemic by 2030. For example, the number of PLWH by country is needed for resource allocation to achieve the 90-90-90 proposed by UNAIDS. If it costs on average $1000 to treat one PLWH per year, a total of $39 billion will be needed to treat all the 39 million PLWH in the world. There were 850,000 PLWH in China in 2015, which meant China needs $850 million per year to treat these infected persons.

Despite great significance, information conveyed by the number of PLWH for individual countries provides limited information about between-country differences in the risk of HIV transition because of population size (Chen, 2017; Chen & Wang, 2017). In addition to risk factors, the total number of PLWH in a country is directly related to the population size. For example, in 2015, there were 850,000 PLWH in China and 830,000 in Brazil (see Appendix to this chapter for detailed data). If larger number of PLWH meant higher risk of HIV transmission, people in China may face a higher risk than people in Brazil. However, the population of Brazil was 208 million, only about 15% of 1.4 billion, the total population in China. We cannot determine whether the risk of HIV transmission is higher in China or in Brazil using only the measure of total headcount of PLWH.

To more accurately assess the risk of HIV transition, a population-based measure has devised by dividing the number of PLWH with total population. In our 4D measurement system, this population-based measure is termed as *p rate* (Chen & Wang, 2017). Epidemiologically, a p rate is more accurate than a headcount to assess between-country differences in risk of HIV transmission because it quantitatively adjusts the differences in population sizes. Following the same example in the previous paragraph, the p rate for Brazil was 3.993/1000 population, 6.4 times higher than 0.630/1000, the p rate for China. Therefore, based on the p rates, we can conclude that the risk of HIV transmission is 6.4 times higher in Brazil than in China.

8.3.2 Two New Measures of G Rate and P Rate

P rate has been one of the most commonly used measures in epidemiology and global health. Despite its advantage in controlling for population size, p rates for different countries are confounded by the geographic area size of a country. Again using PLWH as examples: the total number of PLWH in 2015 was about 220,000 in two countries: Swaziland and Mexico; however, the total area was 172,000 km^2 for Swaziland, much smaller than 19,440,000 km^2, the geographic area size of Mexico. If people from the two countries reside on a same size of a geographic area (say, like Swaziland), the risk of HIV transmission would be 113 times (19,440,000/172,000) higher in Swaziland than in Mexico. To consider difference in geographic area size like the p rate for population size, *a new and geographic area-based measure has been developed and named as g rate* (Chen, 2017; Chen & Wang, 2017).

G rate of a country/place was defined as the ratio of total events over the total geographic area size of the country/place. G rate can be defined for many medical and health events. For example, g rate can be defined and estimated for new infections of a disease to evaluate the risk of disease transmission; g rate can also be defined and estimated for total deaths by country to assess risk of mortality; and certainly g rate can be used to measure PLWH and compare between-country differences in the risk of HIV transmission. While a p rate provides a measure that has epidemiologically adjusted the confounding from different population sizes; a g rate provides another measure that has epidemiologically controlled the confounding from the different geographic area sizes. With a g rate, the significance of geographic areas in disease epidemiology (Sattenspiel, 2009) can be assessed quantitatively.

Inspired by p rate and g rate, a natural extension would be to consider both population size and geographic area to assess the morbidity and mortality of any health conditions. It is based on this line of thought, another new measurement – pg rate has been developed (Chen & Wang, 2017). As the name suggests, a pg rate of a health event for a country is defined as the ratio of total count of the event over both the total population and the total geographic area of the country. Since the confounding effect from both population and geographic areas are adjusted, pg rate provides a measure better than p rate and g rate alone to assess the epidemiology of any medical and health event across countries in the world.

The four epidemiological measures of headcount, p rate, g rate and pg rate consist of a new 4D measurement system. This 4D assessment system extends the conventional measures and can be used in assessing many medical and health conditions to advance both research and practice in global health and epidemiology.

8.4 An Example of Global HIV Epidemic

To demonstrate the 4D measurement System and its application, we analyzed data for PLWH in 2015. The method can be used for study any other diseases.

8.4.1 Materials and Method

Persons living with HIV (PLWH). These data were limited to 2015 and were derived from multi-sources, including the UNAIDS, government websites and different governmental reports. Data for a total of 148 countries with data available on PLWH were included. Of these countries, data for 107 countries were derived from the UNAIDS, and three from the government report or HIV/AIDS data hub, including the United Kingdom, China and Laos (UNAIDS, 2016, 2017b). For the remaining countries with no data in 2015, data for most closed years were used. For example, 2014 data were used for Canada, Fiji, Montenegro, Netherlands, New Zealand, and Singapore were derived from the Progress Report by Country (UNAIDS, 2014a); 2014 data for Estonia were derived from the Evaluation Report of the World Health Organization (WHO Regional Office for Europe, 2014); data for the United States in 2013 were from the Centers for Diseases Control and Prevention (CDC, 2018a); and data for Guinea-Bissau in 2012 were derived from the UNICEF (UNICEF, 2013).

Geographic area size by country. Data for the size of geographic area (km^2) of individual countries are extracted from the World Bank Data Depot (World Bank, 2015a). This is a great official source of geographic data for countries in the world, and has been globally accepted. Data from this source are also widely used in statistical analysis and visualization to address global issues (Redding & Venables, 2004).

Population data by country. The population data by country were also derived from the World Bank Data Depot (World Bank, 2015b). The data stored are compiled by the United Nations Population Division, and the population data in this source are based on multi-official sources, including census reports and other statistical publications, the population and vital statistic report by census bureau of various countries in the world.

8.4.2 Estimation of P Rate, G Rate and PG Rate

P rate, g rate and pg rate for the 148 countries included in this example were computed respectively using the following three equations:

$$p\ rate = \frac{N}{P}\ \text{(per 1000 population)} \tag{8.1}$$

$$g\ rate = \frac{N}{A}\left(\text{per 100 km}^2\right) \tag{8.2}$$

$$pg\ rate = \frac{N}{P \times A}\left(\text{per million population} \cdot 100\ \text{km}^2\right) \tag{8.3}$$

Where N represents the number of PLWH, P represents the number of population, and A represents geographic area size.

The total population and geographic area, the total counts of PLWH, and the calculated p rates, g rates, and pg rates for individual countries were included in Appendix.

8.4.3 Geographic Mapping

The four epidemiologic indicators by country each were mapped globally, including the headcount of PLWH, and the calculated p rates, g rates and pg rates using the software R. Three R packages for mapping were used, including the "maps", "mapproj" and "ggplot2". A dataset "worlddata" was thus created by extracting geographic information of individual countries (country name, longitude, latitude) from the "maps" and merged with the derived data of the population size, geographic area, count of PLWH, calculated p rate, g rate and pg rate by country.

After data preparation, we created a world map using the dataset "worlddata". Following the National Standard Map Services, we used the "ggplot2" with "rectangular" option and orientation (latitude = 90, longitude = 150, rotation = 0) and "mapproj" to create the world map. A color scale was used to represent different levels of each PLWH indicators by *five* percentiles. Greenland located in the far north was not included in the mapping because of the lack of HIV data. R codes for the geographic mapping are available from the author Bin Yu upon request.

8.5 Results

With data from the 148 countries included in this analysis, worldwide an estimate of 35,426,911 persons who were infected and lived with the virus at the time around 2015. The global prevalence rate was 0.51 PLWH per 1000 population.

8.5.1 The Global HIV Epidemic Measured by Headcounts of PLWH

Table 8.1 lists the 15 countries with the largest number of PLWH. Of these 15 countries, the top five were South Africa, Nigeria, India, Kenya and Mozambique with a total of 15,600,000 PLWH, accounting for 44% of that of the total 148 countries included in the analysis.

Figure 8.1 presents the total counts of PLWH by country. Countries with the largest number of PLWH (dark-red) were located, from left to right, in south and middle Africa, Ukraine, India, China and most other Southeast Asian countries, the United States, and Brazil. Overall, the number of PLWH in these countries ranged from 200,000 to 7000,000.

The total number of PLWH provides the information needed for estimating ART cost. One research in South Africa estimates that it costs $119 to maintain ART per

Table 8.1 Top 15 countries with the largest number of persons living with HIV (PLWH) in the world, 2013–2015

Name of the country	Continent	PLWH (in 1000)	Rank
South Africa	Africa	7000	1
Nigeria	Africa	3500	2
India	Asia	2100	3
Kenya	Africa	1500	4
Mozambique	Africa	1500	5
Uganda	Africa	1500	6
Tanzania	Africa	1400	7
Zimbabwe	Africa	1400	8
USA	North America	1242	9
Zambia	Africa	1200	10
Malawi	Africa	980	11
China	Asia	850	12
Brazil	South America	830	13
Ethiopia	Africa	794	14
Indonesia	Asia	690	15
World total	–	35,427	–

PLWH Persons living with HIV

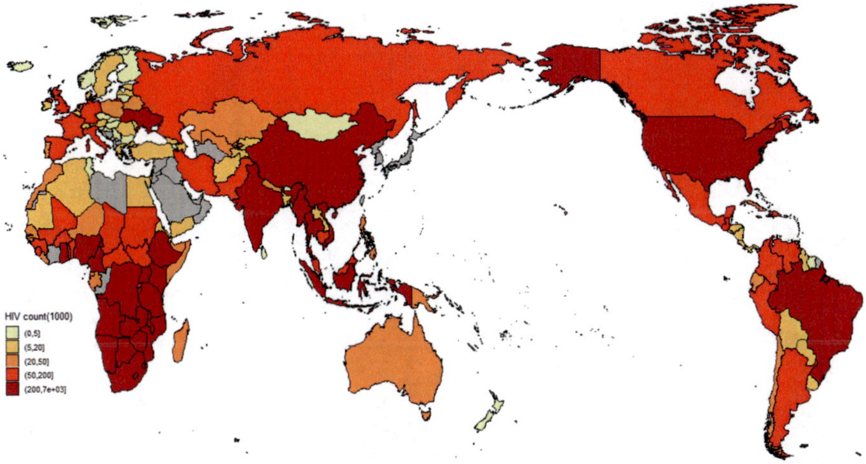

Fig. 8.1 The Global HIV epidemic measured by headcount of PLWH (1000), 2013–2015. Note: *Grey area* data not available

patient per month (Martinson et al., 2009). With this data, for treating one million of PLWH, it will cost $1.44 billion per year to cover the ART cost alone. It is estimated that there are 7000,000 PLWH in South Africa. To provide ART to them, it will cost the country approximately $1 trillion per year. To provide ART for the total 35.4 million of PLWH in the 148 countries, a total of $5+ trillion per year is needed. HIV is by far the one of most expensive diseases (Alistar, Owens, & Brandeau, 2011; CDC, 2017; Martinson et al., 2009).

8.5.2 The Global HIV Epidemic Measured by P Rates of PLWH

There were large variations in the population among the 148 countries varying from 284,000 for Barbados to 1.37 billion in China. The three countries with the smallest populations were Barbados (284,000), Iceland (319,000) and Belize (359,000); and the three countries with largest population were the United States (0.32 billion), India (1.31 billion) and China (1.37 billion). P rate provides a method to consider these between-country differences in population size for comparisons of the HIV epidemic among countries in the globe.

The 15 countries with highest p rates per 1000 population are listed in Table 8.2. Results in the table indicate that all the 15 countries were located in Africa, and with the total five being Swaziland (170.9/1000), Botswana (154.7/1000), Lesotho (145.2/1000), South Africa (127.4/1000) and Zimbabwe (89.7/1000). The p rate for Swaziland was 33.5 times the average rate of 5.1/1000 for the 148 countries.

Table 8.2 Top 15 countries with the highest p rates of PLWH, 2013–2015

Name of the country	Continent	P rate (PLWH/1000)	Rank
Swaziland	Africa	170.9	1
Botswana	Africa	154.7	2
Lesotho	Africa	145.2	3
South Africa	Africa	127.4	4
Zimbabwe	Africa	89.7	5
Namibia	Africa	85.4	6
Zambia	Africa	74.0	7
Malawi	Africa	56.9	8
Mozambique	Africa	53.6	9
Uganda	Africa	38.4	10
Kenya	Africa	32.6	11
Equatorial Guinea	Africa	32.0	12
Gabon	Africa	27.2	13
Cameroon	Africa	26.6	14
Tanzania	Africa	26.2	15
Worldwide	–	5.11	–

PLWH Persons living with HIV

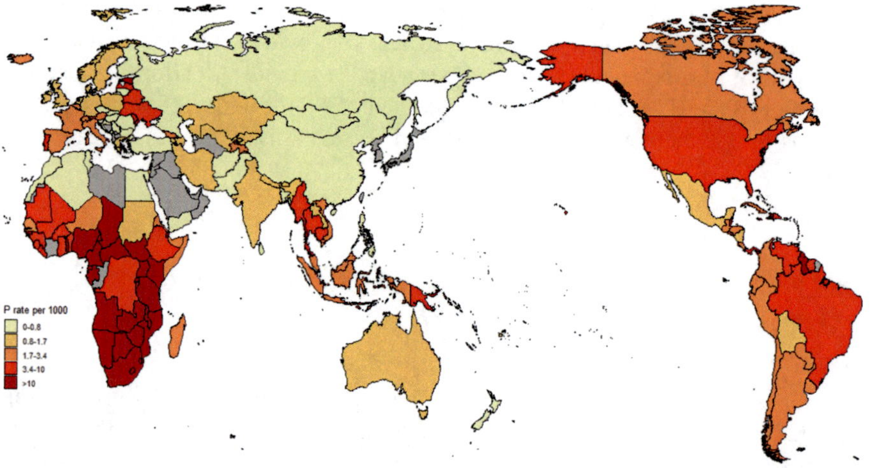

Fig. 8.2 The Global HIV epidemic measured by p rates of PLWH (per 1000 population), 2013–2015. Note: *Grey area* data not available

Figure 8.2 presents the p rate mapping of the global HIV epidemic with population size being adjusted. Thus, the map in this figure provides better data than that Fig. 8.1 (headcount) on the risk of HIV epidemic for cross-country comparison. Compared to Fig. 8.1, the first and most striking difference was that several countries with large population and top headcounts of PLWH were no longer on the top list, such as Brazil, China, India, Mexico, Russia, and USA.

Second, most African countries with highest headcounts of PLWH remained the highest with p rates (dark-red). This result suggests the risk of HIV transmission remained high in these countries after considering the population size. Interestingly, two from the lower PLWH-headcount countries moved to the 20% countries with highest p rates (dark-red): Guyana in South America and Estonia in East Europe. These two countries were rather small with regard to population size but the headcounts of PLWH were higher (see Appendix), resulting in high p rates.

By examining the results in Figs. 8.1 and 8.2 and Table 8.1 together, it can be seen first that a country with high PLWH count may not necessarily be the country with high risk of HIV transmission such as Brazil, China, India, Mexico, Russia, and USA. This is because the high counts of PLWH in these countries were primarily due to the large number of populations.

Second, countries with both high PLWH headcounts and high p rates have high risk of HIV transmission, such as most of the African countries with high ranks of both PLWH headcounts and p rates. With more total PLWH and PLWH per 1000 population in these countries, higher risk of HIV spreading is anticipated.

Last, people living in countries with high p rates are at high risk for HIV transmission regardless of PLWH headcounts, such as Guyana and Estonia.

8.5.3 The Global HIV Epidemic Measured by G Rates of PLWH

The size of geographic area of the 148 countries also varied dramatically from the smallest of 320 km^2 for Malta to the largest of 163,769,000 km^2 for Russia. The total area of the three smallest countries (Malta, Barbados and Singapore) accounted for only 0.001% of the world total; while the total are of the three largest countries (Russia, China and USA) accounts for 28%. Like the p rate for population, g rate provides a measure to gauge the HIV epidemic by adjusting these differences in geographic sizes for cross-country comparisons. This is one of the two new indicators we introduced in this chapter.

The world average and top 15 countries with highest g rates are listed in Table 8.3. The estimated g rate for Swaziland was 1279.1 PLWH/100km^2, 44.4 times that of the world average of 28.8. Of the top five countries, three with g rates greater than 1000 PLWH per unit geographic area of 10×10 km^2.

Figure 8.3 depicts the global HIV epidemic using the estimated g rates of PLWH. Similar to Fig. 8.2, the top 20% countries with highest g rates were colored in dark-red; and these countries were roughly located in three regions of the world. (1) Africa: including a strip of countries from Kenya in the north to South Africa in the south and a small group of countries in the East Africa (Nigeria, Equatorial Guinea, and Cameron); (2) several countries in Southeast Asia (Singapore, Thailand and Vietnam); and (3) several other countries in Caribbean (Costa Rica, Dominican, Hatti and Jamaica).

Table 8.3 Top 15 countries with the highest g rates of PLWH, 2013–2015

Name of the country	Continent	G rate (PLWH/100 km^2)	Rank
Swaziland	Africa	1279.1	1
Malawi	Africa	1039.5	2
Lesotho	Africa	1021.1	3
Rwanda	Africa	810.7	4
Uganda	Africa	748.1	5
Singapore	Asia	697.9	6
Barbados	Africa	604.7	7
South Africa	Africa	577.0	8
Haiti	Africa	471.7	9
Mauritius	Africa	403.9	10
Nigeria	Africa	384.3	11
Zimbabwe	Africa	361.9	12
Burundi	Africa	299.8	13
Jamaica	Gulf of Mexico	267.8	14
Kenya	Africa	263.6	15
Worldwide	–	28.8	–

PLWH Persons living with HIV

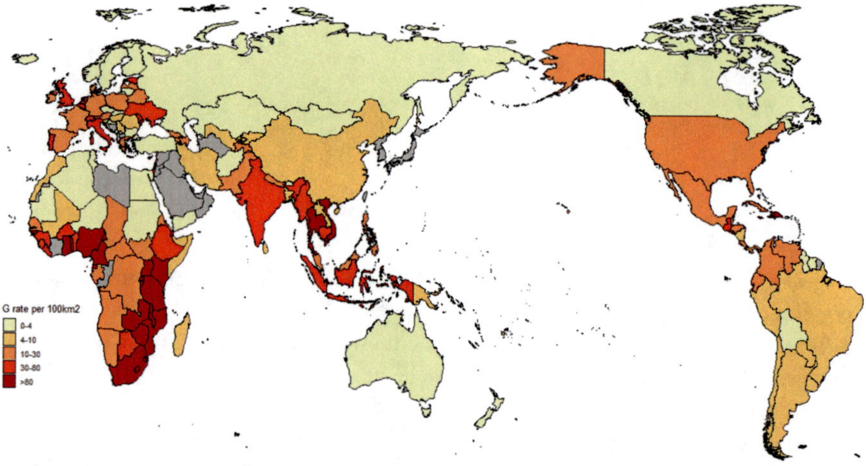

Fig. 8.3 The Global HIV epidemic measured by g rates (PLWH/per 100 km^2). Note: *Grey area* data not available

As expected, g rates were lower for countries with large area sizes even if its PLWH headcount was high, such as Brazil, Canada, China, Russian, and the United States. Given the same area size, higher g rate in a country indicates high risk of HIV transmission because of short distance for personal contact while lower g rate indicates low risk of HIV transmission because of long distance for personal contact.

Table 8.4 Top 15 countries with the highest pg rates of PLWH (per million population per 100 km^2), 2013–2015

Name of the country	Continent	PG rate (/million pop. 100 km^2)	Rank
Barbados	Africa	2127.9	1
Swaziland	Africa	993.8	2
Lesotho	Africa	478.3	3
Malta	Africa	375.0	4
Mauritius	Africa	319.7	5
Bahamas	Caribbean	208.6	6
Trinidad and Tobago	Africa	157.7	7
Cape Verde	Africa	152.6	8
Singapore	Asia	126.9	9
Equatorial Guinea	Africa	113.9	10
Gambia	Africa	104.2	11
Jamaica	Caribbean	98.3	12
Guinea-Bissau	Africa	85.0	13
Luxembourg	Europe	74.5	14
Rwanda	Africa	69.8	15
Worldwide	n/a	0.005	n/a

PLWH Persons living with HIV

More details about individual countries can be found in Appendix to the end of this chapter.

8.5.4 *The Global HIV Epidemic Measured by PG Rates of PLWH*

PG rate is the second new indicator we introduced in this chapter to simultaneously adjust both population size and geographic area. For example, in Fig. 8.3, the United States was categorized into the top 40% countries with the risk of HIV spreading similar to many Caribbean countries, which may not be true, because population size was much large for the United States than for any Caribbean countries. The estimated pg rate indicated that worldwide, there were 0.005 PLWH/million population/100 km^2.

As usual, Table 8.4 lists the top 15 countries with highest pg rates. Barbados was now the country with the highest pg rate in the world with 2127.9 PLWH per million population per 100 km^2. This rate was 425,580 times that of the world average and 30 times that of Rwanda, the last one among the top 15. It was not surprise to see this result because of the small area of Rwanda (24,700 km^2) and population (11,610,000) and a large number of PLWH (an estimate of 200,000).

The global HIV epidemic depicted using pg rates is presented in Fig. 8.4. Results from this figure add addition data better than the headcount, p rate and g rate alone

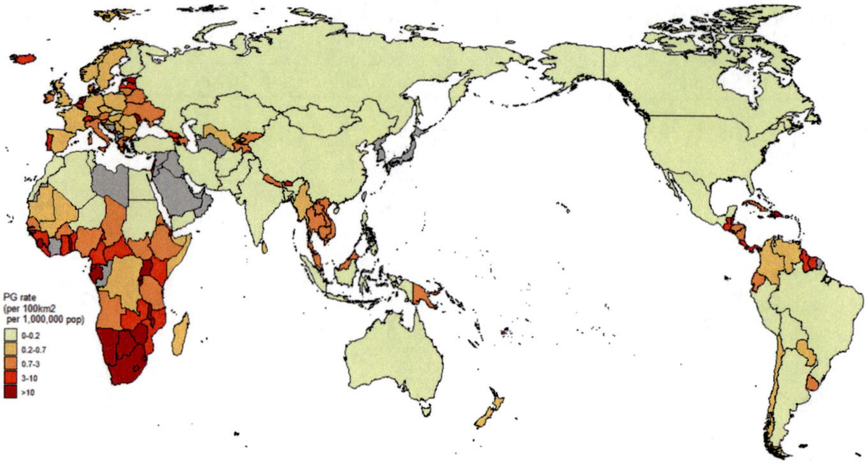

Fig. 8.4 The Global HIV/AIDS epidemic measured by pg rates of PLWH (per million persons per 100 km^2). Note: *Grey area* data not available

to reflect the global pattern of the risk for HIV transmission. Based on the top 40% (colored as dark and light red) with highest pg rates, countries with high threat of HIV epidemic were distributed along with One HIV Hot-Belt and Two HIV Hotspots.

The HIV Hot Belt: This belt comprises a list of countries scattered in a band region, the belt starts with Iceland on the top left of the world map, moves across the Euro-Asian, and ends at Papua New Guinea on the bottom right of the map. Other countries on this HIV Hot Belt region were Estonia, Latvia, Netherlands, Belgium, Luxembourg, Switzerland, Montenegro, Portugal, Moldova, Georgia, Armenia, Azerbaijan, Uzbekistan, Kyrgyzstan, Tajikistan, Nepal, Bhutan, Myanmar, Vietnam, Thailand, Laos, Cambodia, Malaysia, and Singapore.

The HIV Hotspot 1-Africa: These hotspot comprises all countries in South and Middle Africa except Congo (DRC), Angola, and Tanzania. The majority of these countries was also considered as the places where HIV affects people the most using other three measures.

The HIF Hotspot 2-Caribbean: Countries in this hotspot were The Bahamas, Barbados, Belize, Colombia, Costa Rica, Cuba, Dominican Republic, Ecuador, El Salvador, Guatemala, Guyana, Hatti, Honduras, Jamaica, Nicaragua, Panama, Trinidad and Tobago, Suriname, Venezuela.

8.6 Discussion and Conclusion Remarks

In this study, we took a 4D measurement system to describe the global HIV epidemic by adding two newly reported indicators of g rate and pg rate (Chen, 2017; Chen &

Wang, 2017), together with two conventionally used indicators of headcount and p rate. The count and p rate are widely used in research; and the g rate and pg rate add new information, forming a four-dimensional measurement system. We illustrated the utility of the 4D measurement system using HIV data from 148 countries in the world HIV epidemic.

The data about the number of PLWH confirm the conclusion from other studies that it will cost the world a big fortune to end the AIDS epidemic. Providing ART alone for 90% of 36.9 million PLWH in the world will cost \$4.7 trillion per year, based on the estimated cost of \$119 per month for ART in S. African. The estimated lifetime ART cost is \$367,134 per PLWH in the United States (CDC, 2017), which means \$1357 trillion, ~17 times of \$80 trillion, annul GDP produced by all countries in the world. Of the 148 countries included in this study, financial burden will be the greatest for those with highest counts of PLWH, including South African (seven million), Nigeria (3.5million), and India (2.1 million).

Like the p rate to adjust for population size, g rate provides a measure of HIV risk without the influence of the size of a country's geographic area. High g rates suggest greater potentials for close contact between the HIV infected and uninfected persons. Therefore, given the same headcount and p rate, risk of HIV spreading will be higher in countries with high g rates. Singapore provides a best example. This country would be low at HIV transmission if the total number of PLWH (only 4900) and p rate (0.894/1000) were used; however, it became a high-risk country and ranked number 6 in the world when assessed using g rate (126.1 per 1000,000 population per 100 km^2).

On the contrary, g rates will be small for countries with large land area, such as Russia, Canada, Australia, Brazil, the United States and China. Given the same number of PLWH and the same p rate, the risk will be lower for HIV transmission in countries with smaller g rate since small g rate means longer distances for interpersonal contacts. This is consistent with the rural-urban differences in the HIV epidemic with more infections and quicker growths in urban areas where people crowd together than in rural areas where people reside sparsely (Mnyika et al., 1994). Data generated using g rates of PLWH provide direct evidence supporting the role of geographic area in disease epidemiology in general (Sattenspiel, 2009).

Another innovation is the use of pg rate controlling for both population size and the geographic area. It is an index of the number of PLWH in a given number of population and a geographic area. Thus, pg rates provide the most effective measure for cross-country comparison to assess the risk of transmission of HIV as well as many other infectious diseases. Based on the definition, pg rate will be high for countries with large number of headcount of persons suffering from or died of a disease, but a small population and small geographic area. For example, pg rate was 993.861 for Swaziland, which means roughly 1000 PLWH in every million population residing in an area of 100 km^2; while the corresponding pg rate was 0.007 for China, indicating much lower risk of HIV transmission. Given all other conditions the same, the likelihood for HIV (or any other infectious disease) to transmit from one to another in a place with small area and a large number of populations will be greater than in a place with large area and small number of populations.

With pg rate, countries in the region across Middle East and North Africa (MENA) were categorized low risk for HIV transmission. This is consistent with data from different sources (Gokengin, Doroudi, Tohme, Collins, & Madani, 2016) with different interpretations (Abu-Raddad et al., 2010; Gray, 2004). The advantage with our pg rate is that this MENA region looked much smoother and gradually expand to connect with other higher risk regions around, very different from the patterns shown by p rates or headcounts.

Based on pg rates, prevention of HIV transmission should pay particularly high attention to the three regions: One HIV Hot-Belt and two HIV Hotspots to better address the goal set by the UNAIDS to end the AIDS epidemic by 2030 (UNAIDS, 2014b). In general, countries in these high-risk belt and spots are relatively small in geographic area but with a large number of PLWH, in favor of HIV transmission from one to another.

In conclusion, this is the first time a 4D measurement system is formed and tested using the global HIV epidemic. More applications of the same method are highly recommended. For example, the same approach can be used to describe regional differences within a country; and to describe infectious diseases other than HIV. In addition to morbidity, the 4D approach can be used to describe mortality data. The utility of our 4D measurement system integrating headcount, p rate, g rate and pg rate together, providing the most comprehensive measure for researchers and decision makers to grasp the overall pattern of a disease in global health and epidemiology.

A.1 Appendix 1. List of countries with population, land area, total PLWH, P rate, G rate and PG rate

Table A.1 List of countries with population, land area, total PLWH, P rate, G rate and PG rate

Country	Population (1000)	Land area (100 km^2)	PLWH (1000)	P rate (1/1,000)	G rate (1/100 km^2)	PG rate (1/10^6 pop× 100 km^2)
Afghanistan	32527	6,529	6.9	0.212	1.057	0.033
Algeria	39667	23,817	8.8	0.222	0.369	0.009
Angola	25022	12,467	320.0	12.789	25.668	1.026
Argentina	43417	27,367	110.0	2.534	4.019	0.093
Armenia	3018	285	3.6	1.193	12.645	4.190
Australia	23781	76,823	27.0	1.135	0.351	0.015
Austria	8611	825	18.0	2.090	21.812	2.533
Azerbaijan	9651	827	11.0	1.140	13.307	1.379

(continued)

Table A.1 (continued)

Country	Population (1000)	Land area (100 km^2)	PLWH (1000)	P rate (1/1,000)	G rate (1/100 km^2)	PG rate (1/10^6 pop× 100 km^2)
Bahamas	388	100	8.1	20.875	80.919	208.544
Bangladesh	160996	1,302	9.6	0.060	7.375	0.046
Barbados	284	4	2.6	9.148	604.651	2,127.480
Belarus	9513	2,029	35.0	3.679	17.249	1.813
Belgium	11286	303	20.0	1.772	66.050	5.853
Belize	359	228	3.6	10.020	15.783	43.927
Benin	10880	1,128	69.0	6.342	61.192	5.624
Bhutan	775	381	1.0	1.291	2.624	3.386
Bolivia	10725	10,833	18.0	1.678	1.662	0.155
Botswana	2262	5,667	350.0	154.697	61.758	27.296
Brazil	207848	83,581	830.0	3.993	9.930	0.048
Bulgaria	7178	1,086	3.9	0.543	3.592	0.501
Burkina Faso	18106	2,736	95.0	5.247	34.722	1.918
Burundi	11179	257	77.0	6.888	299.844	26.822
Cambodia	15578	1,765	74.0	4.750	41.922	2.691
Cameroon	23344	4,727	620.0	26.559	131.159	5.619
Canada	35852	90,935	75.5	2.106	0.830	0.023
Cape Verde	521	40	3.2	6.148	79.404	152.554
Central African Republic	4900	6,230	120.0	24.488	19.262	3.931
Chad	14037	12,592	170.0	12.110	13.501	0.962
Chile	17948	7,435	32.0	1.783	4.304	0.240
China	1371220	93,882	850.0	0.620	9.054	0.007
Colombia	48229	11,095	150.0	3.110	13.520	0.280
Congo, DR	77267	22,671	370.0	4.789	16.321	0.211
Costa Rica	4808	511	10.0	2.080	19.585	4.074
Croatia	4224	560	1.2	0.284	2.144	0.508
Cuba	11390	1,040	22.0	1.932	21.150	1.857
Czech Republic	10551	772	2.1	0.199	2.720	0.258
Côte d'Ivoire	22702	3,180	460.0	20.263	144.654	6.372
Denmark	5676	423	6.1	1.075	14.434	2.543
Djibouti	888	232	9.4	10.587	40.552	45.674
Dominican	10528	483	68.0	6.459	140.758	13.369
Ecuador	16144	2,484	29.0	1.796	11.677	0.723
Egypt	91508	9,955	11.0	0.120	1.105	0.012
El Salvador	6127	207	20.0	3.264	96.525	15.755
Equatorial Guinea Guinea	845	281	27.0	31.950	96.257	113.905
Eritrea	5169	1,010	14.0	2.708	13.861	2.682
Estonia	1312	424	13.5	10.290	31.847	24.274
Ethiopia	99391	10,000	793.7	7.986	79.370	0.799

(continued)

Table A.1 (continued)

Country	Population (1000)	Land area (100 km^2)	PLWH (1000)	P rate (1/1,000)	G rate (1/100 km^2)	PG rate (1/10^6 pop× 100 km^2)
Fiji	892	183	1.0	1.121	5.473	6.135
Finland	5482	3,039	2.9	0.529	0.954	0.174
France	66808	5,476	160.0	2.395	29.221	0.437
Gabon	1725	2,577	47.0	27.242	18.240	10.572
Gambia	1991	101	21.0	10.548	207.510	104.228
Georgia	3679	695	9.6	2.609	13.815	3.755
Germany	81413	3,489	73.0	0.897	20.923	0.257
Ghana	27410	2,275	270.0	9.850	118.660	4.329
Greece	10824	1,289	16.0	1.478	12.413	1.147
Guatemala	16343	1,072	55.0	3.365	51.325	3.141
Guinea	12609	2,457	120.0	9.517	48.836	3.873
Guinea-Bissau	1844	281	41.0	22.230	145.804	79.055
Guyana	767	1,969	7.8	10.168	3.962	5.166
Haiti	10711	276	130.0	12.137	471.698	44.038
Honduras	8075	1,119	20.0	2.477	17.875	2.214
Hungary	9845	905	4.1	0.416	4.529	0.460
Iceland	331	1,003	1.0	3.023	0.998	3.015
India	1311051	29,732	2,100.0	1.602	70.631	0.054
Indonesia	257564	18,116	690.0	2.679	38.089	0.148
Iran	79109	16,288	73.0	0.923	4.482	0.057
Ireland	4641	689	7.8	1.681	11.322	2.440
Israel	8380	216	8.5	1.014	39.279	4.687
Italy	60802	2,941	140.0	2.303	47.596	0.783
Jamaica	2726	108	29.0	10.639	267.775	98.232
Kazakhstan	17544	26,997	23.0	1.311	0.852	0.049
Kenya	46050	5,691	1,500.0	32.573	263.556	5.723
Kyrgyzstan	5957	1,918	8.1	1.360	4.223	0.709
Laos	6802	2,308	11.0	1.617	4.766	0.701
Latvia	1978	622	6.8	3.437	10.936	5.528
Lebanon	5851	102	2.4	0.410	23.460	4.010
Lesotho	2135	304	310.0	145.198	1021.080	478.253
Liberia	4503	963	30.0	6.662	31.146	6.916
Lithuania	2910	627	1.5	0.515	2.394	0.823
Luxembourg	570	26	1.0	1.755	38.610	67.775
Madagascar	24235	5,818	48.0	1.981	8.250	0.340
Malawi	17215	943	980.0	56.926	1039.457	60.380
Malaysia	30331	3,286	92.0	3.033	28.002	0.923
Mali	17600	12,202	120.0	6.818	9.835	0.559
Malta	431	3	0.5	1.159	156.250	362.252
Mauritania	4068	10,307	14.0	3.442	1.358	0.334
Mauritius	1263	20	8.2	6.494	403.941	319.925
Mexico	127017	19,440	200.0	1.575	10.288	0.081
Mongolia	2959	15,536	0.5	0.169	0.032	0.011

(continued)

Table A.1 (continued)

Country	Population (1000)	Land area (100 km^2)	PLWH (1000)	P rate (1/1,000)	G rate (1/100 km^2)	PG rate (1/10^6 pop× 100 km^2)
Montenegro	622	135	0.5	0.744	3.442	5.531
Morocco	34378	4,463	24.0	0.698	5.378	0.156
Mozambique	27978	7,864	1,500.0	53.614	190.747	6.818
Myanmar	53897	6,531	220.0	4.082	33.687	0.625
Namibia	2459	8,233	210.0	85.406	25.507	10.374
Nepal	28514	1,434	39.0	1.368	27.206	0.954
Netherlands	16937	337	22.1	1.305	65.598	3.873
New Zealand	4596	2,633	2.9	0.631	1.101	0.240
Nicaragua	6082	1,203	9.9	1.628	8.227	1.353
Niger	19899	12,667	49.0	2.462	3.868	0.194
Nigeria	182202	9,108	3,500.0	19.209	384.290	2.109
Norway	5196	3,652	4.5	0.866	1.232	0.237
Pakistan	188925	7,709	100.0	0.529	12.972	0.069
Panama	3929	743	17.0	4.327	22.868	5.820
Papua New Guinea	7619	4,529	40.0	5.250	8.833	1.159
Paraguay	6639	3,973	17.0	2.561	4.279	0.645
Peru	31377	12,800	66.0	2.103	5.156	0.164
Philippines	100699	2,982	42.0	0.417	14.086	0.140
Poland	37999	3,062	35.0	0.921	11.431	0.301
Portugal	10349	916	48.0	4.638	52.399	5.063
Moldova	3554	329	18.0	5.065	54.761	15.408
Romania	19832	2,301	16.0	0.807	6.954	0.351
Russian	144097	163,769	73.0	0.507	0.446	0.003
Rwanda	11610	247	200.0	17.227	810.701	69.830
Senegal	15129	1,925	46.0	3.040	23.892	1.579
Serbia	7098	875	3.5	0.493	4.002	0.564
Sierra Leone	6453	722	51.0	7.903	70.657	10.949
Singapore	5535	7	4.9	0.894	697.884	126.086
Slovakia	5424	481	0.5	0.092	1.040	0.192
Slovenia	2064	201	1.0	0.485	4.965	2.406
Somalia	10787	6,273	30.0	2.781	4.782	0.443
South Africa	54957	12,131	7,000.0	127.372	577.039	10.500
South Sudan	12340	6,197	180.0	14.587	29.044	2.354
Spain	46418	5,002	150.0	3.231	29.987	0.646
Sri Lanka	20966	627	4.2	0.200	6.697	0.319
Sudan	40235	23,760	56.0	1.392	2.357	0.059
Suriname	543	1,560	3.8	6.998	2.436	4.486
Swaziland	1287	172	220.0	170.944	1279.070	993.861
Sweden	9799	4,073	9.1	0.929	2.234	0.228
Switzerland	8287	395	20.0	2.413	50.612	6.108
Tajikistan	8482	1,388	16.0	1.886	11.529	1.359
Thailand	67959	5,109	440.0	6.474	86.124	1.267

(continued)

Table A.1 (continued)

Country	Population (1000)	Land area (100 km^2)	PLWH (1000)	P rate (1/1,000)	G rate (1/100 km^2)	PG rate (1/10^6 pop× 100 km^2)
Togo	7305	544	110.0	15.059	202.243	27.687
Trinidad and Tobago	1360	51	11.0	8.088	214.425	157.655
Tunisia	11108	1,554	2.6	0.234	1.674	0.151
Turkey	78666	7,696	5.5	0.070	0.715	0.009
Uganda	39032	2,005	1,500.0	38.430	748.055	19.165
Ukraine	45198	5,793	220.0	4.867	37.978	0.840
UK	65138	2,419	101.2	1.554	41.830	0.642
Tanzania	53470	8,858	1,400.0	26.183	158.049	2.956
USA	321419	91,474	1,242.0	3.864	13.578	0.042
Uruguay	3432	1,750	10.0	2.914	5.714	1.665
Uzbekistan	31300	4,254	33.0	1.054	7.757	0.248
Venezuela	31108	8,821	110.0	3.536	12.471	0.401
Vietnam	91704	3,101	260.0	2.835	83.852	0.914
Yemen	26832	5,280	9.2	0.343	1.743	0.065
Zambia	16212	7,434	1,200.0	74.020	161.423	9.957
Zimbabwe	15603	3,869	1,400.0	89.728	361.897	23.191

References

Abu-Raddad, L. J., Hilmi, N., Mumtaz, G., Benkirane, M., Akala, F. A., Riedner, G., ... Wilson, D. (2010). Epidemiology of HIV infection in the Middle East and North Africa. *AIDS, 24*(Suppl 2), S5–S23. https://doi.org/10.1097/01.aids.0000386729.56683.33

Alistar, S. S., Owens, D. K., & Brandeau, M. L. (2011). Effectiveness and cost effectiveness of expanding harm reduction and antiretroviral therapy in a mixed HIV epidemic: A modeling analysis for Ukraine. *PLoS Medicine, 8*(3), e1000423. https://doi.org/10.1371/journal.pmed.1000423

AVERT. (2017). *HIV prevention programmes overview*. Retrieved August 15, 2018, from https://www.avert.org/professionals/hiv-programming/prevention/overview

Bautista-Arredondo, S., Gadsden, P., Harris, J. E., & Bertozzi, S. M. (2008). Optimizing resource allocation for HIV/AIDS prevention programmes: An analytical framework. *AIDS, 22*(Suppl 1), S67–S74. https://doi.org/10.1097/01.aids.0000327625.69974.08

Bayer, R., & Galea, S. (2015). Public health in the precision-medicine era. *The New England Journal of Medicine, 373*(6), 499–501. https://doi.org/10.1056/NEJMp1506241

CDC. (2017). *HIV cost-effectiveness*. Retrieved August 8, 2018, from https://www.cdc.gov/hiv/programresources/guidance/costeffectiveness/index.html

CDC. (2018a). HIV in the United States: At a glance. Retrieved August 7, 2018, from https://www.cdc.gov/hiv/statistics/overview/ataglance.html

CDC. (2018b). *HIV transmission*. Retrieved August 15, 2018, from https://www.cdc.gov/hiv/basics/transmission.html

Chen, D. (2017). Comparing geographic area-based and classical population-based incidence and prevalence rates, and their confidence intervals. *Preventive Medical Reports, 7*, 116–118. https://doi.org/10.1016/j.pmedr.2017.05.017

Chen, X. (2014). Understanding the development and perception of global health for more effective student education. *The Yale Journal of Biology and Medicine, 87*(3), 231–240.

Chen, X., & Wang, K. (2017). Geographic area-based rate as a novel indicator to enhance research and precision intervention for more effective HIV/AIDS control. *Preventive Medical Reports, 5*, 301–307. https://doi.org/10.1016/j.pmedr.2017.01.009

Cohen, J. (2011). HIV treatment as prevention. *Science, 334*(6063), 1628–1628. https://doi.org/10.1126/science.334.6063.1628

Courtenay-Quirk, C., Spindler, H., Leidich, A., & Bachanas, P. (2016). Building capacity for data-driven decision making in African HIV testing programs: Field perspectives on data use workshops. *AIDS Education and Prevention, 28*(6), 472–484. https://doi.org/10.1521/aeap.2016.28.6.472

Deeks, S. G., Lewin, S. R., Ross, A. L., Ananworanich, J., Benkirane, M., Cannon, P., ... Zack, J. (2016). International AIDS society global scientific strategy: Towards an HIV cure 2016. *Nature Medicine, 22*(8), 839–850. https://doi.org/10.1038/nm.4108

Ferguson, N. M., Fraser, C., Donnelly, C. A., Ghani, A. C., & Anderson, R. M. (2004). Public health. Public health risk from the avian H5N1 influenza epidemic. *Science, 304*(5673), 968–969. https://doi.org/10.1126/science.1096898

Gokengin, D., Doroudi, F., Tohme, J., Collins, B., & Madani, N. (2016). HIV/AIDS: Trends in the Middle East and North Africa region. *International Journal of Infectious Diseases, 44*, 66–73. https://doi.org/10.1016/j.ijid.2015.11.008

Granich, R., Crowley, S., Vitoria, M., Smyth, C., Kahn, J. G., Bennett, R., ... Williams, B. (2010). Highly active antiretroviral treatment as prevention of HIV transmission: Review of scientific evidence and update. *Current Opinion in HIV and AIDS, 5*(4), 298–304. https://doi.org/10.1097/COH.0b013e32833a6c32

Gray, P. B. (2004). HIV and Islam: Is HIV prevalence lower among Muslims? *Social Science & Medicine, 58*(9), 1751–1756. https://doi.org/10.1016/S0277-9536(03)00367-8

H. I. V. Modelling Consortium Treatment as Prevention Editorial Writing Group. (2012). HIV treatment as prevention: Models, data, and questions—Towards evidence-based decision-making. *PLoS Medicine, 9*(7), e1001259. https://doi.org/10.1371/journal.pmed.1001259

International Aids Society Scientific Working Group on H I V Cure, Deeks, S. G., Autran, B., Berkhout, B., Benkirane, M., Cairns, S., ... Barre-Sinoussi, F. (2012). Towards an HIV cure: A global scientific strategy. *Nature Reviews. Immunology, 12*(8), 607–614. https://doi.org/10.1038/nri3262

Khoury, M. J., Iademarco, M. F., & Riley, W. T. (2016). Precision public health for the era of precision medicine. *American Journal of Preventive Medicine, 50*(3), 398–401. https://doi.org/10.1016/j.amepre.2015.08.031

Lyles, C. M., Kay, L. S., Crepaz, N., Herbst, J. H., Passin, W. F., Kim, A. S., ... HIV Aids Prevention Research Synthesis Team. (2007). Best-evidence interventions: Findings from a systematic review of HIV behavioral interventions for US populations at high risk, 2000-2004. *American Journal of Public Health, 97*(1), 133–143. https://doi.org/10.2105/AJPH.2005.076182

Marsh, J. A., & Farrell, C. C. (2015). How leaders can support teachers with data-driven decision making: A framework for understanding capacity building. *Educational Management Administration & Leadership, 43*(2), 269–289. https://doi.org/10.1177/1741143214537229

Martinson, N., Mohapi, L., Bakos, D., Gray, G. E., McIntyre, J. A., & Holmes, C. B. (2009). Costs of providing care for HIV-infected adults in an urban HIV clinic in Soweto, South Africa. *Journal of Acquired Immune Deficiency Syndromes, 50*(3), 327–330. https://doi.org/10.1097/QAI.0b013e3181958546

Meltzer, M. I., Atkins, C. Y., Santibanez, S., Knust, B., Petersen, B. W., Ervin, E. D., ... Centers for Disease Control and Prevention [CDC]. (2014). Estimating the future number of cases in the Ebola epidemic—Liberia and Sierra Leone, 2014-2015. *MMWR Supplements, 63*(3), 1–14.

Merson, M. H., Black, R. E., & Mills, A. J. (2012). *Global health: Diseases, programs, systems, and policies* (3rd ed.). Jones & Bartlett Learning: Burlington, MA.

Mnyika, K. S., Klepp, K. I., Kvale, G., Nilssen, S., Kissila, P. E., & Ole-King'ori, N. (1994). Prevalence of HIV-1 infection in urban, semi-urban and rural areas in Arusha region, Tanzania. *AIDS, 8*(10), 1477–1481.

National Health and Family Planning Commission of PRC. (2015). *2015 China AIDS Response Progress Report*. Retrieved from http://www.unaids.org/sites/default/files/country/documents/CHN_narrative_report_2015.pdf

Redding, S., & Venables, A. J. (2004). Economic geography and international inequality. *Journal of International Economics, 62*(1), 53–82. https://doi.org/10.1016/j.jinteco.2003.07.001

Rothman, K. J., Greenland, S., & Lash, T. L. (2008). *Modern epidemiology* (3rd ed.). Lippincott, Willimans & Wilkins.

Sattenspiel, L. (2009). *The geographic spread of infectious diseases: Models and applications*. Princeton: Princeton University Press.

Szklo, M., & Nieto, J. (2018). *Epidemiology beyond the basics* (4th ed.). Sudbury, MA: Jones and Bartlett Publishers.

Tanser, F., Barnighausen, T., Grapsa, E., Zaidi, J., & Newell, M. L. (2013). High coverage of ART associated with decline in risk of HIV acquisition in rural KwaZulu-Natal, South Africa. *Science, 339*(6122), 966–971. https://doi.org/10.1126/science.1228160

UNAIDS. (2014a). *2014 Progress reports submitted by countries*. Retrieved August 7, 2018, from http://www.unaids.org/en/dataanalysis/knowyourresponse/countryprogressreports/2014countries

UNAIDS. (2014b). *Fast-Track—Ending the AIDS epidemic by 2030*. Retrieved August 7, 2018, from http://www.unaids.org/en/resources/documents/2014/JC2686_WAD2014report

UNAIDS. (2016). *2016 Progress reports submitted by countries*. Retrieved August 7, 2018, from http://www.unaids.org/en/dataanalysis/knowyourresponse/countryprogressreports/2016countries

UNAIDS. (2017a). *90–90–90—An ambitious treatment target to help end the AIDS epidemic*. Retrieved August 7, 2018, from http://www.unaids.org/en/resources/documents/2017/90-90-90

UNAIDS. (2017b). *People living with HIV*. Retrieved August 7, 2018, from http://aidsinfo.unaids.org/

UNICEF. (2013). *At a glance: Guinea-Bissau*. Retrieved August 7, 2018, from https://www.unicef.org/infobycountry/guineabissau_statistics.html

WHO. (2017). *HIV/AIDS*. Retrieved August 15, 2018, from http://www.who.int/mediacentre/factsheets/fs360/en/

WHO. (2018). *HIV/AIDS data and statistics*. Retrieved August 7, 2018, from http://www.who.int/hiv/data/en/

WHO Regional Office for Europe. (2014). *HIV/AIDS treatment and care in Estonia*. Retrieved August 7, 2018, from http://www.euro.who.int/__data/assets/pdf_file/0008/255671/HIVAIDS-treatment-and-care-in-Estonia.pdf

Wikipedia. (2019). *Timeline of the SARS outbreak*. Retrieved on January 5, 2019, from https://en.wikipedia.org/wiki/Timeline_of_the_SARS_outbreak

World Bank. (2015a). *Land area*. Retrieved August, 2018, from http://data.worldbank.org/indicator/AG.LND.TOTL.K2

World Bank. (2015b). *Total population*. Retrieved August 7, 2018, from http://data.worldbank.org/indicator/SP.POP.TOTL

Chapter 9
Historical Trends in Mortality Risk over 100-Year Period in China with Recent Data: An Innovative Application of Age-Period-Cohort Modeling

Xinguang Chen

Abstract History is the best teacher. It is challenging to learn from history to address contemporary problems in the field of global health and epidemiology. A first challenge is the lack of data to examine medical and health problems in the past. Such challenge is more obvious in developing countries, such as China where no data were collected due to limited resources, wars, plaques, and natural disasters. Theoretical analysis and empirical data from age-period-cohort modeling indicate that recent data by age of a population contains information about the past. For example, mortality rate for people aged 90 in 1990 contains information about mortality risk in 1900 when they were born. Therefore, information contained in mortality by age functions like digital fossil; and the age-period-cohort modeling provides a tool to extract the information from the fossil. In this study we examined the mega-trends in mortality risk for China since 1901 when the 2000-year long feudalism was throughout, to 1949 when the independence was established, and up to 1980s when rapid economic growth emerged. We achieved the goal by analyzing data collected in recent years from 1990 to 2010 with the age-period-cohort modeling method and the intrinsic estimator. Findings of the study suggest the existence of four Sunny Periods and three Cloudy Periods during 1901–2010. These Sunny and Clouding Periods were in close coincident with significant social, cultural, political, economic events in the history of China. Findings of the study revealed that the highest mortality risk was associated with foreign invasion, the second highest risk was associated with civil wars, the third highest risk was associated with economic reform; the lower mortality risk was associated with the post-war period and the establishment of new China, and the longest period with reduced risk of mortality was associated with the Cultural Revolution Period. In

X. Chen (✉)
Department of Epidemiology, College of Public Health and Health Professions, College of Medicine, University of Florida, Gainesville, FL, USA

Global Health Institute, Wuhan University, Wuhan, China
e-mail: jimax.chen@ufl.edu

X. Chen, (Din) D.-G. Chen (eds.), *Statistical Methods for Global Health and Epidemiology*, ICSA Book Series in Statistics,
https://doi.org/10.1007/978-3-030-35260-8_9

conclusion, age-period-cohort modeling provide a powerful tool for researchers to examine medical and health issues in the past with more recent data to advance epidemiology and global health. We highly recommend the use of this method in research in both developed and developing countries.

Keywords Historical epidemiology · APC modeling · Mortality in China · Social economic factors · Global health

9.1 Introduction

The development of global health and epidemiology requires us to investigate significant medical and health issues in the past with a historical perspective. However, it is rather challenging, if not impossible to examine things happened long time ago in the past when no research data were collected. In this chapter, we introduce the age-period-cohort (APC) modeling method, a classic epidemiological modeling tool; demonstrate its use in analyzing more recent data to investigate the time trends in the risk of mortality in China more than 100 years ago since 1906.

9.1.1 Learn from History

History can provide unique information supporting global health and epidemiology to better understand current medical and health problems we are facing. Significant events recorded in history, such as wars, famines, political, socioeconomic changes, often can exert broad and substantial impact on population health. While the majority of published studies use more recent data in research to understand current status of health and diseases; findings from a historical epidemiologic research studies will add new data from a different angle to strengthen current findings and to help clarify controversial issues observed from current studies. In addition to the advancement of our understanding of challenge medical and health issues with a global and temporal perspective, historical data provide information at the macro-level, guiding studies with newly collected data.

To examine historical events in medicine and public health, we often consult qualitative method by reviewing and summarizing events occurred in history and link them to changes in health status. For example, based on mortality recoded in several countries and regions, the epidemiological transition model posts that the life expectancy was rather low for people living in the developed countries in the 1800s when infectious diseases were predominant; and we attribute the rapid increases in life expectancy in modern society to industrialization, economic growth and advancement in medical technology and medicine (McKeown, 2009; Omran, 2005; Zhou et al., 2019). Also, we have no doubt that wars, famine also contributed to high mortality. However, few quantitative and systematic studies in the literature that have associated historical events with changes in health status of a population. Although findings from qualitative studies provide useful information, adding more systematic data will further enhance our mastery of historical events on current health status and better inform decision-making to deal with significant medical and health challenges we are facing today and in the future.

9.1.2 Challenges for Quantitative Historical Research

One reason for the lack of quantitative and systematic investigation of historical events in epidemiology and global health is due to the lack of recorded data to quantify health status of a population in the past. Data are lacking on diseases and deaths during the primitive time for all countries in the world except fossils and grave records from archeology, genealogy records, and church records. Recorded population mortality data are not widely available before World War II because of frequent wars, population migration, and large-scale plaques. More data have gradually become available since the 1950s after the establishment of the World Health Organization (WHO). However, such data are often available primarily for industrialized and developed countries in the Europe and North America.

Collecting health and disease data could not be on agenda for poor countries during the period when people are struggling for survival. Although, changes in the health status of a population during difficult times may contain unique information for researchers to under how natural (i.e., famine, flooding), social (i.e., social movements), political (revolution that moves a country from one system to another), economic, and technical factors may affect health; unfortunately such data are not available. Fortunately, following the developed countries and assisted by WHO and developed countries, many developing countries started to collect data on population health and diseases since the 1980s. China is among one of these countries. If data collected in more recent times contains the information about health status in the past, it may provide an opportunity to quantitatively examine the relationship between significant historical events and the corresponding changes in population health.

In this chapter, we take China as an example to demonstrate how to conduct an historical epidemiologic research with more recent data. We first list the major historical events since 1900s after China abolished the 2000-year long feudalistic society and entered into modern society through long-term frequently social, political, economic, technical and cultural changes. We then demonstrate that the health data collected since 1990 contain the information to measure health status from 1900s to 1990, corresponding to the significant historical events.

9.2 Timeline of Significant Events in China Since 1900

The recent history in China since 1900 presents a good case for epidemiology and global health to examine social, political, cultural and economic factors and population health using APC modeling method with a historical perspective. People in China have experienced a series of historical events with largest scope and highest impact on human kind from the 1900s till today. Relating significant historical events with the risk of population mortality will provide evidence unique for researchers, decision-makers and the general public to objectively assess the history of health policy and changes in population health, to think of the health and disease in the future based on knowledge from the past, and to make evidence-based strategic plans for disease prevention and health promotion.

In this study we focused on the time period since 1900 in China, starting with the period of overthrow of the 2000-year feudalistic society in 1911, the independence of China in 1949, and the open policy and rapid economic reform since 1978. In the following, we list the major historical events that are known to be influential to population health.

9.2.1 Overthrow of the Feudalistic Society

1899–1901: Yehetuan Movement or Boxer Rebellion: Happened in Northcentral China, and described as an anti-foreign invasion, anti-colonial, and anti-western culture, triggered by the power deteriorating of the Qing Dynasty, companied by a growing number of invasions from the earlier industrialized foreign countries.

1901–1911: Abdication of Qing Dynasty, the last feudalism society and the establishment of the Republic of China, the first modern society in Chinese history. The government, also the first time in Chinese history, established the Department of Sanitary in 1905 as the central government agency in charge of health.

1914–1926: The first and second civil wars among major warlords extended from the last administration of Qing Dynasty, after establishment of the Republic of China. The well-known May fourth Movement occurred in 1919 led by students and participated by people from all walks of life against Japanese and warlords.

1927–1934: Ending of the civil war through Northern Anti-Warlord Military Campaign and starting a period of peace and country's reconstruction, particularly the pioneer work of village health workers as part of the Rural Reconstruction Movement for rural uplift. A 3-year famine (1928–1930) occurred during this period, killing millions of people.

1937–1945: The War Anti-Japanese invasion in a full scale as part of the World War II until the Japanese surrendered in 1945. There was also a famine during 1942–1943, killing millions of people.

1945–1949: Start and end of the last Civil Ware and the inauguration of the People's Republic of China.

9.2.2 Early Period After Independence

1949–1957: Reconstruction of the country, including the high-impact Patriotic Health and Hygiene Movement to change the unhealthy lifestyles, to improve environmental health, and to control infectious diseases.

1957–1966: Domestic political movements, 1959–1962 famine, and the Great Leap Forward started and the Campaign of Removing Four Harm Pests (mosquitoes, flies, rats and sparrows) in 1958.

1966–1976: The 10-Year Cultural Revolution with destruction of traditional cultures and cultivation of new culture, national policies and campaigns of "Prevention First", "Shifted the Priority of Healthcare from Urban to Rural", "Barefoot Doctors", "Combination of Traditional Chinese Medicine with Western Medicine", and establishment of the 3-Tier Primary Care System.

9.2.3 The Period of Open Policy and Economic Reform

1978–present: Reform and open policy with unprecedented rural-to-urban population movement, rapid industrialization and economic growth the influence western culture and the 1989 Students Movement, shift from prevention first and free healthcare to market-oriented healthcare with reduced attention to prevention, and shift back in full scope in 2005 to re-emphasis of prevention, the free healthcare for urban residents and collaborative healthcare for rural residents.

9.3 Age-Specific Data and APC Modeling Analysis

9.3.1 Age-Specific Data as Digital Fossils

Epidemiologists are very familiar with mortality data tabulated by age of a population. Figure 9.1 shows how can we think of mortality data tabulated by age as a digital fossil containing information about risk of death in the past. In the figure, it contains a truncated part of population mortality rate per 100,000 by age groups from 25–29 to 60–64 in 1990 in China. For example, the mortality rate for all persons aged 60–64 was 1585.36/100,000 and this rate was the ratio of all persons died in 1990 over the total persons who were born 60–65 years ago in 1925–1930.

This figure tells the mortality rate for persons in an age or age group contains two important pieces of information: mortality risk in the year when the data were collected (the year 1990 as shown in the example), and the mortality risk related to the year of birth, the period 60–65 years ago. Although no data on mortality were collected for China 60–65 years ago during the 1925–1930 period (indicated by the red bracket) when the country were in the wars for domestic division and Japanese

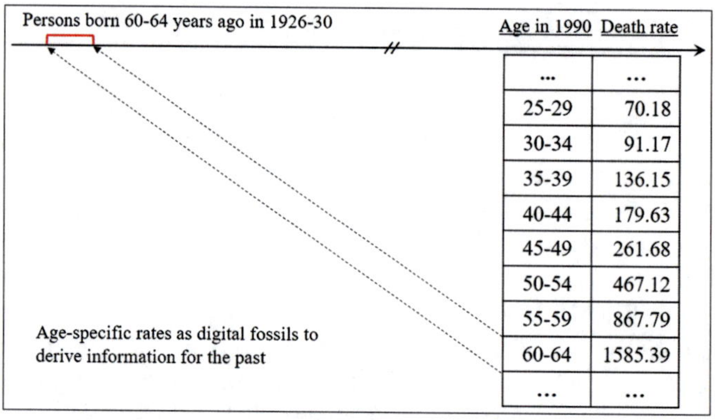

Fig. 9.1 Schematic illustration of age-specific mortality in a current year as digital fossil that contains information about the mortality risk in the past in addition to informing current status. **Note**: Mortality rate for persons aged 60–64 in 1990 contains information related to mortality risk in 1926–1930 when these people were born 60–64 years ago in 1926–1930; likewise, mortality rate for persons aged 80–84 in 1990 contains information of mortality risk in 1906–1910

invasion, it is likely to obtain data to describe the mortality risk during the period using the information contained in the death rate for persons aged 60–65 in 1990 when systematic data are available for use. It is in this regard, we conclude that *age-specific data can be considered as digital fossils* to examine the impact of historical events on mortality and potentially other health outcomes.

Likewise, the higher the age groups for data in more recently years, and further we can describe the past using more recent data. For example, mortality rates for persons aged 80–84 in 1990 contains the mortality risk for the period 80–84 years back during 1906–1910 when these persons were born. Although no data were available for the period long time ago, mortality data from recent times do contain the information to assess the health status during the period. The challenge is how to extract the information from the digital fossil—the age-specific mortality data.

9.3.2 *APC Model to Extract the Historical Information*

APC modeling provides one method to extract information from digital fossils—age-specific mortality data to examine the mortality risk of a population in the past when no systematic data were available for analysis (Chen et al., 2019; Chen & Wang, 2014a, 2014b). The basic principle of APC modeling analysis is to decompose the observed mortality by age of a year into three independent components. Let M_{ij} = the mortality rate for persons in age group i and period j, M_{ij} can be described using a general regression model:

$$f\left(M_{ij}\right) = \mu + \alpha_i + \beta_j + \gamma_k + \epsilon, \tag{9.1}$$

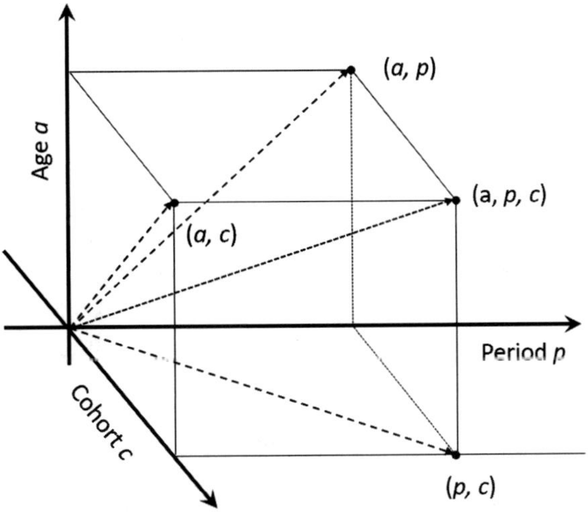

Fig. 9.2 Decomposition of mortality rate into three independent components as age, period and cohort effects. **Note**: In the endless time axis (period), people are continuous born to the world (cohort). At a point in time, one cohort was born. As time goes, this cohort ages. When reaching age a, this these people are corresponding to one point (a, p, c) in a 3D coordinate system. Other three meaningful points are (a, p), (a, c) and (p, c) respectively

where, μ represents the grant mean, α_i represents the impact of age i of the participants or "age effect", β_j represents the impact of the time period j or "period effect", and γ_k represents the impact of birth year k or "cohort effect", and ϵ are residuals. $f()$ is a function that links a mortality measure with the three effects, $f()$ can be identity for linear model, Poison for counting data and logistic for binary data.

From Eq. 9.1 it can be seen that the **cohort effect** $\boldsymbol{\gamma_k}$ is what we need—*information extracted from more recent data to quantify the mortality risk in the past when no data were available.*

Figure 9.2 visually depicts the age, period and cohort effect from Eq. 9.1 in a 3D format. In the chart, the three effects of age α_i, period β_j and cohort γ_k are mutually independent from an APC model as indicated by the three coordinators at the point (a, p, c).

Figure 9.2 also shows other three models routinely used in APC modeling analysis, and they are (1) the age-period model with the age and period effects showing by the two coordinators at the point (a, p); (2) the age-cohort model with the age and cohort effects showing by another two coordinators at the point (a, c); and the period-cohort model with the period and cohort effects showing by two more coordinators at the point (p, c).

9.3.3 Challenges to APC Modeling

Among many challenges to APC modeling, two are critical. The first is that APC modeling method cannot model individual level data and the second is that an APC model is mathematically not identifiable, therefore no valid solution is possible.

Methods are now available for analyzing individual-level data, and more details can be found in the book by Yang and Land (2013). Since modeling individual-level data is beyond the scope of this chapter, we provide some description about the non-identifiablility issue with APC modeling and progress in methodology research to deal with the issue.

Although the APC model described in the previous section is geometrically beautiful and very attractive to many researchers, the defined model is mathematically not identifiable because the three predictor variable age, period and cohort are not independent from each other. Given any two variable, the third one is determined, and can be derived with the other two. For example, if we know the age of a person and the year he/she participated in survey, the year of birth = survey year – age. Namely,

$$\text{Year of birth (c)} = \text{survey year (p)} - \text{age (a)} \tag{9.2}$$

A number of methodologists in demography, public health, and epidemiology have devoted their efforts attempting to find a solution, including the dedicated work by Mason and Winsboro (1973), Fienberg and Mason (1979), Holford (1983, 1991), Hobcraft, Menken, and Preston (1982), Yang and colleagues (Yang, Fu, & Land, 2004; Yang, Schulhofer-Wohl, Fu, & Land, 2008). A more detailed description of the methodology research can be found in O'Brien (2013); Yang and Land (2013), and Chen & Chen in Chap. 10 of this book. Despite much progress, none of the reported methods is very appealing to researchers till the report of the intrinsic estimator (IE) method established by a group of methodologists through a series of mathematical analyses, simulation studies and empirical application as detailed and summarized in the book by Yang and Land (2013).

The invention of the IE method makes it possible the first time to obtain a set of unique solution to an APC model with a minimum number of constraints that do not affect/altering the estimated age, period and cohort effects. After invention, the IE method has been widely used in reported studies on population mortality (Chen & Wang, 2014a, 2014b), chronic disease mortality (Yang, 2008); suicide death (Chen et al., 2019). In this study, we used the IE method for parameter estimation.

9.3.4 *New Data Selection Method to Correctly Estimate Cohort Effect*

In APC modeling analysis, researchers almost always use the following format for data selection: Age-specific data matched and aggregated with the years of data collection (O'Brien, 2013; Yang & Land, 2013). I also used this approach when I conducted my first APC modeling analysis (Chen, Li, Unger, Liu, & Johnson, 2003). Table 9.1 presents an example with hypothetic data to demonstrate the method.

Table 9.1 Hypothetic mortality data (1/100,000) for APC modeling analysis

Age/period	1990–1994	1995–1999	2010–2004	2005–2009	2010–2014
...					
10–14	53	58	54	48	46
15–19	70	73	64	57	51
20–24	88	86	70	64	64
25–29	123	123	90	80	86
30–34	183	185	135	115	119
35–39	275	282	221	186	166
...					

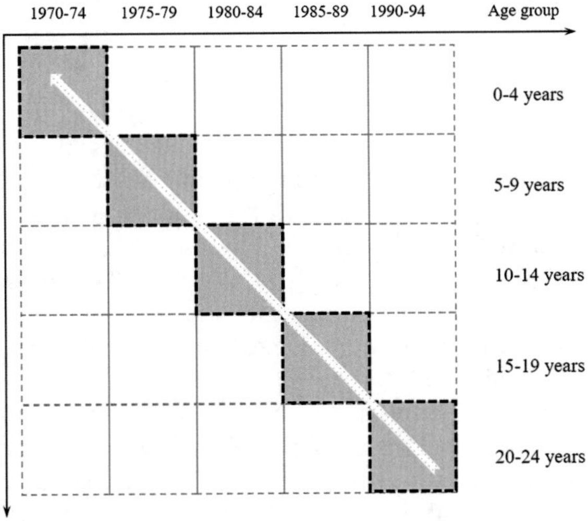

Fig. 9.3 Conventional approach to determine cohort. **Note:** Persons aged 20–24 in 1990–1994 are coded as born in 1970–1975, following the shaded boxes (a synthetic cohort) as in most reported studies using APC modeling, but birth cohort defined using this method is subject to large error

When mortality data are tabulated with 5 years as the age-group interval, the mortality rate must also be tabulated for 5-year period. Even if mortality data by single year are available, such data must be aggregated by summarizing data from five consecutive years into one group. For example, the mortality rate for 1990–1994 for each age group can be calculated by adding all deaths in an age group during this period and divided by summation of total population of the same age group of all 5 years.

In several of my recent studies, I was stopped by a problem using the aggregate-data in the Table 9.1 format in estimating the birth cohort (Chen et al., 2019; Chen & Wang, 2014a, 2014b). Figure 9.3 presents a hypothetic example. Following the conventional method, to calculate the cohort (the years of birth) for people aged 20–24 years in 1990–1994, we simply trace back of this group of persons from the bottom right to the top left (the shaded boxes) as if they were a cohort or synthetic cohort. By tracking, we simple code the years of birth of the persons aged 20–24 in 1990–1994 as if they were born during 1970–1974 for analysis.

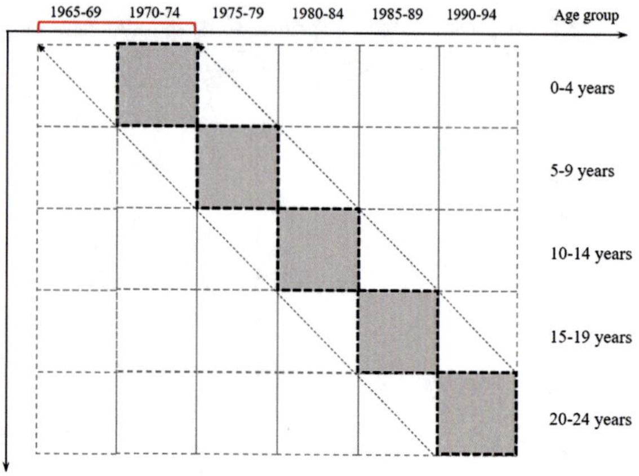

Fig. 9.4 Miss calculation of birth cohort using conventional approach. **Note**: Persons tabulated by 5-year age group and 5-year period were born not in 5 years but 10 years

From Fig. 9.3, at first no one can find anything wrong or want to challenge the method. However, a careful examination of this method, we can see that not all persons aged 20–24 in 1990–1994 were born in 1970–1974. This can be illustrated with Fig. 9.4. Persons aged 20–24 in 1990–1994 including those who were 20–24 years old in 1990, 21–34 in 1991, 22–24 in 1992 and 23–24 in 1993 who were born in 1965–1969 as the second dashed line indicated in the figure. With the conventional methods, these persons are treated as if they were all in the year 1994 rather than the period of 1990–1994.

Obviously, cohort or year of birth determined using the conventional methods have two problems. First, the cohort determined is incorrect using the conventional method because approximately 1/3 (the unshaded upper triangle in the top left of Fig. 9.4) of the persons with the coded year of births not equal the true year of birth. According to Fig. 9.4, the correct cohort for persons aged 20–24 in 1990–1994 should be 1965–1974, rather than 1970–1974 as show in this figure and Fig. 9.3. The second problem because of the first problem of misclassification, is the reduction in time resolution for cohort as seen in reported studies (Wang, Hu, Sang, Luo, & Yu, 2017). With the conventional method, the time resolution for cohort effect is reduced 50% from 5 to 10 years. Consequently significant change in cohort effects over time could be smoothed out when the conventional method is used to code year of birth with tabulated data as shown in a few studies.

9.3.5 *Using Single Year of Data 5 Years Apart as a Solution*

To solve the problem discussed in the previous section, we invented a new method in our previous study—using single year of data that are 5 years apart if the mortality data are aggregated using 5 years as the age interval (Chen et al., 2019; Chen & Wang, 2014a, 2014b). As shown in Fig. 9.5, instead of aggregating data from all 5

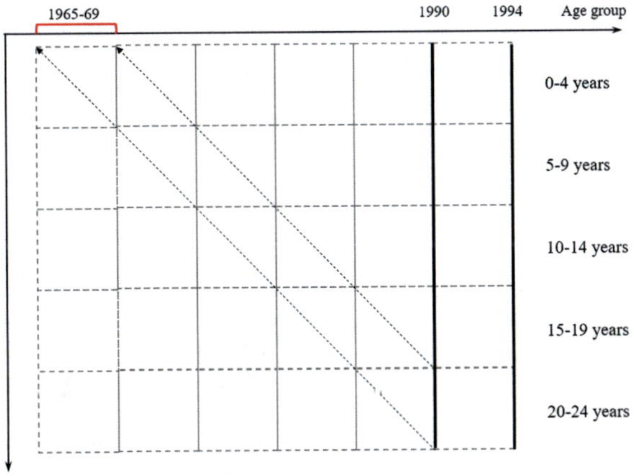

Fig. 9.5 New data selection method to correctly determine birth cohort

years from 1990 to 1994, data in 1990 were used. Clearly, persons aged 20–24 in 1990 were born in 5 years during 1965–1969.

With this approach we solved the two problems at the same time—the cohort is now corrected measured, and the time resolution of the cohort has doubled. In addition, this new approach will increase work efficiency since there is no need to aggregate 5-year data; and there is also no need to have data year by year.

9.4 Materials and Methods

9.4.1 Source of Data

Age-specific mortality rates of urban Chinese population during 1990–2010 were derived from the *China Health Statistical Yearbook*. Mortality data were collected through the Vital Registration System and the Ministry of Health and Hygiene of China and population data were from the National Census of China (Yang et al., 2005). Mortality rates (1/100,000) were computed as the number of deaths over the population, overall and by 5-year age group.

We limited the age-group range from 20–24 to 80–84 years with a total of 13 age groups. Data for people younger than 20 years of age were excluded because the mortality during this period showed a declining trend, different from those 20 years of age and older. The last age group 85+ was excluded because APC model cannot handle open-ended age group (Holford, 1991; Mason & Winsboro, 1973). With data for participants aged 80–84 in 1990, we could assess the risk of mortality as early as 1903–1907 (1990–84 = 1905 and 1990–80 = 1910).

In conventional APC modeling analysis, 5-year average rates are used (Holford, 1991; Mason & Winsboro, 1973; Yang, 2008) (Riggs, McGraw, & Keefover, 1996; Skegg & Cox, 1991; Stack, 2000; Wang et al., 2016). As we discussed early in this

Table 9.2 Age-specific mortality rate (1/100,000) of people living in urban China, 1990–2010

Age group	1990	1995	2000	2005	2010
20–24	64.25	49.08	35.1	42.22	39.27
25–29	70.18	61.08	51.145	51.64	42.46
30–34	91.17	87.37	73.995	84.72	61.91
35–39	136.15	121.33	118.15	138.12	101.79
40–44	179.63	209.75	197.915	209.68	166.06
45–49	261.68	306.02	310.135	306.01	259.72
50–54	467.12	400.97	398.63	502.66	375.04
55–59	867.79	685.52	559.18	738.03	563.96
60–64	1585.39	1434.75	1096.18	1199.14	956.08
65–69	2661.59	2464.04	2145.73	1967.18	1544.13
70–77	4614.63	4311.49	3787.095	3752.49	2766.82
75–79	7455.59	6751.83	6120.66	5938.69	4889.94
80–84	12641.64	11663.7	10043.995	10092.88	8754.1

Data sources and definition: The H*ealth Statistical Yearbook* of China with mortality rates calculated by dividing the number of deaths with the total population. Data were collected through the Vital Registration System and the Ministry of Health and Hygiene of China and population data were from the National Census of China

chapter, with this method, the cohort could not be correctly defined. Also, persons in a 5-year age group within 5-year period were born in a 10-year period, reducing the time resolution to link years of birth with changes in the risk of mortality. To overcome the problem, we used single-year data 5-year apart in 1990, 1995, 2000, 2005, and 2010. With this approach, data for persons in a 5-year age group in 1 year were all born within 5 years—birth cohort (Chen & Wang, 2014a, 2014b). The mortality data were presented in Table 9.2.

9.4.2 APC Modeling Analysis

Let m_{ij} and n_{ij} be the mortality rate and number of persons in age group i and time period j. By definition, the expected number of deaths in age group i and time period j would be $E_{ij} = m_{ij} \times n_{ij}$. Assuming a Poison distribution of the number of deaths, the following log linear model was used to extract cohort effect stretching back to 1905 with data during 1990–2010:

$$\log\left(E_{ij}\right) = \mu + \alpha_i + \beta_j + \gamma_k + \epsilon$$

where E_{ij} = expected number of deaths in age group i and year j; μ denotes the intercept or grant mean; α_i denotes the effect of age-group i (i = 20–24, 25–29, …,80–84); β_j denotes the effect of period j (j = 1990, 1995, …, 2010); and γ_k

denotes the effect of birth cohort k (k = 1906–2010, 1910–1914, ...,1986–1990); and $\epsilon \sim N(0, \sigma)$.

With this model specification, a total of 42 parameters were estimated (one grant mean μ, 13 age effects, 5 period effects, and 17 cohort effects). The 5 period effects plus the 25 cohort effects provided data regarding the risk of mortality among urban Chinese over a period of more than 100 years from 1906–1910 to 2010, with the cohort effects fill in the period from 1906–1989 with no data collection. All the parameters were estimated using the IE method (Fu, 2000; Yang, 2008; Yang et al., 2004). The data-model fit was evaluated using the fit deviance, AIC and BIC. The APC modeling analysis was conducted using the STATA-based software package apc ie with Poisson as the distribution option and *logit* as the link function.

Before the full-scale APC modeling, we fit the data with three 2-component models, including AP (age and period) model, AC (age and cohort) model, and PC (period and cohort) model (see Fig. 9.2). These three models are identifiable, but each of them omitted one predictor. Results from these two-component models were compared with those from the full-scale APC model to show the differences in the estimated effects using different methods and to deepen our understanding of the APC modeling approach.

To effectively describe the historical dynamics of mortality risk change over time through visualization, numerical differentiation was performed over the estimated cohort effect (Chen & Wang, 2014a, 2014b). The numerical differentiations provide an approximate of the changing speed in mortality risk over time. In plotting the changes, y-axis was reversed for the change speed such that any upward trend as a *Sunny Cohort* during which suicide risk was reducing and any downward trend as a *Cloudy Cohort* during which suicide risk was increasing.

As a convention, before statistical modeling analysis, we also plotted the mortality data using several methods to show the potential age, period and cohort effect.

9.5 Main Study Findings

9.5.1 Visual Presentation of the Mortality Data

Figure 9.6 depicts the age-specific mortality by year. Data from the figure indicate that during the 30-year period from 1990 to 2010, there was a progressive decline in the mortality for people from all age groups. Furthermore, the mortality declining was more pronounced for people 60 years of age and older. A careful review of the five curves, we also noted that there were no observable declines in the mortality from 2000 to 2005 for people in all age groups, including the older residents.

We plot the same data from Fig. 9.6 using the age-group and birth-cohort method (Fig. 9.7). Different from Fig. 9.6, a logarithm scale was used for y-axes to better separate the mortality curves for different age groups. In the figure, each line

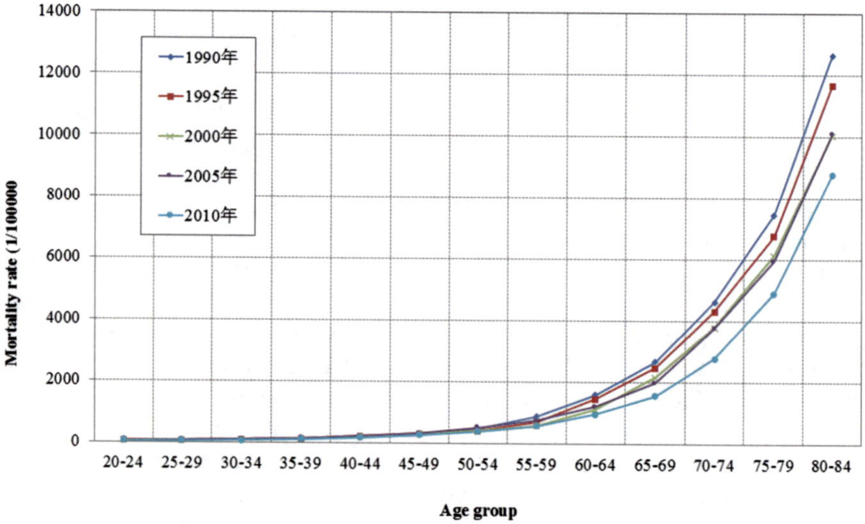

Fig. 9.6 Age-specific mortality of urban Chinese in 1990, 1995, 2000, 2005 and 2010

represents an age group with mortality rates in 1990, 1995, 2000, 2005 and 2010. Results from the figure suggest a progressive decline in mortality associated with year of birth from 1906 to 1990. In addition, the four lines located on the top of the map suggest that the mortality decline was smoother and more consistent for those aged 65 years and older, compared to those in all younger age groups. In fact, the mortality in most of the younger working age groups increased from 2000 to 2005 before it declined.

9.5.2 Comparison of Results from Four Different APC Models

Results in Fig. 9.8 shows that the age, period and cohort effects estimated with the AP, AC and PC models all differed from those estimated with the APC model. This result suggests that the mortality was related to all three predictors. Specifically, with reference to the result from the APC model, the age effect was over estimated with either the AP or the AC model; the PC model resulted in an excaudate increasing trend in period effect while the AP model suppressed the increasing trend. The differences were more dramatic for the cohort effect. Cohort effect obtained from the PC model increased for the first two cohort and then progressively decline to way below the effect from the APC model while the effect from AC model was progressively higher than that from the APC model.

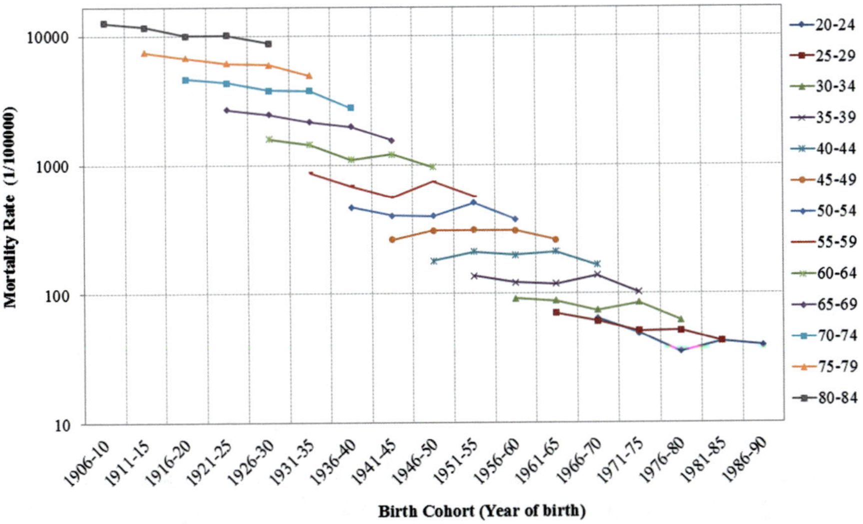

Fig. 9.7 Age-group and birth-cohort plotting of the mortality rate of the urban Chinese in 1990, 1995, 2000, 2005 and 2010

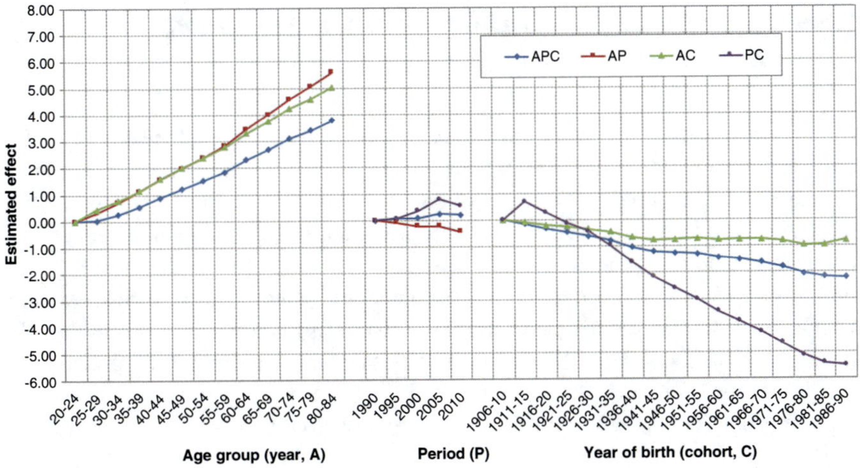

Fig. 9.8 Estimated age, period and cohort effects from different APC models. **Data source**: Mortality data for urban Chinese collected in 1990, 1995, 2000, 2005, and 2010

9.5.3 Period Effect for Mortality Risk Change over 1990–2010

The period effect estimated from the APC modeling over 1990–2010 is presented in Fig. 9.9. Results in the figure indicate a progressive increase in the risk of death from 1990 to 2005 before it declined. This effect was independent from changes in the age composition of the urban population in China and the year of births

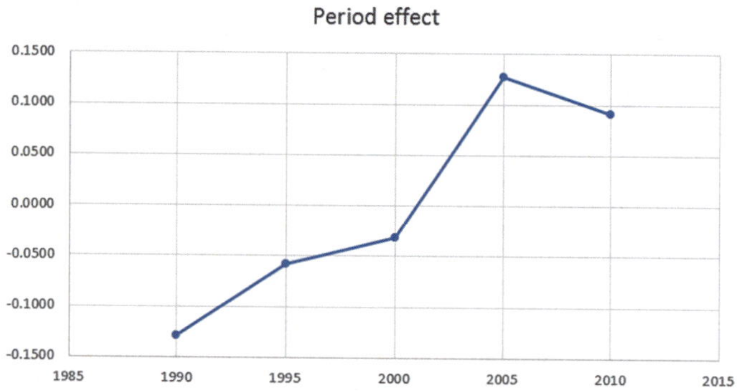

Fig. 9.9 Period effect β assessing the risk of mortality for urban residents of China, 1900–2010

of all urban residents during this period. The period effect extracted through APC modeling reflected the trends in the risk of death all urban residents experienced during the period of 1990–2010.

9.5.4 *Changes in Cohort Effect Through Numerical Differentiation*

Cohort effect is the information this study intended to extract from the mortality data collected during 1990–2010 to describe changes in the mortality risk among urban Chinese since the early 1900s. The estimated cohort effect estimated using the full-scale APC model for the 1905–1990 was presented in Fig. 9.8 (blue line). Despite an overall declining trends with small ups and downs, the estimated cohort effect did not present any more information to associated with significant historical events in China. To better use the historical mortality risk information derived from the APC modeling analysis, Fig. 9.10 presents the estimated cohort effect through numerical differentiation. For example, the number of the 1911–1915 is the differences in the mortality risk (cohort effect) of this cohort relative to the previous cohort of 1905–1910.

For efficient presentation, in Fig. 9.10 we purposefully reversed the y-axes such that an increase in the curve representing a period of *deceleration* in mortality risk (termed as Sunny Period) and a decline in the curve representing a period of *acceleration* in mortality risk (termed as Cloudy Period).

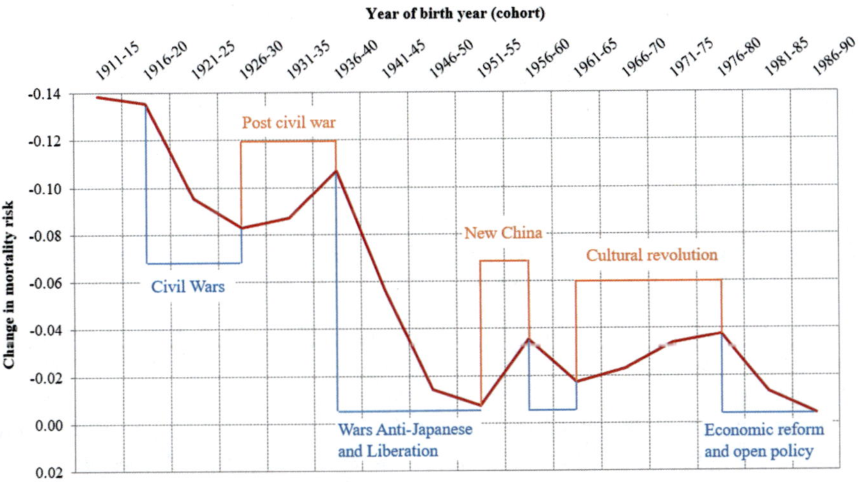

Fig. 9.10 Historical changes in mortality risk among urban Chinese, 1911–1990: Numerical differentiation of the cohort effect extracted using an APC model. Note: The Y-axes is reversed such that an upward trend indicating deceleration in mortality risk and a downward trend indicating acceleration in mortality risk

9.5.5 *Sunny Periods in Historical China*

Results in Fig. 9.10 reveal three obvious Sunny Periods: 1926–1936, 1951–1955, and 1961–1975 during which deceleration in the risk of death was observed. The first Sunny Period (1926–1930) was corresponding to the post-civil wars after the success of the Northern Anti-Warlord Military Campaign. The country returned to peace and started the home reconstruction. The slowing down of the mortality risk reduction during the latter half of the period was associated with the historically recorded famine that lasted for 3 years during 1928–1930.

The second Sunny Period (1951–1955) was corresponding to the time after the liberation of the country and the establishment of the People's Republic of China was established in 1949. Although short, the reduction of mortality risk was reasonable. With a newly liberated and united country after a long period of anti-foreign invasion and domestic war, people started to enjoy peace, reconstruction of the war-broken country and their homes and reconstruction of new lives. Furthermore, the national Patriotic Health and Hygiene Movement was launched during this period for infectious disease control.

The third Sunny Period (1961–1975). This was the longest "healthy period" and overlapped with most part of the 10-year Cultural Revolution from 1966 to 1976. This period is also one of the most controversial periods in contemporary China. Despite the long-standing political and cultural movement, destruction of the traditional Chinese culture, punishment and harsh time for many political leaders and intellectuals, the prolonged declines in the risk of mortality for the whole urban population could be due to the emphasis of prevention and the construction of the three-tier primary healthcare network system and the promotion of the combination of the Traditional Chinese Medicine with Western Medicine. In addition to health and medicine, researchers, politicians, policymakers and historians can learn more from this listen in China.

9.5.6 *Cloudy Period in Historical China*

Results in Fig. 9.10 also showed Four Cloudy Periods: 1916–1925; 1936–1945, 1956–1960, and 1976–1990. The first Cloudy Period (1916–1925) was corresponded with the first and second civil wars (1914–1926) in China after the establishment of the Republic of China in 1911. This was only a part of the long transitions from the 2000-year long feudalistic society to the modern society for a country with the largest population in the world.

The second Cloudy Period (1936–1950). This period was directly related to the Anti-Japanese War as part of the World War II from 1936 to 1945 and the War for Liberation (1946–1949). Among the four cloudy periods, the impact of this one is the largest. China as country dominated with agriculture was invaded by Japan, an industrialized country that attempt to dominate Asia by occupying the largest neighbor country and massacring millions of people with war machines. A recorded famine in 1942–1943 further worsened the survival of the population in China. The cohort effect revealed through this APC modeling provides the first time systematic data showing the increased mortality by Japanese invasion.

The third Cloudy Period (1956–1960). This period, fortunately short, was associated with a number of natural, social and political events, including the Great Leap Forward, the Anti-Righteous Agents Movement, and the sudden destruction of the diplomatic relationship with the former Soviet Union, and another recorded famine in 1959 in the history of China.

The last Cloudy Period (1976–1990). This period was corresponding to the most well-known time in recent China, the Economic Reform and the Open Policy with unprecedented rural-to-urban migration, rapid economic growth, quick industrialization, speedy technological advancement, and dramatic cultural change and diversification. Unfortunately, the estimated cohort effect indicate that risk of mortality accelerated for the urban Chinese during this period, consistent with the recorded mortality rates in the data and the estimated period effect from 1990 to 2005.

9.6 Discussion and Conclusions

In this study, we demonstrated on how to analyze data collected in recent years using APC modeling approach to address historical epidemiological problems. With data collected in more recent years from 1990 to 2010 among urban population, systematic information was extracted from the data to accurately describe the changes in mortality risk since the early 1900s when the country had been torn by civil wars, foreign invasion, natural disasters, political and cultural revolutions, industrialization, and urbanization. The type of data we used is this study are widely available (see Chap. 1 in this book) and the APC modeling is easy to implement with the newly invented IE method (Y. Yang & Land, 2013). The revision to use single year data as well as the introduction to use numerical differentiation further sharpen the APC modeling method for researchers to gain more detailed insight into historical changes with recent data (Chen et al., 2019; Chen & Wang, 2014a, 2014b). In addition to the total mortality, the same analysis can be used to assess individual causes of deaths as well as health behaviors as reported in the literature (Chen et al., 2003).

9.6.1 Findings and Implications for China

Findings about the historical changes in mortality risk among urban population in China since the early 1900s has significant implications.

Good health policies as the best health protection measure.

The first and the most striking finding is the continuous improvement in mortality risk during the 10-year Cultural Revolution. Although substantial damages from Cultural Revolution are reported, the mortality risk persistently declined for the longest period in modern China, but why? A careful review of the related literature indicated that during the Cultural Revolution period, a series of important health policies were established and implemented, including the policy of "Prevention First", "Emphasis of Primary Healthcare", "Establishment of the Three-Tiered Primary Care System", and "Combination of Traditional Chinese Medicine with Modern Medicine". Despite the large-scale and long-standing social and political turmoil with very low levels of economy and medical technology in China during that period, no other factor can convincingly explain the continuous improvement in people's health at the national level except these significant and well-known health policies and programs.

Peace is the best and most efficient guard for population health.

The second important findings of this study is the provision of systematic data document the impact of foreign invasion and domestic wars on increased mortality risk. Although such risk is obvious, but no systematical and valid data has been reported in the literature. In the history of more than 100 years in China since the 1900s, mortality risk was the highest corresponding to the time of Japanese invasion and the anti-Japanese War during the World War II. In addition, the impact of domestic or civil wars was also substantial; and the least was the social political turmoil and natural disasters, which showed the smallest impact in magnitude and lasted short in time.

9.6.2 Economic and Technic Advancement Not Equal to Good Health

Finding from the historical analysis of the data in China indicate that many advancements in recent China, including economy, technology, and culture since the 1970s did not translated into population health by reducing mortality. China has made substantial advancement in economy, technology and culture after implementing the reform and open policy since the 1980. However, evidence from our analysis indicate an increase in risk of mortality for urban Chinese during this period, including the cohort effect derived from age-specific mortality during 1976–1990, and the net period effect (after controlling for age and cohort) during the 1990–2010. This increased mortality occurred in a period when the per capita GDP in China increased from $156 in 1978 to $3838 in 2010 (World Bank); health expenditure increased at 11.32% annually from 1978 to 2010 (China Embassy in the United, 2012).

Fortunately, findings of this study revealed a small decline in the population mortality risk in China since 2005 as the economy of the country continued to grow. This decline was exactly in consistency with the heath policy change in China (Gao, Tang, Tolhurst, & Rao, 2001; Wang, Gusmano, & Cao, 2011) from a market-oriented healthcare back to re-establishing the free health care system, re-emphasizing the prevention first policy and re-building the Three-Tiered Primary Care System that once benefited people's health at the time before the Reform and Open Policy started in China (Hsiao, 1995).

9.6.3 APC Modeling for Historical Epidemiology

By conducting APC modeling analysis and teaching the method to graduate students, I proposed the term historical epidemiology with APC modeling approach (Chen et al., 2019; Chen & Wang, 2014a, 2014b). The idea of historical epidemiology started with the concept that *data by age are digital fossils*, and these fossils contain information regarding the past of an issue we would like to know. Although contained in the age-specific data, the information is indexed by the year of birth—cohort effect. Furthermore, such information can be extracted with APC modeling method, a readily available tool to extract the indexed information. Findings from this study add new evidence to my previous research, supporting the historical epidemiology research with APC modeling method and aggregated data.

Several issues are to be considered when conducting APC modeling for historical epidemiological research. First, your data have not to be in 5-year age group, shorter age groups are even better to describe the risk in the past. For example, if single-year data are available, cohort effect can thus be estimated by single year of birth, more accurate than 5-year interval. Cohort effect estimated by single year will be better than by multi-year to associate the risk with historical events. Second, the older the age in data, the longer the research can trace back to the history. If data are available up to 100 years of age, such data can be used to trace back literately to 100 years back in the past. Third, data for only 1 year cannot be analyzed using APC modeling method; you must have data for multiple years. Mathematically, data for a minimum of 3 years are needed to obtain valid effect estimates.

Application of the APC modeling in research has been hindered for long time because of the non-identifiablity issue inherited with the method. The invention of the IE method has promoted the use of APC modeling in research (Chen et al., 2019; Chung, Yip, Chan, & Wong, 2016; Li, Wang, Gao, Xu, & Chen, 2016; Wang et al., 2017; Yang & Land, 2013). Despite many strengths, commercial software is needed to implement the IE method. Furthermore, the IE method reads complex even for researchers with training in mathematics and statistics, which may reduce the confidence of a researcher to select the for APC modeling. In recent methodology study, we have developed another method to deal with the identifiablity issue inherited with the APC model—Solving APC model using generalized inverse matrix method. This method is based on the well-established Moore and Penrose generalized inverse matrix theory (Moore & Barnard, 1935; Penrose, 1955) and can be executed using R, and software free of charge. Chapter 10 that follows next provides more detailed description about this method.

9.6.4 Implication for Research in Other Countries

One purpose of this chapter is to introduce this method for anyone to conduct research studies in countries all over the world. With research findings from more countries, they will inform local health policy and decision-making with both a historical and a global perspective. The success of this study indicate that similar studies can be conducted for many countries in the world as long as data on population health are available in recent one or two decades. For example, if the earliest data are available for a health measure for people in a country up to 80 years of age in 1980, such data can be used to assess health status since 1900. Such data will help us much to investigate social, political, economic and technological development in affecting population health. As we will see, such information is unique and important for researchers, policy-makers, and the general public to know the health history of their country, to make decisions and to from relevant policies and strategies to handle challenge medical and health issues by adding a historical perspective. When data from many countries are reported in the literature, we can form a historical and global perspective to understand human health and to deal with global and local health challenges with a broader spatiotemporal perspective.

9.6.5 Limitations and Conclusion Remarks

There are several limitations. First, no mortality data by single year of age was available from the data source. This prevented us from using single but 5-year interval to assessing the timing of an observed change in the mortality risk over time. Second, we did not quantify the relationship between the historical events and the mortality risk. Conducting such studies need to have solid methods to code the historical events, which is technically challenging. More methodological research is needed to code these events for quantitative (i.e., correlation and regression) analyses.

Despite the limitations described above, this study is the first one to demonstrate the potentials to examine historical events on population health with APC modeling methods and recent data. It sets an example for researchers in different countries in the world to conduct historical epidemiological research, to obtain new data supporting global health and modern epidemiology.

References

Chen, X., Li, G., Unger, J. B., Liu, X., & Johnson, C. A. (2003). Secular trends in adolescent never smoking from 1990 to 1999 in California: An age-period-cohort analysis. *American Journal of Public Health, 93*(12), 2099–2104.

Chen, X., Sun, Y., Li, Z., Yu, B., Gao, G., & Wang, P. (2019). Historical trends in suicide risk for the residents of mainland China: APC modeling of the archived national suicide mortality rates during 1987-2012. *Social Psychiatry and Psychiatric Epidemiology, 54*(1), 99–110. https://doi.org/10.1007/s00127-018-1593-z

Chen, X., & Wang, P. G. (2014a). Social change and national health dynamics in China. *Chinese Journal of Population Science (in Chinese), 2*, 63–73.

Chen, X., & Wang, P. G. (2014b). Social change and the dynamic change in national health status in China (in Chinese). *Chinese Journal of Population Science (in Chinese), 26*, 63–73.

Chung, R. Y., Yip, B. H., Chan, S. S., & Wong, S. Y. (2016). Cohort effects of suicide mortality are sex specific in the rapidly developed Hong Kong Chinese population, 1976-2010. *Depression and Anxiety, 33*(6), 558–566. https://doi.org/10.1002/da.22431

Fienberg, S. E., & Mason, W. M. (1979). Identification and estimation of age-period-cohort models in the analysis of discrete archival data. *Sociological Methodology, 10*(1979), 1–67.

Fu, W. J. J. (2000). Ridge estimator in singular design with application to age-period-cohort analysis of disease rates. *Communications in Statistics-Theory and Methods, 29*(2), 263–278. https://doi.org/10.1080/03610920008832483

Gao, J., Tang, S., Tolhurst, R., & Rao, K. (2001). Changing access to health services in urban China: Implications for equity. *Health Policy and Planning, 16*(3), 302–312. https://doi.org/10.1093/heapol/16.3.302

Hobcraft, J., Menken, J., & Preston, S. (1982). Age, period, and cohort effects in demography - A review. *Population Index, 48*(1), 4–43. https://doi.org/10.2307/2736356

Holford, T. R. (1983). The estimation of age, period and cohort effects for vital rates. *Biometrics, 39*(2), 311–324.

Holford, T. R. (1991). Understanding the effects of age, period, and cohort on incidence and mortality rates. *Annual Review of Public Health, 12*, 425–457. https://doi.org/10.1146/annurev.pu.12.050191.002233

Hsiao, W. C. (1995). The Chinese health care system: Lessons for other nations. *Social Science & Medicine, 41*(8), 1047–1055.

Li, Z., Wang, P. G., Gao, G., Xu, C. L., & Chen, X. G. (2016). Age-period-cohort analysis of infectious disease mortality in urban-rural China, 1990–2010. *International Journal for Equity in Health, 15*, 55. https://doi.org/10.1186/s12939-016-0343-7

Mason, K. O., & Winsboro, H. (1973). Some methodological issues in cohort analysis of archival data. *American Sociological Review, 38*(2), 242–258. https://doi.org/10.2307/2094398

McKeown, R. E. (2009). The epidemiologic transition: Changing patterns of mortality and population dynamics. *American Journal of Lifestyle Medicine, 3*(1 Suppl), 19S–26S. https://doi.org/10.1177/1559827609335350

Moore, E. H., & Barnard, R. W. (1935). *General analysis part I*. Philadelphia, PA: The American Philosophical Society.

O'Brien, R. M. (2013). Comment of Liying Luo's article, "assessing validity and application scope of the intrinsic estimator approach to the age-period-cohort problem". *Demography, 50*(6), 1973–1975. https://doi.org/10.1007/s13524-013-0250-0

Omran, A. R. (2005). The epidemiologic transition: A theory of the epidemiology of population change. *Milbank Quarterly, 83*(4), 731–757. https://doi.org/10.1111/j.1468-0009.2005.00398.x. (Original work published, 1971).

Penrose, R. A. (1955). Generalized inverse for matrices. *Proceedings of the Cambridge Philosophical Society, 51*, 406–413.

Riggs, J. E., McGraw, R. L., & Keefover, R. W. (1996). Suicide in the United States, 1951-1988: Constant age-period-cohort rates in 40- to 44-year-old men. *Comprehensive Psychiatry, 37*(3), 222–225. https://doi.org/10.1016/S0010-440x(96)90039-5

Skegg, K., & Cox, B. (1991). Suicide in New-Zealand 1957-1986 - The influence of age, period and birth-cohort. *Australian and New Zealand Journal of Psychiatry, 25*(2), 181–190. https://doi.org/10.1080/00048679109077733

Stack, S. (2000). Suicide: A 15-year review of the sociological literature part II: Modernization and social integration perspectives. *Suicide and Life-threatening Behavior, 30*(2), 163–176.

States, China Embassy in the United. (2012). *Medical and Health Services in China (government white paper)*. Embassy of the People's Republic of China in the United States of America.

Wang, H., Gusmano, M. K., & Cao, Q. (2011). An evaluation of the policy on community health organizations in China: Will the priority of new healthcare reform in China be a success? *Health Policy, 99*(1), 37–43. https://doi.org/10.1016/j.healthpol.2010.07.003

Wang, Z. K., Hu, S. B., Sang, S. P., Luo, L. S., & Yu, C. H. (2017). Age-period-cohort analysis of stroke mortality in China: Data from the Global Burden of Disease Study 2013. *Stroke, 48*(2), 271–275. https://doi.org/10.1161/Strokeaha.116.015031

Wang, Z. K., Wang, J. Y., Bao, J. Z., Gao, X. D., Yu, C. H., & Xiang, H. Y. (2016). Temporal trends of suicide mortality in mainland China: Results from the age-period-cohort framework. *International Journal of Environmental Research and Public Health, 13*(8), 784. https://doi.org/10.3390/Ijerph13080784

Yang, G., Hu, J., Rao, K. Q., Ma, J., Rao, C., & Lopez, A. D. (2005). Mortality registration and surveillance in China: History, current situation and challenges. *Population Health Metrics, 3*(1), 3. https://doi.org/10.1186/1478-7954-3-3

Yang, Y. (2008). Trends in US adult chronic disease mortality, 1960-1999: Age, period, and cohort variations. *Demography, 45*(2), 387–416. https://doi.org/10.1353/Dem.0.0000

Yang, Y., Fu, W. J. J., & Land, K. C. (2004). A methodological comparison of age-period-cohort models: The intrinsic estimator and conventional generalized linear models. *Sociological Methodology, 34*, 75–110. https://doi.org/10.1111/j.0081-1750.2004.00148.x

Yang, Y., & Land, K. C. (2013). *Age-period-cohort analysis: New models, methods, and empirical applications*. Boca Raton, FL: Chapman & Hall/CRC.

Yang, Y., Schulhofer-Wohl, S., Fu, W. J. J., & Land, K. C. (2008). The intrinsic estimator for age-period-cohort analysis: What it is and how to use it. *American Journal of Sociology, 113*(6), 1697–1736. https://doi.org/10.1086/587154

Zhou, M., Wang, H., Zeng, X., Yin, P., Zhu, J., Chen, W., ... Liang, X. (2019). Mortality, morbidity, and risk factors in China and its provinces, 1990–2017: a systematic analysis for the Global Burden of Disease Study 2017. *Lancet*. https://doi.org/10.1016/S0140-6736(19)30427-1

Chapter 10
Moore-Penrose Generalized-Inverse Solution to APC Modeling for Historical Epidemiology and Global Health

(Din) Ding-Geng Chen, Xinguang Chen, and Huaizhen Qin

Abstract Age-period-cohort (APC) modeling provides a powerful method for global health research in resource-limited countries and regions with limited data. This method enables researchers to investigate medical and health conditions and influential factors, potentially up to 100+ year in the past with data collected in recent decades. Although widely used in research to examine mortality of various diseases, suicide and quality of life, an APC model is mathematically nonidentifiable. This is because the conlinearity among the three time-related predictors (age, period, and birth cohort). Various methods are reported to deal with this identifiability issue, particularly the intrinsic estimator (IE) that has been most accepted. IE method has been developed through much effort, including mathematical proof, simulations and empirical testing. In this chapter, we introduce the application of Moor-Penrose generalized inverse matrix method (MP) in handling the nonidentifiable issue. Relative to the IE method, the MP method is straightforward to understand and easy to implement. We also show that mathematically MP method is equivalent to IE method.

Keywords APC modeling · M-P generalized inverse · Intrinsic estimator · Historical epidemiology · Mortality risk

(Din) D.-G. Chen (✉)
School of Social Work, University of North Carolina, Chapel Hill, NC, USA
e-mail: dinchen@email.unc.edu

X. Chen (✉)
Department of Epidemiology, College of Public Health and Health Professions, College of Medicine, University of Florida, Gainesville, FL, USA

Global Health Institute, Wuhan University, Wuhan, China
e-mail: jimax.chen@ufl.edu

H. Qin
Department of Epidemiology, University of Florida, Gainesville, FL, USA
e-mail: hqin@ufl.edu

X. Chen, (Din) D.-G. Chen (eds.), *Statistical Methods for Global Health and Epidemiology*, ICSA Book Series in Statistics,
https://doi.org/10.1007/978-3-030-35260-8_10

10.1 Introduction

Age-Period-Cohort (APC) modeling is a classic method widely used in research to address challenge medical and health problems. With the method, researchers can decomposite an observed rate of a medical and health indicators into three independent components: age, period and cohort effect. Another name for APC modeling is cohort analysis based on Dr. Frost's research published in 1939 examining age and cohort differences in tuberculosis mortality (Frost, 1939). The method has been established through continuous efforts by a number of researchers, such as Mason and Winsboro (Mason & Winsboro, 1973), Feinber and Masion (Fienberg & Mason, 1979), Clayton and colleagues (Clayton & Schifflers, 1987a, 1987b), Holfort (Holford, 1991), Robertson and colleagues (Robertson & Boyle, 1998), and Carstensen (Carstensen, 2007). APC modeling method is designed for analyzing aggregate data. Dr. Yong and her colleagues expanded the method to analyze individual-level data (Yang & Land, 2013). Researchers who want to know more about historical development and method application can consult the book by O'Brien with focus on aggregated data analysis (O'Brien, 2015) and Yang & Land with focus on both aggregated and individual-level data analysis (Yang & Land, 2013).

An APC model is designated to model demographic rates, such as mortality, morbidity, fertility observed for a broad age range over a reasonably long time period. The data are tabulated by year of data collection (period) and chronological age when the data were collect; knowing the year of data collection and age at data collection, year of birth (cohort) is derived. For readers who are familiar with demography, the principle of APC modeling can better be understood using a Lexis-diagram which is a coordinate system with data of follow-up along the x-axis, and age along the y-axis with elements on the diagonal as cohort (Carstensen, 2007; Fienberg & Mason, 1979). The purpose of APC modeling is to decomposite the overall rate of an event by year into three independent components of age effect, period effect and cohort effects, describing the contribution of these three time-related factors to the observed trends in the study variables. For example, APC modeling method can be used to computer age and cohort adjusted rate to describe the true time trend in an vital events (as described in Chap. 9) and can used to examine historical trends during a period in the past with no data using the estimated cohort effect as in reported studies (X. Chen et al., 2019; Chen & Wang, 2014) and in Chap. 9 in this book.

APC modeling has been widely used in research to examine many medical and health problems at the population level, including the analysis of morbidity and mortality in general (Holford, 1991; Wang, Hu, Sang, Luo, & Yu, 2017; Yang, 2008), mortality of infectious diseases (Comstock, 1995; Frost, 1939; Li, Wang, Gao, Xu, & Chen, 2016), heart diseases (Chang, Li, Li, & Sun, 2017), stroke (Wang et al., 2017), cancer (Clayton & Schifflers, 1987a, 1987b), and suicide (Chen et al., 2019; Chung, Yip, Chan, & Wong, 2016). Despite widely application, the APC model has an inheretic issue-identifiability. Generally, the APC model can be used to model the (log)rates as a sum of (non-linear) age- period-cohort-effects. The three variables age (at follow-up), a, period (i.e. date of follow-up), p, and cohort (date of birth), c with calculated as $c = p\text{-}a$. Hence the three variables used to describe rates are linearly related, and the model can therefore be parametrized in different ways, and still produce the same estimated rates. In a sense, the development in APC model is a process to find ways to handle this nonidentifiability problem.

One most accepted method to deal with the nonidentifiability problem is the established of a method named as intrinsic estimator (IE) (Yang, Fu, & Land, 2004; Yang & Land, 2013). In this method, among all possible solutions to a constructed APC model, the one with the shortest distance to the origin is selected as the parameter estimates. The validity and efficiency of IE method has been proved mathematically and tested through religious simulation studies (Luo, 2013; Yang & Land, 2013). Although the IE method is now widely used, it is difficult for users to understand this approach analytically. In our own research on unidentified modelling, we found many strengths of Moore-Penrose (MP) generalized inverse method, including its solid mathematically foundation, relative more straight-forward to understand as well as convenient to implement using R, the open-source software free of charge.

In this chapter, we described our work to develop and test the MP-based method to solve for APC model (thereafter referred as "MP-APC"). For better communication, we named the IE method to solve APC as "IE-APC". After a description of the method, we tested MP-APC with Japanese breast cancer data from O'Brien (2015). We then compared results from MP-APC with those from IE-APC also presented in O'Brien (2015). In the last part of this chapter, we mathematically demonstrate the equivalence of the two method.

10.2 APC Model and Its Estimation

10.2.1 An Introduction to APC Model

APC model relates the dependent variable to the effects of age, period and cohort. Corresponding to an aggregated age-period data table with total m age-groups and n time periods, the APC model can be described as follows:

$$y_{ij} = \mu + \alpha_i + \beta_j + \gamma_{m-i+j} + \varepsilon_{ij} \tag{10.1}$$

where y_{ij} is the dependent variable in the ijth cell of the age-period table, μ is the intercept, α_i is the ith age effect, β_j is the jth period effect, γ_{m-i+j} is the $(m - i + j)$th cohort effect. ε_{ij} is the error term associated with the residuals in the age-period table. In matrix form, Model (1) can be re-written as follows:

$$y = Xb + \epsilon \tag{10.2}$$

where y is the vector of observed dependent observations with mn rows, X is the design matrix associated with Model (1) which describe the intercept and the effects of age-period-cohort and therefore has dimension of mn rows and $2(m + n - 3)$ columns (i.e., 1 for intercept, $m - 1$ for age effects, $n - 1$ for period effects and $m + n - 2$ for cohort effects), b is the parameter vector to be estimated which has $2(m + n) - 3$ rows, and ϵ is the vector of residuals with mn rows which is typically assumed to be uncorrelated with the design matrix as $X^{'} \epsilon = 0$. Therefore multiplying X' to Eq. (10.2), we can obtained the normal equation as follows:

$$X'Xb = X'y \tag{10.3}$$

which can be used to estimate the parameter vector, b, if X is full column rank matrix. However, this is not the case in APC modeling where X is not full column rank matrix due to the linear dependences among the age-period-cohort effects. Therefore methods are needed to deal with this problem.

10.2.2 Solving APC Using MP Method

To solve APC described in Eq. (10.3) that is not identifiable, we make use of the generalized-inverse in matrix theory. In general, a generalized-inverse for a matrix A (for APC modeling, $A = X'X$) is defined as: $AA^{-}A = A$, where A^{-} is called the generalized-inverse of A. The purpose of the generalized-inverse is to have a general solution $b = A^{-} X'y$ for any linear system, such as described in Eq. (10.3), regardless of the existence of the inverse of coefficient matrix A.

With this notation, the general solution to the APC Eq. (10.3) can be expressed in $b = A^{-}X^{'}y + (I - A^{-}A)z$ where I is the identity matrix and A^{-} is any fixed generalized-inverse of A, while z represents an arbitrary vector. Therefore, the generalized-inverse A^{-} is not unique which is equivalent to say that the APC in Eq. (10.3) cannot be solved uniquely.

Inspired by the general inverse matrix theory, particularly the work by Moore and Barnard (1935) and Penrose (1955), we make use of a mathematical approach to this problem, i.e. MP-APC.

In his famous paper, Moore and Barnard (1935) proposed three more conditions to the generalized inverse A^{-} defined above. They are as follows:

$$AA^{-}A = A \tag{10.4}$$

The original definition of generalized-inverse matrix is to allow any admissible APC in Eq. (10.3) to be solved easily by matrix representation regardless of the existence of the inverse of coefficient matrix. With this extension, the only requirement is that AA^{-} will map all column vectors of A to the same column vectors, respectively.

$$A^{-}AA^{-} = A^{-} \tag{10.5}$$

This added condition makes A^- a generalized reflexive inverse of A. With this condition A^-A does not need to be an identity matrix, but to map all column vectors of A^- to the same column vectors, respectively.

$$(AA^-)' = AA^- \tag{10.6}$$

The third condition addresses the transpose of AA^- to be itself. It indicates that AA^- is a Hermitian matrix. This is intuitively true that when A is invertible, $AA^- = AA^{-1} = I$ and the transpose of identity matrix I is itself

$$(A^-A)' = A^-A \tag{10.7}$$

The fourth condition is similar to the third condition. It indicates that A^-A is a Hermitian matrix with an intuitive explanation similar to the third condition.

Moore's extended definition did not receive any attention in the mathematics field for 20 years until Penrose (1955) proved the uniqueness of Moore's definition. Since Penrose's work, this definition has been named as Moore-Penrose generalized-inverse and is typically denoted as A^+. The Moore-Penrose generalized inverse has several mathematical properties, and the most relevant one to APC is that the solution of $b = A^+X'y$ is unique as well as being the minimum-norm (i.e. minimum length) solution. It provides a mathematical approach to overcome the challenge in solving a APC model with a non-full rank coefficient matrix. This MP-APC can be very easily implemented in R with function "ginv".

We have used this MP generalized inverse to solve un-identified application in epidemiological and public health problems, such as, to solve PDES for tobacco control (Chen & Chen, 2015; Chen, Yu, & Chen, 2018; Hu, Chen, Cook, Chen, & Okafor, 2016; Yu, Chen, & Wang, 2018). The MP-APC described in this chapter is an extension of our research using MP-theory based method to handle nonidentified systems in research.

10.3 Application with Real Data

10.3.1 Data Source and Arrangement

For illustration, we make use of the data from Clayton and Schifflers (1987a) which described the mortality rates per 100,000 and the number of cases of breast cancer mortality in Japan during the period 1955–1979. The data in Table 10.1 were derived from Table 2.3 in the book by O'Brien (2015, pp. 33). As seen in Table 10.1, the mortality data per 100,000 are organized by 5-year age group with a total of 11 groups, aggregated also by 5-year period with a total of five periods.

Table 10.1 Breast cancer mortality rates (1/100,000) among Japanese women breast cancer

	Period				
Age	1955–1959	1960–1964	1965–1969	1970–1974	1975–1979
25–29	0.44	0.38	0.46	0.55	0.68
30–30	1.69	1.69	1.75	2.31	2.52
35–39	4.01	3.90	4.11	4.44	4.80
40–44	6.59	6.57	6.81	7.79	8.27
45–49	8.51	9.61	9.96	11.68	12.51
50–54	10.49	10.80	12.36	14.59	16.56
55–59	11.36	11.51	12.98	14.97	17.79
60–64	12.03	10.67	12.67	14.46	16.42
65–69	12.55	12.03	12.10	13.81	16.46
70–74	15.81	13.87	12.65	14.00	15.60
75–79	17.97	15.62	15.83	15.71	16.52

Source of the original data: Clayton, D., & Schifflers, E. (1987b). Models for temporal variation in cancer rates. II: Age-period-cohort models. *Stat Med, 6*(4), 469–481

10.3.2 Modeling Analysis with MP-APC

To implement MP-APC, we first reformat the data in Table 10.1 into Eq. (10.2) where y is the vector of log-transformed mortality rates with $m = 11$ age-groups and $n = 5$ period-groups, i.e. y is a $mn = 55 \times 1$ vector.

Similarly, we make the design matrix, X, for MP-APC with dimension $mn = 55$ rows and $2(m + n) - 3 = 29$ columns (i.e., 1 for intercept, 10 for age effects, 4 for period effects and 14 for cohort effects). The model parameter estimates can be obtained as

$$\hat{b} = \left(X'X\right)^{+}X'y. \tag{10.8}$$

This MP-based Eq. (10.8) can be computed to solve for b with R program as *b* = *ginv*(*t*(*X*) % $*$ % *X*) % $*$ % *t*(*X*) % $*$ % y, where t(X) is the transpose of matrix X, "%$_*$%" is the matrix product and "ginv" is the Moore-Penrose generalized inverse. The detail implementation of the entire analysis can be seen from the R program in Appendix A.

With this computation, Fig. 10.1 illustrates the MP-APC fitted log-mortality rates with respect to the observed log-mortality rates. It can be seen that they are very close with $R^2 = 0.9994$, which indicates a very satisfactory MP-APC model fitting.

We further performed a Shapiro-Wilk normality test on the residuals and yielded a p-value of 0.9796. This result indicated that the residuals from MP-APC modeling of the data are normally distributed. Figure 10.2 graphically illustrated the QQ-

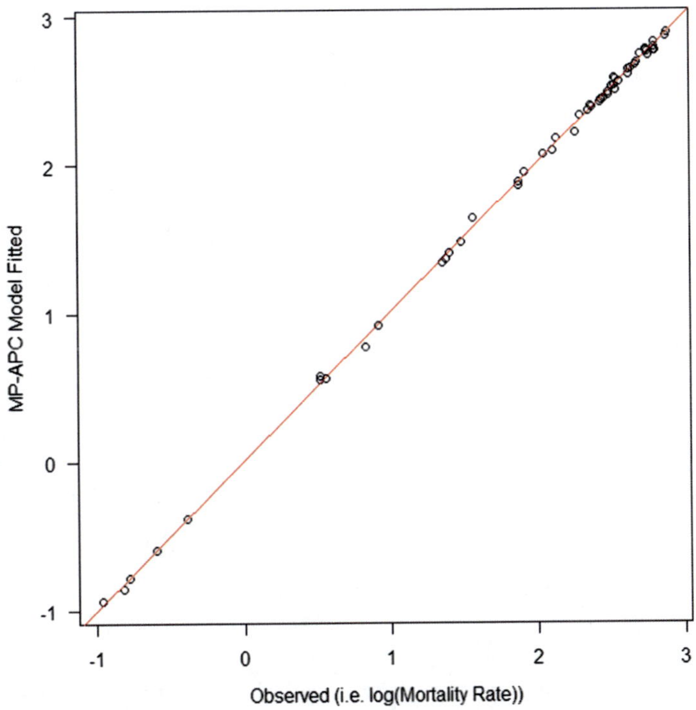

Fig. 10.1 The observed log-mortality rates and the MP-APC fitted log-mortality rates

plot of the residual and again confirmed that the residuals are normally distributed. This residual diagnostic analysis validated the assumption of normally distributed residuals of APC model in Eq. (10.1).

For further statistical inference, we programmed the computations of standard error, t-statistics and the associated p-values for statistical hypothesis testing. The estimates for the 52 parameters of the constructed APC model using the MP-APC modeling analysis are presented in Table 10.2 (last four columns, including the estimated model coefficients, standard error, t-values and the associated p-values).

The estimated parameters in Table 10.2 describe the relationship between the three time-related variables, age, time period and birth cohort and the risk of death due to breast cancer among women in Japan. For example, the estimated age effects indicate the risk of breast cancer death increased progressively since age 25, peaked at ages 55–59, followed by a declining trends. The estimated period effects indicated a continuous increasing trends in breast cancer mortality among Japanese women from 1955 to 1979. The estimated cohort effect indicate varying risk of breast cancer death for Japanese women born in different periods.

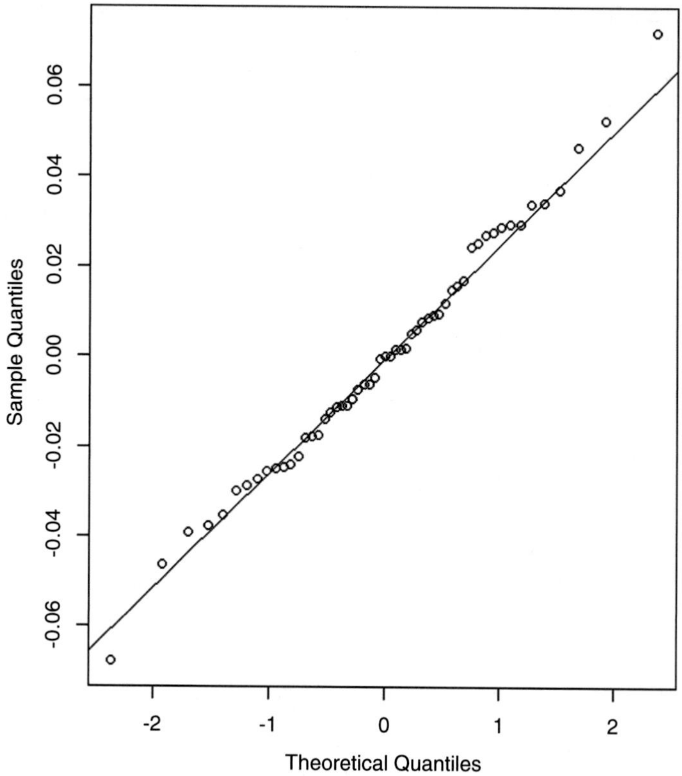

Fig. 10.2 QQ-normal plot on the residuals from MP-APC

10.3.3 Comparison with Results from IE-APC

As reported by O'Brien (2015), the first column (IE-APC) in Table 10.2 are the estimates for the same 52 parameters using the same data in Table 10.1. This result was reported in Table 2.5 from O'Brien original work (2015, pp. 37). By comparing the results presented in the first and second column of Table 10.2, we noted that parameters estimated using the MP-APC are identical with those from the IE-APC.

10.4 Relationship Between IE-APC and MP-APC

To explore potential reasons why the estimated results from our MP-APC modeling method and those from the IE-APC method, we conducted mathematical analysis to understand potential underlying relationships between the two methods in handling the non-identifiability issue for APC modeling.

Table 10.2 Results from MP-APC with comparison to IE-APC from O'Brien (2015)

		IE-APC	MP-APC			
		Est	Est.	Std.Err	t-value	Pr(>|t|)
Intercept		1.9887	1.9887	0.0338	58.9255	0.0000
Age	25–29	−2.3302	−2.3303	0.0967	−24.1022	0.0000
	30–30	−0.9899	−0.9899	0.0866	−11.4336	0.0000
	35–39	−0.2885	−0.2885	0.0877	−3.2904	0.0014
	40–44	0.1636	0.1636	0.0896	1.8262	0.0397
	45–49	0.4533	0.4533	0.0915	4.9556	0.0000
	50–54	0.6057	0.6057	0.0926	6.5400	0.0000
	55–59	0.6147	0.6147	0.0916	6.7147	0.0000
	60–64	0.5248	0.5248	0.0898	5.8440	0.0000
	65–69	0.4529	0.4529	0.0880	5.1446	0.0000
	70–74	0.4070	0.4070	0.0870	4.6756	0.0000
	75–79	0.3866	0.3866	0.0945	4.0924	0.0002
Period	1955–59	−0.2636	−0.2636	0.0536	−4.9151	0.0000
	1960–64	−0.1977	−0.1977	0.0543	−3.6421	0.0006
	1965–69	−0.0432	−0.0432	0.0543	−0.7953	0.2168
	1970–74	0.1674	0.1674	0.0535	3.1262	0.0022
	1975–79	0.3371	0.3371	0.0558	6.0363	0.0000
Cohort	1875–79	0.7770	0.7770	0.1848	4.2052	0.0001
	1880–84	0.5997	0.5998	0.1336	4.4907	0.0001
	1885–89	0.4044	0.4044	0.1124	3.5974	0.0007
	1890–94	0.2194	0.2194	0.1005	2.1826	0.0191
	1895–99	0.0809	0.0810	0.0918	0.8822	0.1929
	1900–04	0.0314	0.0314	0.0972	0.3225	0.3748
	1905–09	−0.0077	−0.0077	0.1004	−0.0768	0.4697
	1910–14	−0.0277	−0.0277	0.1011	−0.2737	0.3933
	1915–19	−0.0727	−0.0727	0.0993	−0.7323	0.2353
	1920–24	−0.1638	−0.1638	0.0948	−1.7270	0.0480
	1925–29	−0.2511	−0.2511	0.0883	−2.8439	0.0043
	1930–34	−0.3945	−0.3945	0.0955	−4.1309	0.0002
	1935–39	−0.3965	−0.3965	0.1070	−3.7073	0.0005
	1940–44	−0.4177	−0.4177	0.1284	−3.2530	0.0016
	1945–49	−0.3812	−0.3812	0.2111	−1.8055	0.0413

10.4.1 IE-APC Modeling

In IE-APC modeling, it deals with the same APC model as described in Eq. (10.2) with the X matrix being not a full rank but one column short. Consequently, Eq. (10.3) has an infinite number of solutions, each of which can be written as

$$\hat{b} = B + tB_0, \tag{10.9}$$

where t is a real number, vector B_0 the unique unit-length ($B_0'B_0 = 1$) eigenvector of X with respect to the eigenvalue 0 ($XB_0 = 0$), and B is the intrinsic estimator (IE) B, which is orthogonal to B_0 and is *uniquely* determined by Y and matrix X (Yang et al., 2004; Yang, Schulhofer-Wohl, Fu, & Land, 2008). However, a *unique* singular-value decomposition of the matrix X exists (Golub & Reinsch, 1970):

$$X = U \times \text{diag}\,(\sigma_1, \ldots, \sigma_{r-1}, 0) \times V', \tag{10.10}$$

where $r = 2(m + n) - 4$ is the ranked of X, $\sigma_1 > \cdots > \sigma_{r-1} > 0$, $U'U = V'V = I_r$, the identify matrix of order r. It follows that

$$\begin{aligned} A &= X'X \\ &= V \times \text{diag}\,(\sigma_1, \ldots, \sigma_{r-1}, 0) \times U'U \times \text{diag}\,(\sigma_1, \ldots, \sigma_{r-1}, 0) \times V' \\ &= V \times \text{diag}\left(\sigma_1^2, \ldots, \sigma_{r-1}^2, 0\right) \times V'. \end{aligned} \tag{10.11}$$

10.4.2 MP-APC Modeling

When using MP-APC method, the Moore-Penrose inverse of A is

$$A^+ = V \times \text{diag}\left(\frac{1}{\sigma_1^2}, \ldots, \frac{1}{\sigma_{r-1}^2}, 0\right) \times V'. \tag{10.12}$$

This MP matrix is unique and satisfies all the three Eqs. (10.4), (10.5), and (10.6). It can be shown that

$$\hat{b}_I \overset{\text{def}}{=} A^+X'y = V \times \text{diag}\left(\frac{1}{\sigma_1}, \ldots, \frac{1}{\sigma_{r-1}}, 0\right) \times U'y \tag{10.13}$$

Equation (10.13) is exactly the same as Eq. (10.11) for IE method. First, it is *uniquely* determined by X and y according to the uniqueness of the SVD of matrix X. Second,

$$\begin{aligned} \hat{b}_I'B_0 &= y'U\,\text{diag}\left(\tfrac{1}{\sigma_1}, \ldots, \tfrac{1}{\sigma_{r-1}}, 0\right) V'B_0 \\ &= y'U\,\text{diag}\left(\tfrac{1}{\sigma_1^2}, \ldots, \tfrac{1}{\sigma_{r-1}^2}, 0\right) \times \text{diag}\,(\sigma_1, \ldots, \sigma_{r-1}, 0) \times V'B_0 \\ &= y'U\,\text{diag}\left(\tfrac{1}{\sigma_1^2}, \ldots, \tfrac{1}{\sigma_{r-1}^2}, 0\right) U'U \times \text{diag}\,(\sigma_1, \ldots, \sigma_{r-1}, 0) \times V'B_0 \\ &= y'U\,\text{diag}\left(\tfrac{1}{\sigma_1^2}, \ldots, \tfrac{1}{\sigma_{r-1}^2}, 0\right) U'XB_0 = 0. \end{aligned} \tag{10.14}$$

Third, it follows from Eqs. (10.13) and (10.14) that

$$
\begin{aligned}
X'X\hat{b}_I &= V \times \text{diagdiag}\left(\sigma_1, \ldots, \sigma_{r-1}, 0\right) \times U'U \times \text{diag}\left(\sigma_1, \ldots, \sigma_{r-1}, 0\right) \times V'\,V \\
&\quad \times \text{diag}\left(\frac{1}{\sigma_1}, \ldots, \frac{1}{\sigma_{r-1}}, 0\right) \times U'y \\
&= V \times \text{diagdiag}\left(\sigma_1, \ldots, \sigma_{r-1}, 0\right) \times U'y \\
&= X'y.
\end{aligned}
\tag{10.15}
$$

In other words, $\hat{b}_I$ is a solution to Eq. (10.3). According to Eqs. (10.12) and (10.13), for an arbitrary t, $\hat{b} = \hat{b}_I + tB_0$ is an also solution to Eq. (10.3).

10.5 Discussion and Conclusions

In this chapter, we first briefly introduced the APC modeling method and listed its application research. We then introduced in detail about the MP-APC modeling method, including its principle, and application in handling the nonidentifiability issue, test the method with real data, and compared the results from MP-APC we proposed with those from the widely accepted IE-APC method. After we observed the identical results from the two methods, we further demonstrate that these two approaches are mathematically identical.

There are several advantages with our MP-APC modeling method than the IE-APC modeling and so as for many other methods previously reported. The MP-APC modeling method is based on a well-established Moore-Penrose generalized inverse matrix theory (Moore & Barnard, 1935; Penrose, 1955). We also used this approach in our previous research to dealing with under-defined systems (Chen & Chen, 2015; Chen et al., 2018; Hu et al., 2016; Yu et al., 2018).

Relative to the IE-APC, the MP-APC modeling approach is mathematically more straight forward. It simply mimic the method to solve for a linear matrix system but with a X matrix short of one column to be a full-ranked matrix. This will be much easier for researchers with limited mathematical background to understand the method, therefore may be more confident to use it in their own research. No one wants to use a method he/she has little understanding of it.

Relative to IE-APC, MP-APC can be implemented using the well-tested and widely available packages/functions from the free software R. In addition to facilitating programing and statistical computing, this advantage will allow researchers in middle- and low-income countries with limited sources to use the powerful APC modeling method in advancing their research to promote global health and epidemiology. To facilitate application of the MP-APC modeling method, in the Appendix, a set of R programming codes is provided for use.

It is worth mentioning that the MP-APC method provides a method for us to obtain an unique solutions for a constructed APC model, this does not mean that the nonidentifiability of the APC model has been solved. It is likely a solution obtained using the MP-APC modeling may be biased in some special conditions when a large number of information carried by the missed column cannot be represented by the rest of the data.

Appendix: R Program for MP-APC

```
### 1. Get the data in Table 2.3 from O'Brian, page 33:
# Note: a. data should be in .csv format
#       b. The 1st col is the "Age"
#       c. The rest cols are the mortality rates by "period"
dd = read.csv("table2.3.csv", row.names="Age",header=T)
# get the data dimension
dat.dim = dim(dd); a = dat.dim[1];a; p = dat.dim[2];p;
# age/period
# make the y-vector corresponding to the parms
y = matrix(t(as.matrix(dd)), ncol=1)
# log-transformation to the mortality rate
y = log(y); nobs = length(y)
# Call the apcmat to make the parameters with constraints
source("apc_fun.r")
xmat = apcmat(a, p); nparm = dim(xmat)[2]
### 2. MP now #####
library(MASS)
# parm estimates
estparm = ginv(t(xmat)%*%xmat)%*%t(xmat)%*%y
# calculate the parm estimates for the last effects
muhat = estparm[1]; alphahat1=estparm[2:a];
betahat1=estparm[(a+1):(a+p-1)];gammahat1=estparm[(a+p):
(2*a+2*p-3)]
alphahat = c(alphahat1, -sum(alphahat1))
betahat  = c(betahat1,-sum(betahat1))
gammahat = c(gammahat1,-sum(gammahat1))
# put all the parm together for MP-APC
estparm.vec = c(muhat, alphahat,betahat,gammahat)
round(estparm.vec,4) # compare this to Table 2.5 at page 37

############################################
## The subroutine function of "apc_fun.r"
apcmat <- function(a, p){
## matrix for APC model, see Fu (1998)
    alpha <- rbind(diag(rep(1, a - 1)), rep(-1, a - 1))
    beta <- rbind(diag(rep(1, p - 1)), rep(-1, p - 1))
    gamma <- rbind(diag(rep(1, a + p - 2)), rep(-1, a + p - 2))
    x <- rep(0, 2 * (a + p) - 3)
    for(i in 1:a) {
        for(j in 1:p) {
            rr <- c(1, alpha[i, ], beta[j, ], gamma[a - i + j, ])
            x <- rbind(x, rr)
        }
    }
    x <- x[-1, ]
    x
}    # end of "apcmat"
```

References

Carstensen, B. (2007). Age-period-cohort models for the Lexis diagram. *Statistics in Medicine, 26*(15), 3018–3045. https://doi.org/10.1002/sim.2764

Chang, J., Li, B., Li, J., & Sun, Y. (2017). The effects of age, period, and cohort on mortality from ischemic heart disease in China. *International Journal of Environmental Research and Public Health, 14*(1), 50. https://doi.org/10.3390/ijerph14010050

Chen, D., & Chen, X. (2015). Solving probabilistic discrete event systems with Moore–Penrose generalized inverse matrix method to extract longitudinal characteristics from cross-sectional survey data. In D. Chen & J. Wilson (Eds.), *Innovative statistical methods for public health data* (pp. 81–94). Springer.

Chen, X., Sun, Y., Li, Z., Yu, B., Gao, G., & Wang, P. (2019). Historical trends in suicide risk for the residents of mainland China: APC modeling of the archived national suicide mortality rates during 1987-2012. *Social Psychiatry and Psychiatric Epidemiology, 54*(1), 99–110. https://doi.org/10.1007/s00127-018-1593-z

Chen, X., & Wang, P. G. (2014). Social change and national health dynamics in China. *Chinese Journal of Population Science (in Chinese), 2*, 63–73.

Chen, X., Yu, B., & Chen, D. G. (2018). Probabilistic discrete event systems modeling of nonlinear transitions between electronic and combustible cigarette smoking with the 2014 National Youth Tobacco Survey Data. *Nonlinear Dynamics, Psychology, and Life Sciences, 22*(3), 289–312.

Chung, R. Y., Yip, B. H., Chan, S. S., & Wong, S. Y. (2016). Cohort effects of suicide mortality are sex specific in the rapidly developed Hong Kong Chinese population, 1976-2010. *Depression and Anxiety, 33*(6), 558–566. https://doi.org/10.1002/da.22431

Clayton, D., & Schifflers, E. (1987a). Models for temporal variation in cancer rates. I: Age-period and age-cohort models. *Statistics in Medicine, 6*(4), 449–467.

Clayton, D., & Schifflers, E. (1987b). Models for temporal variation in cancer rates. II: Age-period-cohort models. *Statistics in Medicine, 6*(4), 469–481.

Comstock, G. W. (1995). Re: "The age of selection of mortality from tuberculosis in successive decades". *American Journal of Epidemiology, 141*(8), 790.

Fienberg, S. E., & Mason, W. M. (1979). Identification and estimation of age-period-cohort models in the analysis of discrete archival data. *Sociological Methodology, 10*(1979), 1–67.

Frost, W. H. (1939). The age selection of mortality from tuberculosis in successive decades. 1939. *American Journal of Hygiene, 30*, 91–96. (Reprinted in Am J Epidemiol 1995; 11141: 11994–11999).

Golub, G. H., & Reinsch, C. (1970). Singular value decomposition and least squares solutions. *Numerische Mathematik, 14*(5), 403–420. https://doi.org/10.1007/Bf02163027

Holford, T. R. (1991). Understanding the effects of age, period, and cohort on incidence and mortality rates. *Annual Review of Public Health, 12*, 425–457. https://doi.org/10.1146/annurev.pu.12.050191.002233

Hu, X., Chen, X., Cook, R. L., Chen, D. G., & Okafor, C. (2016). Modeling drinking behavior progression in youth with cross-sectional data: Solving an under-identified probabilistic discrete event system. *Current HIV Research, 14*(2), 93–100.

Li, Z., Wang, P. G., Gao, G., Xu, C. L., & Chen, X. G. (2016). Age-period-cohort analysis of infectious disease mortality in urban-rural China, 1990-2010. *International Journal for Equity in Health, 15*, 55. https://doi.org/10.1186/s12939-016-0343-7

Luo, L. Y. (2013). Assessing validity and application scope of the intrinsic estimator approach to the age-period-cohort problem. *Demography, 50*(6), 1945–1967. https://doi.org/10.1007/s13524-013-0243-z

Mason, K. O., & Winsboro, H. (1973). Some methodological issues in cohort analysis of archival data. *American Sociological Review, 38*(2), 242–258. https://doi.org/10.2307/2094398

Moore, E. H., & Barnard, R. W. (1935). *General analysis Part I*. Philadelphia: The American Philosophical Society.

O'Brien, R. M. (2015). *Age-Period-Cohort models: Approaches and analysis with aggregate data*. Boca Raton, FL: Chapman & Hall/CRC.

Penrose, R. A. (1955). Generalized inverse for matrices. *Proceedings of the Cambridge Philosophical Society, 51*, 406–413.

Robertson, C., & Boyle, P. (1998). Age-period-cohort analysis of chronic disease rates. I: Modelling approach. *Statistics in Medicine, 17*(12), 1305–1323. https://doi.org/10.1002/(Sici)1097-0258(19980630)17:12<1305::Aid-Sim853>3.0.Co;2-W

Wang, Z. K., Hu, S. B., Sang, S. P., Luo, L. S., & Yu, C. H. (2017). Age-period-cohort analysis of stroke mortality in China: Data from the Global Burden of Disease Study 2013. *Stroke, 48*(2), 271–275. https://doi.org/10.1161/Strokeaha.116.015031

Yang, Y. (2008). Trends in US adult chronic disease mortality, 1960-1999: Age, period, and cohort variations. *Demography, 45*(2), 387–416. https://doi.org/10.1353/Dem.0.0000

Yang, Y., Fu, W. J. J., & Land, K. C. (2004). A methodological comparison of age-period-cohort models: The intrinsic estimator and conventional generalized linear models. *Sociological Methodology, 34*, 75–110. https://doi.org/10.1111/j.0081-1750.2004.00148.x

Yang, Y., & Land, K. C. (2013). *Age-Period-Cohort analysis: New models, methods, and empirical applications*. Chapman & Hall/CRC.

Yang, Y., Schulhofer-Wohl, S., Fu, W. J., & Land, K. C. (2008). The intrinsic estimator for Age-Period-Cohort analysis: What it is and how to use it. *American Journal of Sociology, 113*(6), 1697–1736.

Yu, B., Chen, X. G., & Wang, Y. (2018). Dynamic transitions between marijuana use and cigarette smoking among US adolescents and emerging adults. *American Journal of Drug and Alcohol Abuse, 44*(4), 452–462. https://doi.org/10.1080/00952990.2018.1434535

Chapter 11
Mixed Effects Modeling of Multi-site Data-Health Behaviors Among Adolescents in Hong Kong, Macao, Taipei, Wuhan and Zhuhai

Xinguang Chen

Abstract An important approach for global health and epidemiology research is to collect and use data from multiple study-sites within one or between various cultures to address high impact medical and health issues. When multisite data are used, it is challenge to deal with data heterogeneity, since such heterogeneity cannot be efficiently addressed using conventional multivariate regression methods. In this chapter, we describe application of mixed effects modeling, a statistical method designated for analyzing longitudinal trials, in analyzing cross-sectional multisite data. We demonstrate the application using data collected among middle and high school students in five Chinese cities (n = 13,950), including Hong Kong, Macau, Taipei, Wuhan, and Zhuhai. Data for lifestyle (sedentary, dietary, physical activity) and addictive behaviors (cigarette smoking, alcohol consumption and participation in gamble) were analyzed as outcomes. Factors at the individual and contextual level, as well as interventions between the two were associated with the outcome variables. Findings of this study indicate that although sharing a similar mainstream Chinese culture, these adolescent participants were significantly different from each other with regard to engagement in health-related behavior and the differences were associated with both individual- and contextual-level factors.

Keywords Mixed effects modeling · Cross-cultural research · Global health · Adolescent health · Lifestyle factors · Addictive behaviors

---

X. Chen (✉)
Department of Epidemiology, College of Public Health and Health Professions, College of Medicine, University of Florida, Gainesville, FL, USA

Global Health Institute, Wuhan University, Wuhan, China
e-mail: jimax.chen@ufl.edu

X. Chen, (Din) D.-G. Chen (eds.), *Statistical Methods for Global Health and Epidemiology*, ICSA Book Series in Statistics,
https://doi.org/10.1007/978-3-030-35260-8_11

11.1 Introduction

Rapid globalization since the last century presents a challenge to today's health problems for all people across the globe (Blum & Nelson-Mmari, 2004; Woodward, Drager, Beaglehole, & Lipson, 2001; Yu, Chen, & Li, 2014). It is challenge for many of us to adapt to the rapid economic and social changes along with the globalization (Labonte, Mohindra, & Schrecker, 2011; Martens, Akin, Maud, & Mohsin, 2010; Taylor, 2009). The unevenly-paced development, a major driving force for population migration, leads to health disparities not only among countries across the globe but also across different regions within a country (Charlson et al., 2015; Lopez, Mathers, Ezzati, Jamison, & Murray, 2006; Walker, Mcgee, & Druss, 2015). The unevenly-paced development also leads to increased frequency of traveling and large-scale population migration, while rapid advancement in technologies gives people more options to adopt different cultures and lifestyles. In addition to accelerating the spread of infectious diseases such as HIV/AIDS, tuberculosis, and Dengue (Cain, Benoit, Winston, & Mac Kenzie, 2008; Chen, Yu, Zhou, et al., 2015; Fredericks & Fernandez-Sesma, 2014), globalization and population migration put migrants under stress (Chen, Yu, Gong, Zeng, & MacDonell, 2015; Hertz, 1993; Yu et al., 2019) and make more people adopt unhealthy lifestyles, including reductions in physical activities, increases in unhealthy diet with more calories and less vegetables and fruits, increases in abuse of internet, tobacco, alcohol, and illicit drugs (Chen, Unger, Cruz, & Johnson, 1999; Gil, Wagner, & Vega, 2000; McLeod, Buscemi, & Bohnert, 2016). Although many of us may already be aware that it is unwise to *risk health for money*, but we often forget health. Evidence from empirical research study is needed to inform all individuals and the society as a whole to make wise choices for healthy life.

Despite numerous challenges, globalization also provides opportunities to address these challenges. The rapid economic and technological development make it possible for researchers to assess medical, health, and behavioral problems across different cultures and countries distant apart (Sperber, 2009). For example, many researchers from the World Health Organization and the United States have conducted collaborative international and global studies to understand tobacco use and to test and implement evidence-based intervention programs for tobacco use prevention and cessation (Global Youth Tobacco Survey Collaborating Group, 2003; Warren, Jones, Eriksen, Asma, and Global Tobacco Surveillance System (GTSS) Collaborative Group, 2006; Yach, 2014). In addition to healthy lifestyles, collective effort for international and global research, intervention and control of the HIV/AIDS epidemic becomes a mainstream in global health and epidemiology (Decker et al., 2014; Gouws, Cuchi, and International Collaboration on Estimating HIV Incidence by Modes of Transmission, 2012; Mathers et al., 2010).

Globalization also makes it possible to conduct global epidemiological research without traveling to different countries. One consequence from globalization is that it brings people from different cultures, regions and countries together in one place. Colleges and universities with international students represent best examples in favor of conducting global health research without traveling. International students, particularly graduate students bring with them much of their native culture, beliefs, and lifestyles. Data collected from them provide a very useful source for epidemiology and global health research. This approach has been widely used in studing stress, depression, smoking, dietary factors, and physical activities with a cross-cultural and global perspective (Haase, Steptoe, Sallis, & Wardle, 2004; Steptoe et al., 2002; Wang & Mallinckrodt, 2006).

Industrial zones in both developed and developing countries present another example for international and global health research without traveling. In these settings, data can be collected among people come from multiple countries who join the workforce in one location. Capitalizing on this advantage, researchers can investigate medical and health issues related to population migration (such as vulnerability to poor health, tuberculosis, HIV spreading and control, and migration stress) with a cross-cultural/country data without cross-country traveling (Chen, Yu, Zhou, et al., 2015; Jia et al., 2008; Organista et al., 2013; Quesada, Hart, & Bourgois, 2011).

11.2 Methodology Challenge and Alternatives

Relative to commonly reported studies, research with a global focus must deal with data heterogeneity—data for participants coming from different countries and places with greater between-group difference than within group difference. In this case, using conventional statistical methods designated for homogenous samples will lead to false conclusions. Therefore, the commonly used statistical methods such as student t-test, ANOVA, linear correlation and regression will no longer be appropriate. Fortunately, there is an alternative—the mixed effects modeling method. This advanced statistical method was originally devised for analyzing multi-center randomized controlled trials with longitudinal data; and it can be adopted to analyze multi-site cross-sectional data collected among participants from different countries and places.

11.2.1 Heterogeneity Data for Global Health Research

A study with data collected from participants in different cultures, countries and/or regions is somewhat like a natural experimental design to examine medical and health issues with a cross-cultural or global perspective. For example, by comparing women living in Japan with Japanese American women who migrated to or born in the United States, one can examine the role of genetic factors, diet and lifestyle factors for breast cancer (Severson, Nomura, Grove, & Stemmermann, 1989). The advantage of such design is obvious. It provides an ideal approach for researchers to exam the complex genetic, environmental factors and interactions between the two; and findings from such research will provide unique data supporting culturally appropriate cancer prevention interventions.

However, a "side-effect" from this cross-country approach is that data collected from a cross-country sample are highly heterogeneous. Relative to data collected from a homogenous sample of one country (site), the between-site variance in a study variable is often greater than the within-site variance (McGraw & Wong, 1996; Verbeke & Lesaffre, 1996). This data heterogeneity, if not considered, will result in underestimate of variance and inflation of type I error, leading to false statistical inferential conclusion (Bonett, 2002; Verbeke & Lesaffre, 1996). That is, *a non-significant result could be mistakenly concluded as statistically significant.*

11.2.2 Understand Multi-site and Multi-level Data

With a multi-site (i.e., cities, states, or countries) design, data can be collected at both the individual participant level and the study site-level. Table 11.1 presents a data structure for a five-city study project we used in this chapter (detailed in next section). As shown in the table, data will be collected among middle and high school students from five Chinese cities, Hong Kong, Macau, Taipei, Wuhan and Zhuhai. With the design we can collect data for five individual participating cities: the site-level data **Xj** (j = 1, 2,..., 5). Any data in all J study cites that may affect the study problems can be collected. Typical data include population size, geographic area, economy, healthcare systems, physicians, nurses, hospital beds, and health expenditure. We listed two variables (population and per capita GDP) as an example in the table. In addition to describing the study site, these variables can be used as predictors in statistical analysis for other study purposes.

When site-level data are not available, an alternative approach is to calculate the mean of the individual level data as a proxy of the site-level measure. The calculated mean provides an unbiased estimate for the site if individual participants of a site are randomly selected. For example, the amount of money students spend per week

Table 11.1 Multi-site two-level data structure for a five-city school-based survey study

Site/variable	Hong Kong J = 1	Macau J = 2	Taipei J = 3	Wuhan J = 4	Zhuhai J = 5
Site level (Xj)					
Population					
Per capita GDP					
...					
Individual level (Xij)					
Age					
Sex					
Grade					
Smoking					
...					

can be estimated using data collected from individual participants of a city and used as a proxy of the site-level socioeconomic status.

In addition to site-level data, individual-level data are collected. As shown also in Table 11.1, individual-level data are expressed using **X**ij for individual participant i (i = 1, 2, ..., nj) in site j (j = 1, 2, ..., 5). Obviously, the individual participant-level data are simply an aggregation of a single-site study to a multi-site study by adding more sites with the same or similar variables across all sites. In practice, individual sites with slightly different variables can be used to accommodate actual situations and different needs. More details about multi-site study with slightly different variables are discussed in Chap. 5 in this book.

11.3 A Study Across Five Chinese Cities: An Example

11.3.1 Purposes and Rational

Differences between a developing and a developed country (such as China and United States) may provide unique data to assess the impact of economic and technological factors on the risk of health and diseases (Strong et al., 2015; Turbin et al., 2006; Yoshino et al., 2006). However, results from cross-country comparisons can be confounded by differences in the mainstream cultures if participants are recruited from countries with different cultural traditions and practices (Dummer & Cook, 2008; Michaud, Blum, & Slap, 2001; Weinehall et al., 2001). To understand the impact of contextual factors on health behavior while avoid confounding by mainstream cultures, this example study take another approach, comparing participants from different cities but share a similar mainstream culture.

The study was a part of the Chinese Student Health Project (CSHP), and it was conducted by a group of researchers from the United States and the five Chinese cities, including Hong Kong, Macau, Taipei, Zhuhai and Wuhan (Chen et al., 2016). A fundamental hypothesis of this project is that people living in these five cities share the mainstream Chinese culture but the five cities are located in different geographic regions (Fig. 11.1) with different subcultures and large variations in socioeconomic development (Table 11.1)—the contextual factors. Therefore, a research study with such a cross-Chinese city design will enable researchers to investigate the impact of contextual factors such as economic growth and technological development and their interaction with individual-level factors on many health outcomes, including health related behaviors in adolescents; but with little or no worry about confounding effect from differences in the mainstream culture.

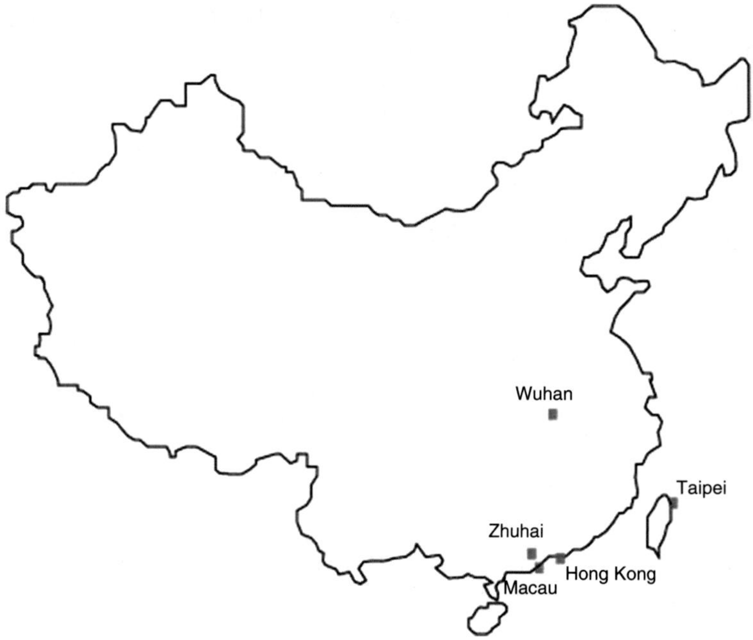

Fig. 11.1 Location of the five study sites

11.3.2 Participants and Procedure

The study targeted students in grades 7 through 9. The participants were selected randomly using the following schedule. A project leader in each participating city first selected schools that agreed to participate. From each school agreed to participate, one single grade was selected using the random digits method, and all classes of the selected grade in the school were invited to participate. The study was approved by IRB in the corresponding cities. Informed consents were first obtained from the schools in which they acted as loco parentis.

The paper-pencil survey was administered in classroom settings. All students were well-informed that their participation in the survey was voluntary. The students were also informed that they had the rights not to participate and to quit during any time of the survey. Data were collected using the Chinese Students Health Survey Questionnaire (CSHSQ). This questionnaire was developed by the CSHP investigators based on previous studies among Chinese youth in China and the United States (Chen et al., 2006; Jessor, 1992) and survey questions used in the Global School-based Student Health Survey (Centers for Disease Control and Prevention & World Health Organization, 2011).

Since students in the five Chinese cities speak different dialects, the CSHSQ was developed in two steps. Step 1, a master copy of the questionnaire was developed by the leading investigators of the CSHP, together with all other investigators through several cycles of a draft-revision to obtain the finalized copy. Step 2, investigators at individual participation sites created their own questionnaire in local dialect by rewording/translating the survey questions from the master copy. The finalized CSHSQ contains 50 questions with a brief introduction sheet to the survey. The survey can be completed in approximately 15–20 min for a typical middle and high school student.

11.3.3 Measurement of Lifestyle Behavior

Three lifestyle behaviors were measures: (1) *Time spent on sitting position.* This variable was assessed using the question: "In general, how much time do you often used to watch TV, play electronic games, chatting with friends or any other sedentary activities (e.g., reading, play cards, etc.)?" Answer options were: <1 h, 1–2, 3–4, 5–6, 7–8, and 8 or more hours per day. A student was coded as sedentary if he/she reported spending 3 or more hours on siting position in a day. (2) *Frequency of eating vegetables.* This variable was assessed using the question: "Please recall the past 30 days. How many times do you often have vegetables in a day, including salad and other vegetables?" Answer options were: none, <1 time a day, once a day, twice a day, 3 times a day, 4 times a day, and 5 or more times a day. A student was coded as eating vegetables if he/she reported having had vegetables at least once daily. (3) *Frequency of having fruits.* This variable was assessed using the question: "Please recall the past 30 days. How many times do you have fruits in a day, including apples, oranges, etc.?" Answer options were: none, <1 time a day, once a day, twice a day, 3 times a day, 4 times a day, and 5 or more times a day. Likewise, a student was coded as having fruits if he/she reported having had fruits at least once daily.

11.3.4 Measurement of Addictive Behaviors

Three addictive behaviors were measured. (1) Alcohol consumption. This variable was assessed using the question: "In the past 30 days, on how many days did you drink at least one couple of alcoholic beverage?" (Answer options were: 0, 1–2 days, 3–5 days, 6–9 days, 10–19, days, 20–29 days, and every day). Students who reported having a drink at least on one day in the past 30 days were coded as a drinker. (2) Cigarette smoking. This variable was assessed using the question: "In the past 30 days, on how many days did you smoke cigarette?" (Answer options: Never smoked, no smoking in the past 30 days, smoked in 1–2 days, in 3–5 days, 6–9 days, 10–19 days, 20–29 days, daily). Students who reported having smoked at least on one day were coded as a smoker. (3) Ever participation in gambling. This variable was assessed using the question: "How many times have you participated in gambling in your whole life?" (Answer options were: 0 times, 1–2 times, 3–9 times, 10 times or more). Students who reported having participated at least one to two times were coded as ever participated in gambling.

11.3.5 Measurement of Student-Level Factors

Demographic factors were age (in years), gender (male/females), school performances (below average, average and above average, self-report), parental monitoring (scale scores), and parental education (from no formal education to college or above, student reported). Perceived parental monitoring was assessed using a 3-item instrument with 5-point Likert scale (alpha = 0.67) (Centers for Disease Control and Prevention & World Health Organization, 2011; Lau, Chen, & Ren, 2012). Parental monitoring scores were calculated by adding up the scores for the three items such that higher scores meaning closer monitoring from parents as perceived by youth.

11.3.6 Measurement of Site-Level Factors

Three site-level factors were assessed, including total population (as measure of the scale of a city), per capita GDP (as a measure of economic development) and literacy rates (as a measure of education). Data for these variables were extracted from official statistics for the corresponding cities, up to, or close to the time period when the survey was conducted.

11.4 Statistical Analysis and Results

11.4.1 Data Analysis

As an example for analyzing multi-site study, the following statistical analysis was conducted. A descriptive analysis was conducted to summarize the sample, overall and by individual study site (i.e., the five participating cities). Following the sample description, prevalence rates of the six behavior measures were computed and compared among the five cities. Lastly, the variable time spent on siting position in predicting the outcome variables was analyzed using both linear regression and mixed effects modeling analyses. In the mixed effects modeling, intraclass correlation was calculated to assess the with- and between-site variance differences. Statistical analysis was conducted using the commercial software SAS version 9.4 (SAS Institute Inc., Cary, NC).

11.4.2 Study Site and Sample

The basic characteristics of the study sites and the samples by sites were presented in Table 11.2. There were substantial differences in per capita GDP and rate of illiteracy across the five study sites. Per capita GDP was USD $40,000 for Macau,

Table 11.2 Basic information for the five study sites and sample characteristics of the Chinese Student Health Survey, 2008–2009

Variables	Participation cities where students were sampled					Total n (%)
	Hong Kong n (%)	Macau n (%)	Taipei n (%)	Zhuhai n (%)	Wuhan n (%)	
Population (1000)[a]	7098	552	2618	1481	8100	–
Literacy rate[b]	93.5%	91.3%	96.1%	95.9%	93.9%	91.3–96.1%
GDP per capita[c]	$30,000	$40,000	$16,000	$10,000	$6000	
Sample size	6466 (46.4)	547 (3.9)	1782 (12.8)	1774 (12.7)	3381 (24.2)	13,950
Gender						
Male	3298 (51.0)	341 (62.3)	885 (49.7)	955 (53.8)	1812 (53.6)	7291 (52.3)
Female	3168 (49.0)	206 (37.7)	897 (50.3)	819 (46.2)	1569 (46.4)	6659 (47.7)
Age						
≤12	1826 (28.2)	152 (27.8)	65 (3.7)	15 (0.9)	549 (19.2)	2707 (19.4)
13	1824 (28.2)	173 (31.6)	500 (28.1)	93 (5.2)	1095 (32.4)	3685 (26.4)
14	2081 (32.2)	118 (21.6)	660 (37.0)	772 (43.5)	1060 (31.4)	4691 (33.6)
≥15	735 (11.4)	104 (19.0)	557 (31.3)	894 (50.4)	577 (17.1)	2867 (20.6)
Mean (SD)	13.3 (1.0)	13.3 (1.1)	14.0 (0.9)	14.4 (0.6)	13.5 (1.0)	13.6 (1.0)
P. monitoring, Mean (SD)	2.68 (0.96)	2.55 (1.00)	2.91 (0.95)	2.86 (1.03)	3.18 (1.14)	2.85 (1.04)
School grade						
>Average	1783 (17.8)	96 (18.0)	673 (37.9)	707 (40.0)	1370 (40.7)	4629 (33.4)
Average	2594 (40.4)	239 (44.8)	499 (28.1)	461 (26.1)	879 (26.1)	4672 (33.7)
<Average	2044 (31.8)	199 (37.3)	603 (34.0)	599 (33.9)	1115 (33.2)	4560 (32.9)

(continued)

Table 11.2 (continued)

Variables	Participation cities where students were sampled					Total n (%)
	Hong Kong n (%)	Macau n (%)	Taipei n (%)	Zhuhai n (%)	Wuhan n (%)	
Maternal edu.						
≤Primary	828 (12.8)	96 (17.7)	62 (3.5)	369 (20.9)	610 (18.1)	1965 (14.1)
Middle school	3333 (51.6)	237 (43.8)	923 (51.9)	742 (42.0)	1945 (57.6)	7180 (51.6)
≥College	672 (10.4)	20 (3.7)	614 (34.5)	393 (22.3)	379 (11.2)	2078 (14.9)
Don't know	1622 (25.1)	188 (34.8)	181 (10.2)	262 (14.8)	442 (13.9)	2695 (19.4)
Paternal edu.						
≤Primary	685 (10.6)	92 (17.0)	72 (4.0)	207 (11.7)	300 (8.9)	1356 (9.8)
Middle school	3110 (48.2)	191 (35.2)	796 (44.7)	769 (43.5)	2176 (64.5)	7042 (50.6)
≥College	856 (13.3)	27 (5.0)	719 (40.4)	537 (30.4)	498 (14.8)	2637 (19.0)
Don't know	1800 (27.9)	232 (42.8)	193 (10.8)	255 (14.4)	397 (11.8)	2877 (20.68)

[a]2010 Chinese census data, National Bureau of Statistics of China

[b]Data for Hong Kong, Macau and Taiwan are from CIA factbook 2010. Data for Zhuhai and Wuhan are from 2000 China census

[c]Data for Hong Kong and Macau are from World Bank 2009 database. Data for Taiwan is from IMF 2009. Wuhan and Zhuhai data is provided by National bureau of Statistics of China 2009. All rounded to 1000

the highest among the five study sites while the per capita GDP was only USD $6000 for Wuhan, the difference between the two was 6.7 times.

Data for a total of 13,950 students (52% male and 48% female) were included in the analysis. Among these participants, 6466 (46.4%) were from Hong Kong, 547 (3.9%) from Macau, 1782 (12.8%) from Taipei, 3381 (24.2%) from Wuhan, and 1774 (12.7%) from Zhuhai. Different sample sizes were used for different cities mainly because of the limitations of funds available for the research. Gender composition also differed across study sites with the largest difference for Macau (62.3% boys and 37.7% girls) and the smallest difference for Taipei (49.7% boys and 50.3% girls) and Hong Kong (51% boys and 49% girls). On average, participants were 13.6 (SD = 1.0) years of age and the mean age slightly different across study sites. More detailed data are presented in Table 11.2.

11.4.3 Prevalence of Life Style Variables

The age-standardized prevalence rates in Fig. 11.2 indicate that the percentage of participants in sedentary positions (yellow bars) for 3 or more hours per day was the highest for Hong Kong sample (75.2%), and the lowest for Wuhan sample (45.2%). For dietary behaviors, approximately 90% of students reported having had vegetables at least once daily (blue bars) and approximately 70% reported having had fruit at least once daily (green bars). The highest rates of vegetable and fruit intake were for youth in Taipei (94.9% for vegetables and 81.1% for fruits) while the lowest rates for youth in Macau (88.5% for vegetables and 65.7% for fruits).

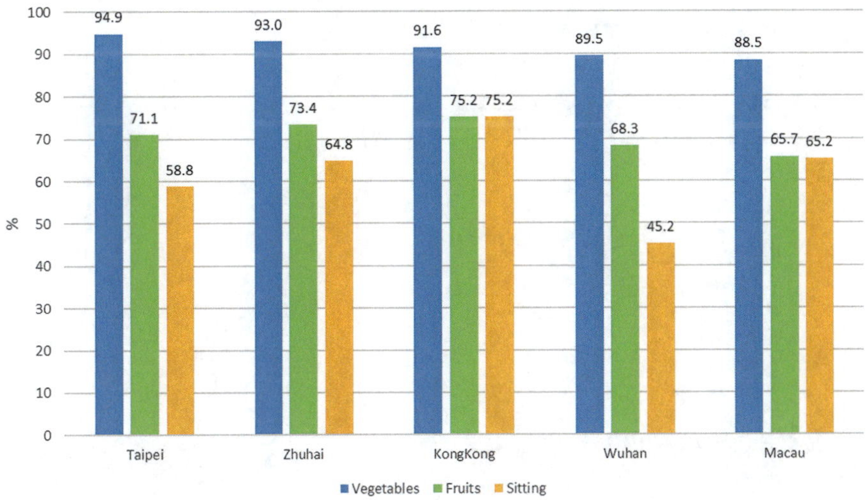

Fig. 11.2 Standardized prevalence rate of three lifestyle behaviors among students in Hong Kong, Macau, Taipei, Zhuhai and Wuhan

11.4.4 Prevalence of Addictive Behaviors

The age-standardized prevalence rates in Fig. 11.3 indicate that the percentage of youth used alcoholic beverage in the past month was the highest for youth in Hong Kong (39.5%), the lowest in Wuhan (23.2%), with other three cities in in between. The past 30-day smoking rate varied from 4 to 5% across the study sites except Macau where the rate was 9.8%, the highest among all five sites. The percentage of youth participation in gambling was the highest in Taipei (37.1%) and Hong Kong (35.9%) but not Macau, while the lowest was Wuhan (20.7%).

11.4.5 Intraclass Correlation for the Variable Time on Siting Position

To demonstrate on how to quantitatively assess the data heterogeneity, the intraclass correlation (ICC) was calculated. ICC represents the proportion of the variance explained by the group variable (city in this study) over the total variance. ICC was estimated by fitting the data to an empty mixed effect model (no predictors, see the SAS code below). With data in this study, the estimated ICC was 0.06 for the variable time on sitting position. It means that 6% of the total variance of the sitting time variable was explained by the between-city difference. This is a relatively small ICC, suggesting certain homogeneity among the five participating cities. This result appears reasonable since the five cities share the same mainstream Chinese culture.

SAS code for ICC calculation:

```
*EMPTY MODEL FOR ICC;
PROC MIXED DATA = A;
CLASS CITY;
MODEL SITHOUR = /SOLUTION;
RANDOM INTERCEPT/SUB=CITY;
RUN;
```

Covariance Parameter Estimates		
Cov Parm	Subject	Estimate
Intercept	CITY	0.1045
Residual		1.7204

ICC = 0.1045 / (0.1045+1.7204) = 0.06

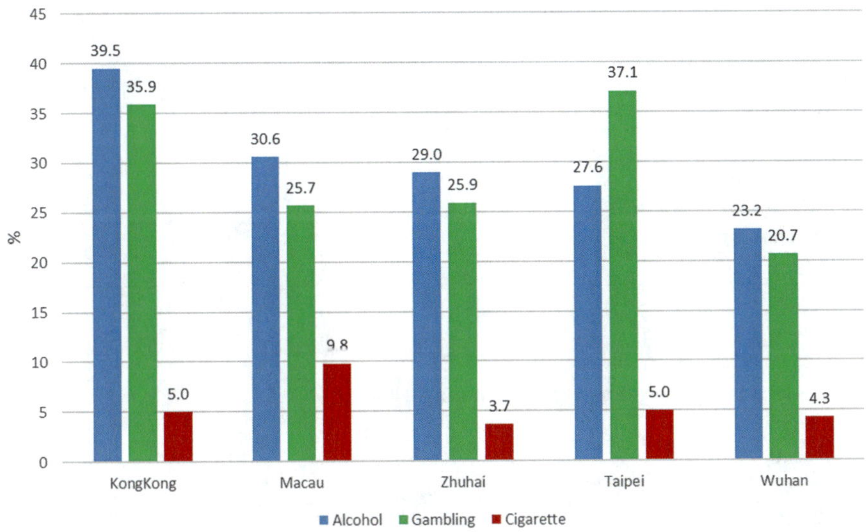

Fig. 11.3 Standardized prevalence rate of three addictive behaviors among students in Hong Kong, Macau, Taipei, Zhuhai and Wuhan

11.4.6 Results from Mixed Effects Model and Linear Regression

Results from the multilevel mixed effects modeling analysis are presented in second column of Table 11.3. Data in the table indicate that at the site level, higher GDP was positively associated with hours of sitting. At the individual level, age was positively associated with hours of sitting; self-rated school performance and perceived parental monitory each were negatively associated with hours of sitting.

Results in the mid-panel of Table 11.3 indicate significant interactions between the two individual levels factors (e.g., perceived parental monitory and self-rated school performance) and the five participation cities. For example, compared to students in Hong Kong, perceived paternal monitoring was associated with longer hours of sitting positions for students in Macau (regression coefficient = 0.1832, $p < 0.01$) and Wuhan (regression coefficient = 0.1213, $p < 0.01$), although parental monitoring overall was negatively associated with hours of sitting positions.

The third column of Table 11.3 presents the results from linear regression analysis in which city was included as a covariate. Similar results were found as the mixed effects model for most parts except some differences. In addition to the small magnitude change of the coefficients, the significance level has changed differed for several variables, including the city level variable population size, and individual level variables and the interaction term between school performance and city. We also compared the R square between the two models used in Table 11.3, and found

Table 11.3 Association of individual and city-level variables on *Time spending on siting position* among Chinese Students in Hong Kong, Macau, Taipei, Wuhan, and Zhuhai

Variables at city and student levels	Mixed effects model	Linear regression model
City level		
Population (million)	0.0333	0.0305**
Literacy rate (%)	0.1194	0.0544
GDP per capita ($10,000)	0.4278**	0.5008**
Individual student level		
Age (years)	0.0761**	0.0762**
If female	0.0286	0.0285
Perceived parental monitoring	−0.1911**	−0.1929**
Self-rated school performance	−0.0781**	−0.0800**
Cross-level interaction of parental monitoring with city		
Hong Kong	Ref	Ref
Macau	0.1832**	0.1852**
Taipei	0.0063	0.0106
Zhuhai	0.0499	0.0531
Wuhan	0.1213**	0.1227**
Cross-level interaction of school performance with city		
Hong Kong	Ref	Ref
Macau	−0.1558*	−0.1357
Taipei	−0.0387	−0.0347
Zhuhai	0.1657**	0.1691**
Wuhan	0.0229	0.0245
Data-model fit		
R^2	0.11	0.08

Results (Standard Regression Coefficients) from Multilevel Modeling Analysis and Linear Regression

Note: *p < 0.5 and **p < 0.01; Ref: Reference group

that the variance explained by the mixed effects model was higher than the linear regression model (0.11 vs. 0.08).

SAS Code for the results in Table 11.3:

```
*LINEAR MODEL;
PROC GLM DATA = A;
CLASS GENDER(REF='1') CITY(REF='1');
MODEL SITHOUR = POPU LITERACY GDP AGE GENDER MONSCALE SCORE MONSCALE*CITY SCORE*CITY CITY/SOLUTION;
RUN;


*MIXED EFFECTS MODEL;
PROC MIXED DATA = A COVTEST;
CLASS CITY(REF='1');
MODEL SITHOUR  =POPU LITERACY GDP AGE GENDER MONSCALE SCORE MONSCALE*CITY SCORE *CITY /SOLUTION;
RANDOM INTERCEPT /SUBJECT = CITY;
RUN;
```

11.5 Discussion and Conclusions

In this chapter, we demonstrated the significance to conduct cross-culture and multi-site studies in addressing significant medical and public health issues in global health and epidemiology. We introduced the multilevel mixed effects method to analysis multisite studies using a five-city project as an example. This example project collected cross-sectional data in Hong Kong, Macau, Taipei, Zhuhai, and Wuhan with a total sample size of 13,950 students in grades 7–9. In addition to handling the multisite design for correct variance estimation and statistical inference, factors at the students and city level as well as the interaction between the two are analyzed to assess their impact on health behaviors among these students.

11.5.1 Significance of the Mixed Effects Modeling Methods

Multisite cross-cultural design is a powerful and useful approach for global health and epidemiology. In addition to influential factors at the individual, contextual factors characterizing different communities, cities, states and countries can be examined. Furthermore, it provide a tool to investigate the interactions between the individual and contextual level factors. As we demonstrated in this study, factors for individual students (i.e., age, gender, perceived parental monitoring) and participating cities (i.e., population size, GDP) as well as the interactions for some variables between the two levels were modeled simultaneously.

With a multi-site design, the mixed effects modeling method provides one of the most relevant approaches for data analysis to address many epidemiological and global health issues. Although the method was originate for analyzing longitudinal data, it can be used to handle data collected using cross-sectional designs. The big threat to the internal validity of a study with multi-site design is ICC. In a multisite study, the between-study site variance is often greater than the within-study site variance, showing as an increase in ICC. Large ICC will result in inflated variance, leading to invalid statistical inference if data from multisite studies are analyzed using methods that cannot handle this design effect such as the student t-test, chi-square test, correlation and regression analyses. In addition to handling the design effect for internal validity, the mixed effects modeling analysis provide an approach to assess cross-level interactions.

11.5.2 Implications of the Findings from This Study

Findings of this study provide useful information to understand the difference in adolescent health behaviors and the influential factors. Previous studies on Chinese adolescent health behaviors were all individually undertaken in the Mainland China

(Chen et al., 2006; Tian, Zhang, & Qian, 2007; Unger et al., 2001; Xing, Ji, & Zhang, 2006), Taiwan (Chen, Tang, & Huang, 2008; Wang et al., 2005; Yeh, Chiang, & Huang, 2006), Hong Kong (Lai, Ho, & Lam, 2004; Lau & Kan, 2010; Lee, Tsang, Lee, & To, 2001), and Macau (Wong, 2010). This study was the first to document health behaviors among Chinese youth across different cities, informing further etiological and intervention research. Age- and gender-standardized rates indicate that sedentary behaviors are most prevalent among students in Hong Kong, such as watching TV, playing games, and the lowest for students in Wuhan. The highest rate of vegetable and fruit consumption is for students in Taipei and the lowest rate for youth in Macau.

With regard to addictive behaviors, the standardized prevalence rates of past 30-day alcohol consumption was the highest among students in Hong Kong and the lowest in Wuhan; the standardized 30-day smoking rate was the highest for students in Macau and the lowest was for Zhuhai; and the rate of participation in gambling was the highest for students in Taipei and Hong Kong and the lowest for students in Wuhan.

Findings of this study showed the impact of city-level factors. The scale of a city (as measured with population size) was associated with higher frequencies of vegetable consumption; literacy rates were associated with longer hours of sitting position (e.g. playing electronic games or surfing the internet) and higher rates of participation in gambling; higher per capita GDP was associated with longer sitting hours and more frequent of alcohol use. An increase in sedentary behavior may be attributable to increased urbanization with a high population density, lack of public leisure facilities, high-density traffic and population (Centers for Disease Control and Prevention & World Health Organization, 2011). Besides, GDP growth and rise of information and communications technology have significantly changed people's lifestyles. A high prevalence of public Wi-Fi internet service and increasing affordability of home computer with internet connection may contribute to longer sitting hours as people can accomplish their daily work online (like online shopping) and play online games for leisure (Centers for Disease Control and Prevention & World Health Organization, 2011; Mythily, Qiu, & Winslow, 2008). The GDP growth also corresponds to people's daily consumption patterns (like food and alcohol consumption) (Centers for Disease Control and Prevention & World Health Organization, 2011; Li & Zhou-ping, 2012). Data derived from the city-level findings are of great significance for public health planning and decision making.

Findings of this study also indicate the significance of factors at the individual student level. Overall, perceived parental monitoring was consistently associated with protective behaviors, including reductions in sitting position, increases in frequency of vegetable and fruit intake, declines in cigarette smoking, alcohol drinking and gambling. However, the perceived parental monitoring-student behavior associations varied substantially across the five study sites. Relative to Hong Kong, the association was stronger for students in other sites with regard to lifestyle and addictive behaviors, except vegetable and fruit consumption in Macau.

Likewise, overall students self-rated school performance was positively associated with long-hour sitting position, vegetables and fruit consumption, and negatively associated with cigarette smoking and gambling. However, when compared with Hong Kong, students with better school performance in Macau were less likely to be in sitting position for longer time but more likely to consume more fruits; while a reverse pattern existed for students in Wuhan. In the aspect of addictive behaviors, the associations between student's school performance and their involvement in cigarette smoking and gambling in Wuhan were weak when comparing with Hong Kong.

Acknowledgements Data used as example in this chapter are part of the Chinese Student Health project that was carried out with site project leaders in five cities (in alphabetic order): (1) Hong Kong: Ming Yue Kan from Hong Kong Institute of Education and Maggie Lau from City University of Hong Kong; (2) Macau: Lue Li from Macau Polytechnic Institute; (3) Taipei: I-Chyun Chiang from Yuanpei University and Yin-Jin Hu from National Taiwan Normal University; (4) Wuhan: Jie Gong from Wuhan Center for Disease Prevention and control; and (5) Zhuhai: King-Lun Ngok from Sun Yat-Sen University of Guangzhou.

This study was co-funded by the Wuhan Center for Disease Prevention and Control; Hong Kong Centraline Charity Fund, the 2010 New Century Talents Scholarship from the Chinese Ministry of Education to Sun Yat-Sen University, Taiwan Department of Health Bureau of Health Promotion, and Wayne State University School of Medicine, USA.

Approvals were obtained from all the participation agencies before the project was implemented. The researchers had no conflict of interest associated with the project.

References

Blum, R. W., & Nelson-Mmari, K. (2004). The health of young people in a global context. *The Journal of Adolescent Health, 35*(5), 402–418. https://doi.org/10.1016/j.jadohealth.2003.10.007

Bonett, D. G. (2002). Sample size requirements for estimating intraclass correlations with desired precision. *Statistics in Medicine, 21*(9), 1331–1335. https://doi.org/10.1002/sim.1108

Cain, K. P., Benoit, S. R., Winston, C. A., & Mac Kenzie, W. R. (2008). Tuberculosis among foreign-born persons in the United States. *JAMA-Journal of the American Medical Association, 300*(4), 405–412. https://doi.org/10.1001/jama.300.4.405

Centers for Disease Control and Prevention & World Health Organization. (2011). *Global school-based student health survey (GSHS).* Atlanta and Geneva: Centers for Disease Control and Prevention, and World Health Organization. Retrieved January 3, 2011, from http://www.cdc.gov/gshs/questionnaire/index.htm

Charlson, F. J., Baxter, A. J., Dua, T., Degenhardt, L., Whiteford, H. A., & Vos, T. (2015). Excess mortality from mental, neurological and substance use disorders in the Global Burden of Disease Study 2010. *Epidemiology and Psychiatric Sciences, 24*(2), 121–140. https://doi.org/10.1017/S2045796014000687

Chen, C. Y., Tang, G. M., & Huang, S. L. (2008). Transition from alcohol to other drugs among adolescents in Taiwan: The first drinking context matters. *Journal of Studies on Alcohol and Drugs, 69*(3), 378.

Chen, X., Lau, M., Kan, M. Y., Chiang, I. C., Hu, Y. J., Gong, J., . . . Ngok, K. L. (2016). Lifestyle and addictive behaviors among Chinese adolescents in Hong Kong, Macau, Taipei, Wuhan, and Zhuhai—A first cross-subculture assessment. *International Journal of Behavioral Medicine, 23*(5), 561–570. https://doi.org/10.1007/s12529-016-9548-9

Chen, X., Unger, J. B., Cruz, T. B., & Johnson, C. A. (1999). Smoking patterns of Asian-American youth in California and their relationship with acculturation. *Journal of Adolescent Health, 24*(5), 321–328. https://doi.org/10.1016/S1054-139x(98)00118-9

Chen, X., Yu, B., Gong, J., Zeng, J., & MacDonell, K. K. (2015). The Domestic Migration Stress Questionnaire (DMSQ): Development and psychometric assessment. *Journal of Social Science Studies, 2*(2), 117–133.

Chen, X., Yu, B., Zhou, D. J., Zhou, W., Gong, J., Li, S. Y., & Stanton, B. (2015). A Comparison of the number of men who have sex with men among rural-to-urban migrants with non-migrant rural and urban residents in Wuhan, China: A GIS/GPS-assisted random sample survey study. *PLoS One, 10*(8), e0134712. https://doi.org/10.1371/journal.pone.0134712

Chen, X., Stanton, B., Fang, X., Li, X., Lin, D., Zhang, J., ... Yang, H. (2006). Perceived smoking norms, socioenvironmental factors, personal attitudes and adolescent smoking in China: A mediation analysis with longitudinal data. *The Journal of Adolescent Health, 38*(4), 359–368.

Decker, M. R., Peitzmeier, S., Olumide, A., Acharya, R., Ojengbede, O., Covarrubias, L., ... Brahmbhatt, H. (2014). Prevalence and health impact of intimate partner violence and non-partner sexual violence among female adolescents aged 15-19 years in vulnerable urban environments: A multi-country study. *Journal of Adolescent Health, 55*(6), S58–S67. https://doi.org/10.1016/j.jadohealth.2014.08.022

Dummer, T. J., & Cook, I. G. (2008). Health in China and India: A cross-country comparison in a context of rapid globalisation. *Social Science & Medicine, 67*(4), 590–605. https://doi.org/10.1016/j.socscimed.2008.04.019

Fredericks, A. C., & Fernandez-Sesma, A. (2014). The burden of dengue and chikungunya worldwide: Implications for the southern United States and California. *Annals of Global Health, 80*(6), 466–475. https://doi.org/10.1016/j.aogh.2015.02.006

Gil, A. G., Wagner, E. F., & Vega, W. A. (2000). Acculturation familism, and alcohol use among Latino adolescent males: Longitudinal relations. *Journal of Community Psychology, 28*(4), 443–458. https://doi.org/10.1002/1520-6629(200007)28:4<443::Aid-Jcop6>3.0.Co;2-A

Global Youth Tobacco Survey Collaborating Group. (2003). Differences in worldwide tobacco use by gender: Findings from the global youth tobacco survey. *Journal of School Health, 73*(6), 207–215.

Gouws, E., Cuchi, P., & International Collaboration on Estimating HIV Incidence by Modes of Transmission. (2012). Focusing the HIV response through estimating the major modes of HIV transmission: A multi-country analysis. *Sexually Transmitted Infections, 88*, I76–I85. https://doi.org/10.1136/sextrans-2012-050719

Haase, A., Steptoe, A., Sallis, J. F., & Wardle, J. (2004). Leisure-time physical activity in university students from 23 countries: Associations with health beliefs, risk awareness, and national economic development. *Preventive Medicine, 39*(1), 182–190. https://doi.org/10.1016/j.ypmed.2004.01.028

Hertz, D. G. (1993). Bio-psycho-social consequences of migration stress—A multidimensional approach. *Israel Journal of Psychiatry and Related Sciences, 30*(4), 204–212.

Jessor, R. (1992). Reply—Risk behaviors in adolescence: A psychosocial framework for understanding and action. *Developmental Review, 12*, 374–390.

Jia, Z. W., Jia, X. W., Liu, Y. X., Dye, C., Chen, F., Chen, C. S., ... Liu, H. L. (2008). Spatial analysis of tuberculosis cases in migrants and permanent residents, Beijing, 2000-2006. *Emerging Infectious Diseases, 14*(9), 1413–1419. https://doi.org/10.3201/eid1409.071543

Labonte, R., Mohindra, K., & Schrecker, T. (2011). The growing impact of globalization for health and public health practice. *Annual Review of Public Health, 32*, 263–283. https://doi.org/10.1146/annurev-publhealth-031210-101225

Lai, M. K., Ho, S. Y., & Lam, T. H. (2004). Perceived peer smoking prevalence and its association with smoking behaviours and intentions in Hong Kong Chinese adolescents. *Addiction, 99*(9), 1195–1205. https://doi.org/10.1111/j.1360-0443.2004.00797.x

Lau, M., Chen, X., & Ren, Y. (2012). Increased risk of cigarette smoking among immigrant children and girls in Hong Kong: An emerging public health issue. *Journal of Community Health, 37*(1), 144–152. https://doi.org/10.1007/s10900-011-9428-9

Lau, M., & Kan, M. (2010). Prevalence and correlates of problem behaviors among adolescents in Hong Kong. *Asia-Pacific Journal of Public Health, 22*(3), 354–364.

Lee, A., Tsang, C. K., Lee, S., & To, C. (2001). A YRBS survey of youth risk behaviors at alternative high schools and mainstream high schools in Hong Kong. *Journal of School Health, 71*(9), 443–447.

Li, J. P., & Zhou-ping, S. G. (2012). Food consumption patterns and per capita calorie intake of China in the past three decades. *Journal of Food, Agriculture and Environment, 10*(2), 201–206.

Lopez, A. D., Mathers, C. D., Ezzati, M., Jamison, D. T., & Murray, C. J. L. (2006). Global and regional burden of disease and risk factors, 2001: Systematic analysis of population health data. *Lancet, 367*(9524), 1747–1757. https://doi.org/10.1016/S0140-6736(06)68770-9

Martens, P., Akin, S. M., Maud, H., & Mohsin, R. (2010). Is globalization healthy: A statistical indicator analysis of the impacts of globalization on health. *Globalization and Health, 6*, 16. https://doi.org/10.1186/1744-8603-6-16

Mathers, B. M., Degenhardt, L., Ali, H., Wiessing, L., Hickman, M., Mattick, R. P., ... 2009 Reference Group to the UN on HIV and Injecting Drug Use. (2010). HIV prevention, treatment, and care services for people who inject drugs: A systematic review of global, regional, and national coverage. *Lancet, 375*(9719), 1014–1028. https://doi.org/10.1016/S0140-6736(10)60232-2

McGraw, K. O., & Wong, S. P. (1996). Forming inferences about some intraclass correlation coefficients. *Psychological Methods, 1*(1), 30–46. https://doi.org/10.1037/1082-989x.1.1.30

McLeod, D. L., Buscemi, J., & Bohnert, A. M. (2016). Becoming American, becoming obese? A systematic review of acculturation and weight among Latino youth. *Obesity Reviews, 17*(11), 1040–1049. https://doi.org/10.1111/obr.12447

Michaud, P. A., Blum, R. W., & Slap, G. B. (2001). Cross-cultural surveys of adolescent health and behavior: Progress and problems. *Social Science & Medicine, 53*(9), 1237–1246. https://doi.org/10.1016/S0277-9536(00)00423-8

Mythily, S., Qiu, S., & Winslow, M. (2008). Prevalence and correlates of excessive internet use among youth in Singapore. *Annals Academy of Medicine, 37*(1), 9–14.

Organista, K. C., Worby, P. A., Quesada, J., Arreola, S. G., Kral, A. H., & Khoury, S. (2013). Sexual health of Latino migrant day labourers under conditions of structural vulnerability. *Culture, Health & Sexuality, 15*(1), 58–72. https://doi.org/10.1080/13691058.2012.740075

Quesada, J., Hart, L. K., & Bourgois, P. (2011). Structural vulnerability and health: Latino migrant laborers in the United States. *Medical Anthropology, 30*(4), 339–362. https://doi.org/10.1080/01459740.2011.576725

Severson, R. K., Nomura, A. M., Grove, J. S., & Stemmermann, G. N. (1989). A prospective study of demographics, diet, and prostate cancer among men of Japanese ancestry in Hawaii. *Cancer Research, 49*(7), 1857–1860.

Sperber, A. D. (2009). The challenge of cross-cultural, multi-national research: Potential benefits in the functional gastrointestinal disorders. *Neurogastroenterology and Motility, 21*(4), 351–360. https://doi.org/10.1111/j.1365-2982.2009.01276.x

Steptoe, A., Wardle, J., Cui, W. W., Bellisle, F., Zotti, A. M., Baranyai, R., & Sanderman, R. (2002). Trends in smoking, diet, physical exercise, and attitudes toward health in European university students from 13 countries, 1990-2000. *Preventive Medicine, 35*(2), 97–104. https://doi.org/10.1006/pmed.2002.1048

Strong, V. E., Wu, A. W., Selby, L. V., Gonen, M., Hsu, M., Song, K. Y., ... Brennan, M. F. (2015). Differences in gastric cancer survival between the U.S. and China. *Journal of Surgical Oncology, 112*(1), 31–37. https://doi.org/10.1002/jso.23940

Taylor, S. (2009). Wealth, health and equity: Convergence to divergence in late 20th century globalization. *British Medical Bulletin, 91*, 29–48. https://doi.org/10.1093/bmb/ldp024

Tian, B., Zhang, W., & Qian, L. (2007). Health behaviors and protective factors of school students aged 13-15 years old in four cities of China. *International Electronic Journal of Health Education, 10*, 35–59.

Turbin, M. S., Jessor, R., Costa, F. M., Dong, Q., Zhang, H., & Wang, C. (2006). Protective and risk factors in health-enhancing behavior among adolescents in China and the United States: Does social context matter? *Health Psychology, 25*(4), 445–454. https://doi.org/10.1037/0278-6133.25.4.445

Unger, J. B., Yan, L., Chen, X., Jiang, X., Azen, S., Qian, G., ... Anderson Johnson, C. (2001). Adolescent smoking in Wuhan, China: Baseline data from the Wuhan Smoking Prevention Trial. *American Journal of Preventive Medicine, 21*(3), 162–169. https://doi.org/10.1016/s0749-3797(01)00346-4

Verbeke, G., & Lesaffre, E. (1996). A linear mixed-effects model with heterogeneity in the random-effects population. *Journal of the American Statistical Association, 91*(433), 217–221. https://doi.org/10.2307/2291398

Walker, E. R., Mcgee, R. E., & Druss, B. G. (2015). Mortality in mental disorders and global disease burden implications: A systematic review and meta-analysis. *JAMA Psychiatry, 72*(4), 334–341. https://doi.org/10.1001/jamapsychiatry.2014.2502

Wang, C. C. D. C., & Mallinckrodt, B. (2006). Acculturation, attachment, and psychosocial adjustment of Chinese/Taiwanese international students. *Journal of Counseling Psychology, 53*(4), 422–433. https://doi.org/10.1037/0022-0167.53.4.422

Wang, Y. C., Lee, C. M., Lew-Ting, C. Y., Hsiao, C. K., Chen, D. R., & Chen, W. J. (2005). Survey of substance use among high school students in Taipei: Web-based questionnaire versus paper-and-pencil questionnaire. *The Journal of Adolescent Health, 37*(4), 289–295. https://doi.org/10.1016/j.jadohealth.2005.03.017

Warren, C. W., Jones, N. R., Eriksen, M. P., Asma, S., & Global Tobacco Surveillance System (GTSS) Collaborative Group. (2006). Patterns of global tobacco use in young people and implications for future chronic disease burden in adults. *Lancet, 367*(9512), 749–753. https://doi.org/10.1016/S0140-6736(06)68192-0

Weinehall, L., Lewis, C., Nafziger, A. N., Jenkins, P. L., Erb, T. A., Pearson, T. A., & Wall, S. (2001). Different outcomes for different interventions with different focus!—A cross-country comparison of community interventions in rural Swedish and US populations. *Scandinavian Journal of Public Health. Supplement, 56*, 46–58.

Wong, L. K. (2010). Internet gambling: A school-based survey among Macau students. *Social Behavior and Personality: An International Journal, 38*(3), 365–371.

Woodward, D., Drager, N., Beaglehole, R., & Lipson, D. (2001). Globalization and health: A framework for analysis and action. *Bulletin of the World Health Organization, 79*(9), 875–881.

Xing, Y., Ji, C., & Zhang, L. (2006). Relationship of binge drinking and other health-compromising behaviors among urban adolescents in China. *The Journal of Adolescent Health, 39*(4), 495–500. https://doi.org/10.1016/j.jadohealth.2006.03.014

Yach, D. (2014). The origins, development, effects, and future of the WHO Framework Convention on Tobacco Control: A personal perspective. *Lancet, 383*(9930), 1771–1779. https://doi.org/10.1016/S0140-6736(13)62155-8

Yeh, M. Y., Chiang, I. C., & Huang, S. Y. (2006). Alcohol use and problem drinking in Taiwanese adolescents: Comparison of the Han and indigenous populations. *International Psychiatry, 3*(2), 32–33.

Yoshino, M., Kuhlmann, M. K., Kotanko, P., Greenwood, R. N., Pisoni, R. L., Port, F. K., ... Levin, N. W. (2006). International differences in dialysis mortality reflect background general population atherosclerotic cardiovascular mortality. *Journal of the American Society of Nephrology, 17*(12), 3510–3519. https://doi.org/10.1681/ASN.2006020156

Yu, B., Chen, X., Elliott, A. L., Wang, Y., Li, F., & Gong, J. (2019). Social capital, migration stress, depression and sexual risk behaviors among rural-to-urban migrants in China: A moderated mediation modeling analysis. *Anxiety, Stress & Coping, 32*(4), 362–375. https://doi.org/10.1080/10615806.2019.1596673

Yu, B., Chen, X., & Li, S. (2014). Globalization, cross-culture stress and health. *Zhonghua Liu Xing Bing Xue Za Zhi, 35*(3), 338–341.

Chapter 12
Geographically Weighted Regression

Yang Yang

Abstract The family of geographically weighted regression (GWR) methods has seen its wide applications in a variety of fields including ecology, agriculture, social science, and public health. The popularity of these methods stems from their ability to depict spatial heterogeneity, easy interpretation of outputs, and the availability of user-friendly software tools. These methods have evolved extensively in the recent decade to address the challenges of multicolinearity in predictors and variable selection in the era of big data, and a comprehensive review is needed to raise both awareness and practical validation of these progresses. Equally needed is an up-to-date introduction to the associated software packages, especially those developed on the popular statistical software platform R. This chapter provides a systematic overview of the foundation and recent development of the methodology of GWR, with a balance between rigidity and practicality. Via a case study, this chapter also offers step-by-step guideline to the use of three major GWR-dedicated R packages, including their facilities for multicolinearity diagnosis and variable selection. We hope a broadened user group of these methods will in turn motivate more methodological advances and improve the contribution of GWR methods to global health.

Keywords Geographically weighted regression · Spatial heterogeneity · Variable selection · Multicolinearity · GWR software

12.1 Introduction

Health outcomes such as chronic conditions and infectious diseases typically exhibit spatial and temporal variation, driven by both risk factors and random errors. While

Y. Yang (✉)
Department of Biostatistics, School of Public Health and Health Professions & Emerging Pathogens Institute, University of Florida, Gainesville, FL, USA
e-mail: yangyang@ufl.edu

X. Chen, (Din) D.-G. Chen (eds.), *Statistical Methods for Global Health and Epidemiology*, ICSA Book Series in Statistics,
https://doi.org/10.1007/978-3-030-35260-8_12

changes in risk factors explain a significant amount of variations in health outcomes, it is quite often they do not explain all. Additional variation may be accounted for by spatial or temporal heterogeneity in the effects of risk factors. An example is shown in Fig. 12.1, where the effects of drug infection history (left) and drug rehabilitation history (right) on the risk of HCV infection in a Yi Ethnicity Autonomous Prefecture in Southwestern China were estimated using the geographically weighted regression (GWR) approach (Zhou et al. 2016). This figure clearly demonstrates spatial heterogeneity in the estimated effects. Such heterogeneity is more prominent at larger spatial scales, e.g., states, countries or continents.

Figure 12.2 shows the spatial distributions of local R-squares (upper left) and selected GWR-estimated regression coefficient estimates for teenage birth rate in rural counties of the United States during 2003 (Shoff & Yang, 2012). The effects of some factors such as clinic rate have opposite signs across different regions. If such heterogeneity is ignored and the covariate effects are assumed spatially homogeneous, the effects could be estimated as null and are thus very misleading.

A natural and widely used solution to spatial heterogeneity is to group data points by spatial regions, where the regions are usually defined as administrative units, e.g., counties or states, or as ecological zones. A categorical variable indicating the regions is then incorporated into the analysis. As a main effect, this variable can capture spatial variation in the intercept, i.e., the mean level of the dependent variable. Spatial variation in the effects of other predictors can be investigated by formulating interaction terms between these predictors and the region indicator variables. Assuming that n individuals are observed in a total of J spatial regions, a typical statistical presentation of the model is

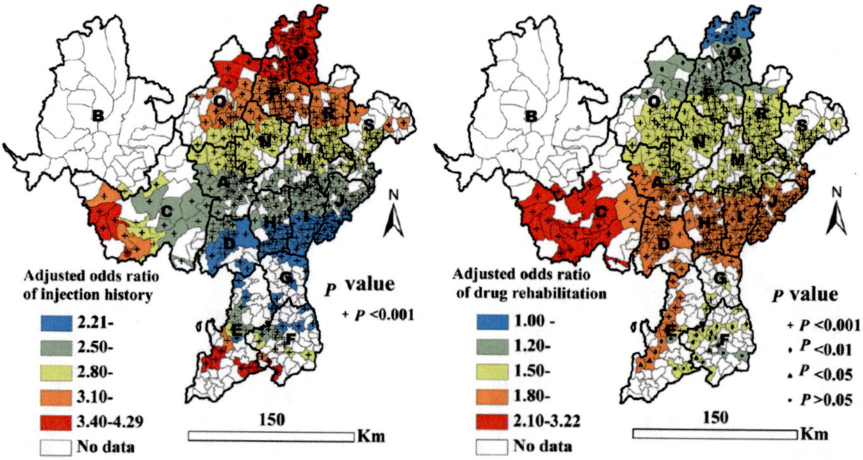

Fig. 12.1 Spatial distribution of GWR-fitted adjusted odds ratios for drug injection history (left) and drug rehabilitation history (right) with regard to their effects on HCV infection in Southwestern China (Zhou et al. 2016)

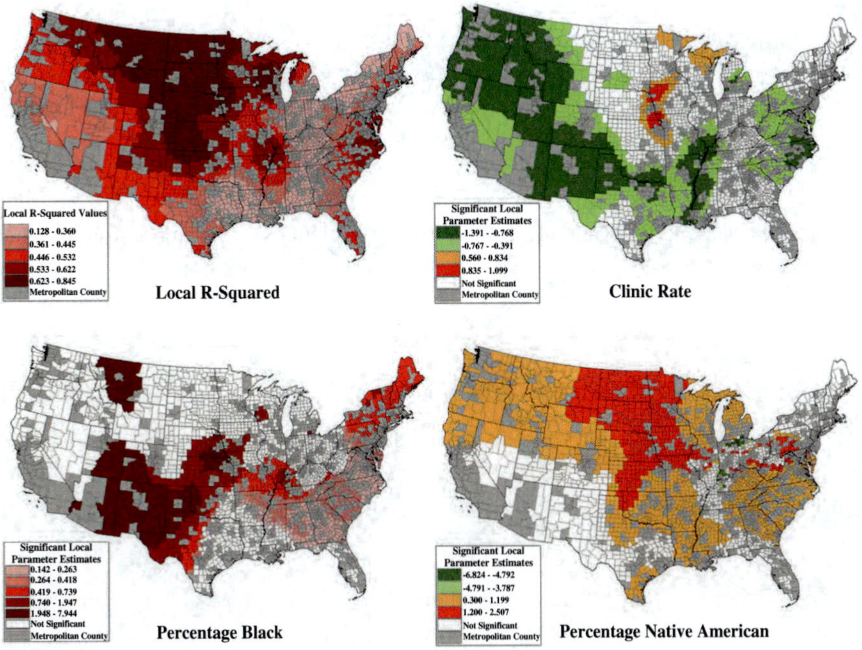

Fig. 12.2 Spatial distribution of GWR-fitted local R-squares and estimated coefficients of predictors for average teenage birth rates during 1999–2001 among non-metropolitan counties in the United States (Shoff & Yang, 2012)

$$y_i = \alpha + \beta x_i + \sum_{j=1}^{J-1} \eta_j z_{ij} + \sum_{j=1}^{J-1} \xi_j z_{ij} x_i + \epsilon_i, \quad i = 1, \ldots, n,$$

where, for individual i, y_i is the response, x_i is a risk factor of interest, z_{ij} indicates whether observation i is in region j (1=yes, 0=no), $j = 1, \ldots, J-1$, and ϵ_i is the error term that is often assumed identically and independently distributed (i.i.d.) as normal with mean 0 and an unknown variance σ^2. We assume only one risk factor for illustrative purpose. The coefficients α and β are the intercept and slope for the reference region defined by $z_{i1} = \ldots = z_{i(J-1)} = 0$. For the region associated with $z_{ij} = 1$, the intercept and slope are $\alpha + \eta_j$ and $\beta + \xi_j$, respectively. Several disadvantages of this approach are worth noting. First, the grouping of data points into regions is often a choice of convenience, not necessarily matching the true geographic pattern in data-generating mechanism. For example, the spatial variation of data-generating mechanism may be smooth over the whole study area rather than with abrupt changes at boundaries of regions as assumed by the grouping approach. Second, there is no widely accepted guideline on choosing the level and number of spatial regions. A few large regions may not be adequate to delineate the spatial heterogeneity, creating issues such as ecological fallacy, whereas too many small regions may encounter the identifiability issue because of sparse data in some regions. Ecological fallacy refers to the phenomenon that heterogeneous individual trends within a region are represented by a homogeneous but misleading trend for the whole region when individual data are aggregated by region for analysis (Wakefield 2008).

An extension of the grouping approach is the expansion method (Casetti 1972; Jones 1992), which models the regression coefficients as continuous functions of the geocoordinates. A general presentation of the expansion method is

$$y_i = \alpha(u_i, v_i) + \beta(u_i, v_i)x_i + \epsilon_i,$$

where (u_i, v_i) are the geocoordinates of individual i, e.g., longitude and latitude. A simple example is the linear mapping

$$\alpha_i = \alpha_0 + \alpha_1 u_i + \alpha_2 v_i,$$

$$\beta_i = \beta_0 + \beta_1 u_i + \beta_2 v_i.$$

Higher orders of u_i and v_i as well as their interactions can be added when needed. A major limitation of the expansion method is that spatial patterns in real life are often much more complex and cannot be satisfactorily captured by polynomials of geocoordinates. In addition, the interpretation of the estimated coefficients can be very difficult. Fotheringham, Charlton, and Brunsdon (1998) compared the expansion method and the geographically weight regression (GWR) using the data of limiting long-term illness (LLTI) in Northeastern England. Risk predictors under consideration were unemployment rate, household crowdedness, proportion of single-parent families among children <5 years, social class and population density. All predictors were modeled as linear effects in all models. Figure 12.3 shows the spatial distribution of (a) standardized LLTI in the study area; (b) intercept under the expansion method when linear expansion was applied to intercept and all slopes; (c) intercept under the expansion method when quadratic expansion (including interaction) was applied to intercept and all slopes; and (d) intercept under the GWR approach. The gradients of intercept under linear expansion (Fig. 12.3b) is largely consistent with the observed pattern of LLTI, although the direction of decrease appeared more from northeast to southwest for the model than from north to south as shown by the data. Under the quadratic expansion (Fig. 12.3c), however, the direction of gradients flipped, now increasing from northeast to southwest. The distribution of the intercept term of the GWR (Fig. 12.3d) reflects the spatial pattern observed in the data and reserves some non-directional spatial differences compared to the linear expansion method.

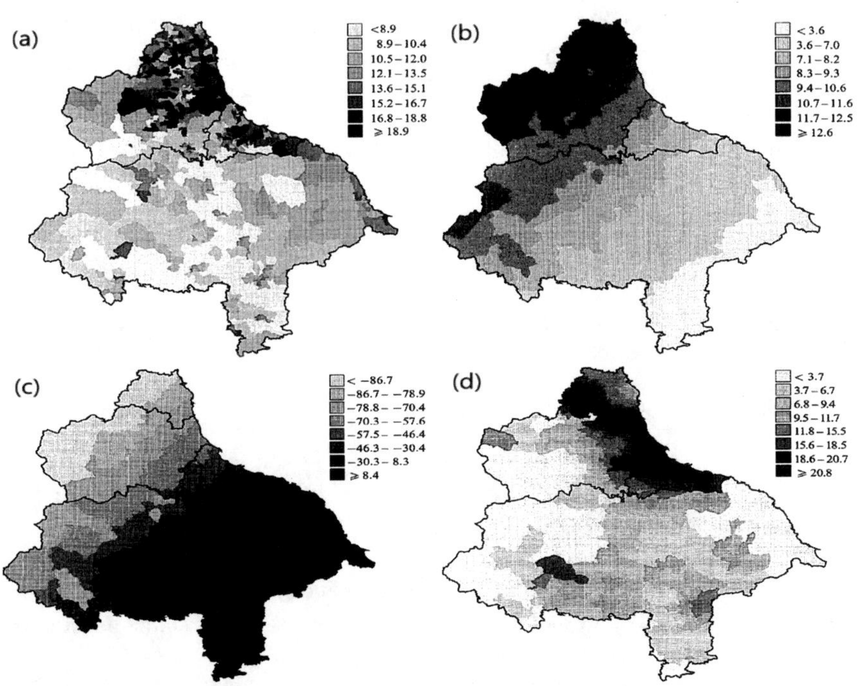

Fig. 12.3 (**a**) Spatial distribution of limiting long-term illness data in Northeastern England; (**b**) distribution of the intercept term under linear expansion; (**c**) distribution of the intercept term under quadratic expansion; (**d**) distribution of the intercept term fitted by the GWR method. The subfigures are adapted from Fotheringham et al. (1998)

12.2 Theory

12.2.1 Basic Model Structure and Inference

The model expression of GWR is very similar to that of the expansion method, except that no specific functional form is assumed for the dependence of coefficients on geocoordinates. Suppose we are regressing an dependent variable on p predictors. For notional simplicity, define $s = (u, v)$ for the geocoordinates. For a given individual i at location $s_i = (u_i, v_i)$, the model to be fitted is

$$y_i = \beta_0(s_i) + \sum_{k=1}^{p} \beta_k(s_i)x_{ik} + \epsilon_i = \boldsymbol{X}_i^\tau \boldsymbol{\beta}(s_i) + \epsilon_i, \tag{12.1}$$

where $\boldsymbol{X}_i = (1, x_{i1}, \ldots, x_{ip})^\tau$ and $\boldsymbol{\beta}(s_i) = (\beta_0(s_i), \ldots, \beta_p(s_i))^\tau$ are the vectors of covariates and coefficients, respectively, and τ denotes transpose of vectors or matrices. As usual, we assume $\epsilon_1, \ldots, \epsilon_n \overset{i.i.d.}{\sim} Normal(0, \sigma^2)$. The coefficients,

$\beta_0(s), \ldots, \beta_p(s)$ can be viewed as continuous spatial functions defined at any point s in the study area rather than only at the observed locations $s_1, \ldots, s_n$. The essence of GWR is the construction of the diagonal weight matrix $\boldsymbol{W}(s_i)_{n\times n} = \text{diag}\big(w_1(s_i), \ldots, w_n(s_i)\big)$, where each diagonal element $w_j(s_i)$ is determined by a predefined distance between s_i and s_j, $j = 1, \ldots, n$. Let $\boldsymbol{X}$ be a $n \times (p+1)$ matrix with $\boldsymbol{X}_i$ as its ith row, $i = 1, \ldots, n$, and let $\boldsymbol{Y} = (y_1, \ldots, y_n)^\tau$ be the column vector of the dependent variable. Following standard linear model theory, minimizing the sum of weighted squares of residuals chosen as the objective function

$$\arg\min_{\boldsymbol{\beta}(s_i)} ||\boldsymbol{W}(s_i)^{1/2}(Y - \boldsymbol{X}\boldsymbol{\beta}(s_i))||^2 = \arg\min_{\boldsymbol{\beta}(s_i)} \sum_{j=1}^{n} w_j(s_i)\big(y_j - \boldsymbol{X}_j^\tau \boldsymbol{\beta}(s_i)\big)^2 \quad (12.2)$$

yields the WLS estimates for the coefficients

$$\hat{\boldsymbol{\beta}}(s_i) = \boldsymbol{B}(s_i)\boldsymbol{Y}, \quad \text{where } \boldsymbol{B}(s_i) = \big(\boldsymbol{X}^\tau \boldsymbol{W}(s_i)\boldsymbol{X}\big)^{-1}\boldsymbol{X}^\tau \boldsymbol{W}(s_i).$$

This is also the maximum likelihood estimate (MLE) of $\boldsymbol{\beta}(s_i)$ under the normal assumption for ϵ_i's with a correlation matrix $\boldsymbol{W}(s_i)$. Model (12.1) is to be fitted n times, one at each individual location in the data. It can also be fitted at an arbitrary location s in the study area, but the model need to be restated in a more general form

$$y(s) = \beta_0(s) + \sum_{k=1}^{p} \beta_k(s)x_k(s) + \epsilon(s) = \boldsymbol{X}(s)^\tau \boldsymbol{\beta}(s) + \epsilon(s).$$

However, $y(s)$ and $\boldsymbol{X}(s)$ are observed only at the locations of the study-sampled individuals, i.e., s_i, $i = 1, \ldots, n$.

To obtain a variance estimate for $\hat{\boldsymbol{\beta}}(s_i)$ so that we can construct confidence intervals for all the local coefficients, we need to estimate σ^2, the variance of the error term. Let $\hat{y}_i = \boldsymbol{X}_i^\tau \hat{\boldsymbol{\beta}}(s_i)$ be the model-fitted value at s_i, and let $\hat{\boldsymbol{Y}} = (\hat{y}_1, \ldots, \hat{y}_n)^\tau$. We can write $\hat{\boldsymbol{Y}} = \boldsymbol{H}\boldsymbol{Y}$, where

$$\boldsymbol{H} = \begin{pmatrix} \boldsymbol{X}_1^\tau \boldsymbol{B}(s_1) \\ \boldsymbol{X}_2^\tau \boldsymbol{B}(s_2) \\ \vdots \\ \boldsymbol{X}_n^\tau \boldsymbol{B}(s_n) \end{pmatrix}$$

is analogous to the *hat* matrix in the ordinary linear regression setting. Let $\hat{\boldsymbol{\epsilon}} = \boldsymbol{Y} - \hat{\boldsymbol{Y}}$ be the vector of residuals. An important statistic is the residual sum of square

$$\begin{aligned} \text{RSS} &= \sum_{i=1}^{n} \big(y_i - \hat{y}_i\big)^2 = \hat{\boldsymbol{\epsilon}}^\tau \hat{\boldsymbol{\epsilon}} \\ &= (\boldsymbol{Y} - \hat{\boldsymbol{Y}})^\tau(\boldsymbol{Y} - \hat{\boldsymbol{Y}}) = \boldsymbol{Y}^\tau(\boldsymbol{I} - \boldsymbol{H})^\tau(\boldsymbol{I} - \boldsymbol{H})\boldsymbol{Y}, \end{aligned}$$

where $\boldsymbol{I}$ is the $n \times n$ identity matrix. Following Leung, Mei, and Zhang (2000), under the assumption that $\mathbb{E}(\hat{\boldsymbol{Y}}) = \mathbb{E}(\boldsymbol{Y})$, RSS can further written as

$$\begin{aligned}\text{RSS} &= \big[\boldsymbol{Y} - \mathbb{E}(\boldsymbol{Y})\big]^{\tau}(\boldsymbol{I} - \boldsymbol{H})^{\tau}(\boldsymbol{I} - \boldsymbol{H})\big[\boldsymbol{Y} - \mathbb{E}(\boldsymbol{Y})\big] \\ &= \boldsymbol{\epsilon}^{\tau}(\boldsymbol{I} - \boldsymbol{H})^{\tau}(\boldsymbol{I} - \boldsymbol{H})\boldsymbol{\epsilon}\end{aligned}$$

Note that

$$\begin{aligned}\mathbb{E}(\text{RSS}) &= \mathbb{E}\big[\boldsymbol{\epsilon}^{\tau}(\boldsymbol{I} - \boldsymbol{H})^{\tau}(\boldsymbol{I} - \boldsymbol{H})\boldsymbol{\epsilon}\big] \\ &= \mathbb{E}\Big[trace\big(\boldsymbol{\epsilon}^{\tau}(\boldsymbol{I} - \boldsymbol{H})^{\tau}(\boldsymbol{I} - \boldsymbol{H})\boldsymbol{\epsilon}\big)\Big] \\ &= \mathbb{E}\Big[trace\big((\boldsymbol{I} - \boldsymbol{H})^{\tau}(\boldsymbol{I} - \boldsymbol{H})\boldsymbol{\epsilon}\boldsymbol{\epsilon}^{\tau}\big)\Big] \\ &= trace\Big[(\boldsymbol{I} - \boldsymbol{H})^{\tau}(\boldsymbol{I} - \boldsymbol{H})\mathbb{E}\big(\boldsymbol{\epsilon}\boldsymbol{\epsilon}^{\tau}\big)\Big] \\ &= \sigma^2\nu_1\end{aligned}$$

where $\nu_1 = trace\big((\boldsymbol{I} - \boldsymbol{H})^{\tau}(\boldsymbol{I} - \boldsymbol{H})\big) = n - \big[2tr(\boldsymbol{H}) - tr(\boldsymbol{H}^{\tau}\boldsymbol{H})\big]$ is the degree of freedom of the RSS, and $2tr(\boldsymbol{H}) - tr(\boldsymbol{H}^{\tau}\boldsymbol{H})$ represents the effective number of parameters (Fotheringham, Brunsdon, & Charlton, 2002). The trace function of a matrix is simply the sum of diagonal elements of that matrix. An unbiased estimate for σ^2 is then $\hat{\sigma}^2 = \text{RSS}/\nu_1$, and the variance-covariance matrix of $\hat{\boldsymbol{\beta}}(s_i)$ can then be estimated as

$$\widehat{\text{Cov}}\big[\hat{\boldsymbol{\beta}}(s_i)\big] = \boldsymbol{B}(s_i)\boldsymbol{B}(s_i)^{\tau}\hat{\sigma}^2. \tag{12.3}$$

The Wald-type 95% confidence interval for each coefficient can be established as

$$\hat{\beta}_k(s_i) \pm 1.96 \times \sqrt{\widehat{\text{Var}}\big[\hat{\beta}_k(s_i)\big]},$$

where $\widehat{\text{Var}}\big[\hat{\beta}_k(s_i)\big]$ is the kth diagonal element of $\widehat{\text{Cov}}\big[\hat{\boldsymbol{\beta}}(s_i)\big]$, $k = 0, 1, \ldots, p$.

12.2.2 Constructing Weights

The choices of the weights $w_j(s_i)$ depends on the nature of the data. When the individuals under observation are relatively large spatial units such as zip codes, counties or states, the neighbor indicator is a reasonable choice, i.e., $w_j(s_i) = 1$ if units i and j share a common border and 0 otherwise. The concept of adjacency-based weighting can be generalized to k-order neighbors (Zhang & Murayama, 2000). The neighbor structure can be viewed as an undirected graph with directly neighbored units connected by edges. If the shortest path between two units has k edges, then the two units are k-order neighbors. Consequently, a more general adjacency-based weighting scheme is to let $w_j(s_i) = 1$ if units i and j are k-order neighbors for any $k \leq h$, where h is called the bandwidth. When it is appropriate to consider predefined geographic distances between individuals, a kernel function of the distance subject to a bandwidth constraint is often used, e.g., the bisquare function

$$w_j(s_i) = \begin{cases} \left(1 - d_{ij}^2/h^2\right)^2, & \text{if } d_{ij} < h, \\ 0, & \text{otherwise} \end{cases},$$

where h is the bandwidth. Two other popular choices are the Gaussian density kernel, $w_j(s_i) = \exp(-d_{ij}^2/h^2)$, and the exponential kernel, $w_j(s_i) = \exp(-d_{ij}/h)$. Any kernel function, $K(d)$, of distance d that satisfies (1) $K(0) = 1$, (2) $K(\infty) = 0$, (3) $K(d) > 0$ for $d > 0$ and (4) non-increasing can be considered. A monotone decreasing kernel function ensure that higher weights are put on observations that are closer to the current location s_i. The bandwidth, h, further controls how fast the weight should decay according to the distance, and its choice is crucial for the inferential performance of the method. If h is large so that the decay is slow, then distant observations contributed almost equally as the nearby ones. On one hand, the effective sample size increases and thus the estimates will be more stable and less variant; on the other hand, however, if the coefficients vary substantially over the space, severe bias is likely to occur. This is a large-bias-small-variance situation. Conversely, if h is too small, only close-by observations will contribute, leading to small bias but large variance. Consequently, the choice of h is actually an issue of balance between bias and variance, and cross-validation (CV) procedure is recommended to choose the bandwidth (Brunsdon, Fotheringham, & Charlton, 1996). Let $\hat{y}_{(i)}(h) = \boldsymbol{X}_i^T \hat{\boldsymbol{\beta}}(s_i, h)$ be the fitted value at the location of individual i with a given value of h, where the model is fitted with individual i excluded. We use the notation $\hat{\boldsymbol{\beta}}(s_i, h)$ instead of $\hat{\boldsymbol{\beta}}(s_i)$ to reflect its dependence on h. Then, h is chosen by minimizing the sum of squares of residuals:

$$h^\star = \arg\min_h \sum_{i=1}^n \left[y_i - \hat{y}_{(i)}(h)\right]^2.$$

Another popular objective function for bandwidth calibration is related to the Akeike Information Criterion (AIC) that balances between goodness-of-fit and model parsimony,

$$AIC_c(h) = \log\left[RSS/n\right] + \frac{n + trace(H)}{n - 2 - trace(H)},$$

where both RSS and H depend on h (Fotheringham et al. 2002). The optimal bandwidth is then $h^\star = \arg\min_h AIC_c(h)$. In practice, empirical data or expert opinions may also inform the choice of h.

12.2.3 Testing Spatial Nonstationarity

Two questions naturally arise with the use of GWR:

1. Is the GWR fitting the data better than the ordinary least squares (OLS) regression that assumes spatial stationarity in covariate coefficients?
2. Which covariate coefficients have significant spatial heterogeneity?

The first question is about testing the global presence of spatial nonstationarity, while the second is about testing spatial variation for each individual predictor. Statistically, the null hypotheses to be tested are

1. H_{0a}: $\boldsymbol{\beta}(s_1) = \boldsymbol{\beta}(s_2) = \cdots = \boldsymbol{\beta}(s_n)$.
2. H_{0b}: $\beta_k(s_1) = \beta_k(s_2) = \cdots = \beta_k(s_n)$ for a given k.

For the global testing, Brunsdon et al. (1996) suggested the CV-derived bandwidth parameter $h^\star$ as a test statistic, as the smaller the bandwidth the larger the spatial heterogeneity. A GWR with $h^\star = \infty$ is equivalent to the OLS. For the testing of specific coefficients, Brunsdon et al. (1996) recommended the sample variance (or standard deviation) of each location-specific coefficient, i.e., $S_k = \frac{1}{n}\sum_{i=1}^{n}\left(\hat{\beta}_k(s_i) - \frac{1}{n}\sum_{j=1}^{n}\hat{\beta}_k(s_j)\right)^2$. As the theoretical distribution under each null hypothesis is not easy to derive, a permutation-based approach was proposed (Brunsdon et al. 1996). Under the global null hypothesis H_{0a}, the data $(y_i, \boldsymbol{X}_i)$ can be randomly permuted across all locations. Suppose M permuted sample data sets are generated, and let the bandwidth derived based on the mth sample dataset by h_m. The p-value of the observed value $h^\star$ from the original data for testing H_{0a} is given by

$$\Pr(h \le h^\star) = \frac{1}{M}\sum_{j=1}^{M}\mathcal{I}(h_m \le h^\star),$$

where $\mathcal{I}(c)$ is the indicator function taking 1 if condition c is true and 0 otherwise. Although $h = \infty$ corresponds to spatial stationarity theoretically, the meaningful null distribution of h in reality is bounded by the size of the study area. Brunsdon et al. (1996) suggested using the sample permutation approach to find the null distribution of S_k; however, the obtained distribution is under H_{0a} instead of H_{0b}. As the parameter space under H_{0a} is a subspace of that under H_{0b}, using the distribution of S_k under the global null will not necessarily yield a valid type I error, and will likely lack sufficient statistical power.

The computational burden of the permutation approach is heavy for large n, especially for the calculation of h_m which itself involves a search for the optimal bandwidth for each sample dataset. Leung et al. (2000) explored the possibility of asymptotical tests for the two hypotheses. The test statistic they proposed for H_{0a} is $F_a = \frac{\text{RSS}_{gwr}/\nu_1}{\text{RSS}_{ols}/(n-p-1)}$, where $\text{RSS}_{gwr} = \boldsymbol{Y}^\tau(\boldsymbol{I} - \boldsymbol{H})^\tau(\boldsymbol{I} - \boldsymbol{H})\boldsymbol{Y}$ and $\text{RSS}_{ols} = \boldsymbol{Y}^\tau(\boldsymbol{I} - \boldsymbol{X}(\boldsymbol{X}^\tau\boldsymbol{X})^{-1}\boldsymbol{X}^\tau)\boldsymbol{Y}$ are the residual sums of squares based on GWR and OLS, respectively. Leung et al. (2000) suggested the null distribution of F_1 be approximated by the $F(\nu_1/\nu_2, n-p-1)$ distribution, where $\nu_2 = trace\Big[\big((\boldsymbol{I} - \boldsymbol{H})^\tau(\boldsymbol{I} - \boldsymbol{H})\big)^2\Big]$. H_{0a} is rejected if the observed value of F_1 is less than the $\alpha \times 100\%$ percentile for a given type I error α. To test H_{0b}, the suggested test statistic is $F_b = \frac{S_k^2/\gamma_1}{\hat{\sigma}^2}$, where $\gamma_1 = \frac{1}{n} trace\Big[\boldsymbol{B}^\tau(\boldsymbol{I} - \frac{1}{n}\boldsymbol{J})\boldsymbol{B}\Big]$, $\boldsymbol{J}$ is a $n \times n$ matrix with all elements equal to one,

$$\boldsymbol{B}_k = \begin{pmatrix} \boldsymbol{e}_k^\tau \boldsymbol{B}(s_1) \\ \boldsymbol{e}_k^\tau \boldsymbol{B}(s_2) \\ \vdots \\ \boldsymbol{e}_k^\tau \boldsymbol{B}(s_n) \end{pmatrix},$$

and $\boldsymbol{e}_k$ is a vector of zeros of length $p+1$ except for the $(k+1)$th element being one. The null distribution of F_b is approximated by $F(\gamma_1^2/\gamma_2, \nu_1^2/\nu_2)$, where $\gamma_2 = trace\Big[\big(\frac{1}{n}\boldsymbol{B}^\tau(\boldsymbol{I} - \frac{1}{n}\boldsymbol{J})\boldsymbol{B}\big)^2\Big]$. H_{0b} is rejected if the observed F_b exceeds the $(1-\alpha) \times 100\%$ percentile of the null distribution.

These approximate asymptotic null distributions, however, remain to be rigorously justified in the sense that the numerators and denominators are not necessarily independent. In addition, Fotheringham et al. (2002) noted that the computation load of these asymptotic tests is as heavy as the permutation tests in practice. Finally, the F_1 statistic could be used as an alternative to h in the permutation test for the global null hypothesis H_{0a}, in particular when h is fixed rather than calibrated in cross-validation, e.g., the binary neighbor indicator matrix.

Mei, Wang, and Zhang (2006) proposed a resampling based approach to test the hypotheses in a more general form

- H_0: $\beta_k(s_1) = \beta_k(s_2) = \cdots = \beta_k(s_n)$ for $k \in \Delta$, where Δ is a given subset of $\{1, \ldots, p\}$.
- H_1: All coefficients vary over space.

The set Δ could be a single coefficient, a subset of or all of the coefficients. This bootstrap procedure goes with the following steps:

1. Fit the unrestricted model to obtain the residuals $\hat{\boldsymbol{\epsilon}} = (\hat{\epsilon}_1, \ldots, \hat{\epsilon}_n)^\tau = (\boldsymbol{I} - \boldsymbol{H}_1)\boldsymbol{Y}$ and the residual sum of squares $RSS_1 = \boldsymbol{Y}^\tau(\boldsymbol{I} - \boldsymbol{H}_1)^\tau(\boldsymbol{I} - \boldsymbol{H}_1)\boldsymbol{Y}$, where H_1 is the hat matrix. Let $\hat{\boldsymbol{\epsilon}}_c = (\hat{\epsilon}_{c1}, \ldots, \hat{\epsilon}_{cn})^\tau$ be the centered residuals, i.e., $\hat{\epsilon}_{ci} = \hat{\epsilon}_{ci} - \frac{1}{n}\sum_{j=1}^n \hat{\epsilon}_j$.

2. Fit the null model using the two-step method of Fotheringham et al. (2002) to obtain the residual sum of squares $RSS_0 = \boldsymbol{Y}^\tau(\boldsymbol{I} - \boldsymbol{H}_0)^\tau(\boldsymbol{I} - \boldsymbol{H}_0)\boldsymbol{Y}$, where H_0 is the hat matrix under the null.
3. Compute the observed statistic $T = \frac{RSS_0 - RSS_1}{RSS_1}$.
4. For $m = 1, \ldots, M$, draw with replacement random samples $\tilde{\boldsymbol{\epsilon}}^{(m)} = (\tilde{\epsilon}_1^{(m)}, \ldots, \tilde{\epsilon}_n^{(m)})^\tau$ from the centered residuals $\hat{\boldsymbol{\epsilon}}_c$, formulate new responses as $\tilde{\boldsymbol{Y}}^{(m)} = (\tilde{y}_1^{(m)}, \ldots, \tilde{y}_n)^{(m)})^\tau = \boldsymbol{H}_0\boldsymbol{Y} + \tilde{\boldsymbol{\epsilon}}^{(m)}$, and calculate the statistics $\tilde{T}^{(m)} = \frac{\widetilde{RSS}_0^{(m)} - \widetilde{RSS}_1^{(m)}}{\widetilde{RSS}_1^{(m)}}$, where $\widetilde{RSS}_k^{(m)} = (\tilde{\boldsymbol{Y}}^{(m)})^\tau(\boldsymbol{I} - \boldsymbol{H}_k)^\tau(\boldsymbol{I} - \boldsymbol{H}_k)\tilde{\boldsymbol{Y}}^{(m)}$, $k = 0, 1$.
5. The p-value is calculated as $p = \frac{1}{M}\sum_{m=1}^{M} \mathcal{I}(\tilde{T}^{(m)} \geq T)$.

12.2.4 Geographically Weighted Generalized Linear Models

Analogous to the generalized linear global models (GLM) for fitting binary and count data, geographically weighted generalized linear models (GWGLM) have also been developed. The GLM theory is based on the exponential family of statistical distributions in the form

$$f(y|\theta, \phi) = \exp\left\{\frac{y\theta - b(\theta)}{a(\phi)} - c(y, \phi)\right\},$$

to which many commonly seen distributions such as normal, binomial, Poisson and negative binomial (when the overdispersion parameter is assumed known) belong. Parameters θ and ϕ are called the canonical parameter and the dispersion parameter, respectively, and the functions $a(\cdot)$, $b(\cdot)$ and $c(\cdot, \cdot)$ are assumed known. For example, the Poisson distribution with parameter λ can be written as

$$f(y|\lambda) = \exp\left\{\frac{y\log(\lambda) - \lambda}{1} - \log\Gamma(y+1)\right\},$$

with $\theta = \log(\lambda)$, $b(\theta) = \exp(\theta)$, $a(\phi) = 1$, and $c(y, \phi) = \log\Gamma(y+1)$. The mean and variance of y are related to this parameterization via $\mathbb{E}(Y) = \mu = b'(\theta)$ and $\text{Var}(Y) = a(\phi)b''(\theta)$, where $b'(\theta)$ and $b''(\theta)$ are the first and second derivatives of $b(\theta)$. The mean μ is related to linear predictors $\eta = \beta_0 + \beta_1 x_1 + \ldots + \beta_p x_p = \boldsymbol{x}^\tau\boldsymbol{\beta}$ via the link function $\eta = g(\mu)$. Table 12.1 lists the model components for several distributions in the exponential family.

A general Iteratively Reweighted Least Squares (IRLS) algorithm is available to fit these models (Nelder & Wedderburn, 1972), which can be adapted to the GWGLM setting (da Silva & Rodrigues, 2014; Fotheringham et al. 2002; Nakaya, Fotheringham, Brunsdon, & Charlton, 2005). The following algorithm is modified from Fotheringham et al. (2002). The algorithm is applied to the local fitting at

Table 12.1 GLM components for selected distributions

Distribution	θ	ϕ	$a(\phi)$	$b(\theta)$	$c(y,\phi)$	$g(\mu)$
$Normal(\mu,\sigma^2)$	μ	σ^2	ϕ	$\theta^2/2$	$-\frac{1}{2}\left[\frac{y^2}{\phi}+\log(2\pi\phi)\right]$	μ
$Binomial(n,p)$[a]	$\log\left(\frac{p}{1-p}\right)$		$1/n$	$\log(1+e^{\theta})$	$\log\left[\binom{n}{ny}\right]$	$\log\left(\frac{\mu}{1-\mu}\right)$
$Poisson(\mu)$	$\log(\mu)$		1	e^{θ}	$-\log(y!)$	$\log(\mu)$
$NB(\mu,\alpha)$[b]	$\log\left(\frac{\mu}{r+\mu}\right)$		1	$-r\log\left(1-e^{\theta}\right)$	$\log\frac{\Gamma(r+y)}{y!\Gamma(r)}$	$\log(\mu)$

[a] y/n is viewed as the random variable
[b] For negative binomial to be in exponential family, r is assumed known

each location s_i separately, i.e., all parameters $(\boldsymbol{\beta}, \eta, \mu, \theta, \phi)$ depend on s_i, but we suppress such dependence in notation for simplicity. η, μ and θ further depend on $\boldsymbol{x}_j$ at all observation locations when we fit the local model centered around s_i, and thus we use η_j, μ_j and θ_j, $j = 1, \ldots, n$ to reflect such dependence.

1. Choose initial estimate $\boldsymbol{\beta}^{(0)}$ and $\phi^{(0)}$, and obtain $\eta_j^{(0)} = \boldsymbol{x}_j^{\tau}\boldsymbol{\beta}^{(0)}$, $\mu_j^{(0)} = g^{-1}(\eta_j^{(0)})$, and $\theta_j^{(0)} = b'^{-1}(\mu_j^{(0)})$, where $g^{-1}(\cdot)$ and $b'^{-1}(\cdot)$ are inverse functions of $g(\cdot)$ and $b'(\cdot)$ respectively. For iterations $k = 0, 1, \ldots$, do the following steps:
2. Derive the adjusted dependent variable $z_j^{(k)} = \eta_j^{(k)} + g'(\mu_j^{(k)})(y_j - \mu_j^{(k)})$.
3. Construct a diagonal matrix $\boldsymbol{A}^{(k)}$ with its jth diagonal element being
$$a_{jj}^{(k)} = \left\{\left[g'(\mu_j^{(k)})\right]^2 a(\phi^{(k)})b''(\theta_j^{(k)})\right\}^{-1}.$$
4. Update the coefficients as
$$\boldsymbol{\beta}^{(k+1)} = (\boldsymbol{X}^{\tau}\boldsymbol{W}\boldsymbol{A}^{(k)}\boldsymbol{X})^{-1}\boldsymbol{X}^{\tau}\boldsymbol{W}\boldsymbol{A}^{(k)}\boldsymbol{Z}^{(k)},$$
where $\boldsymbol{X}$ and $\boldsymbol{W}$ are the covariate matrix (including first column of 1s) and weight matrix as defined before, and $\boldsymbol{Z}^{(k)}$ is the column vector $(z_1^{(k)}, \ldots, z_n^{(k)})^{\tau}$.
5. Estimate the dispersion parameter using the Newton Raphson approach, i.e.,
$$\phi^{(k+1)} = \phi^{(k)} - \left\{\left[\frac{\partial^2 l(\phi, \boldsymbol{\beta}^{(k+1)})}{\partial\phi^2}\right]^{-1}\frac{\partial l(\phi, \boldsymbol{\beta}^{(k+1)})}{\partial\phi}\right\}_{\phi=\phi^{(k)}},$$
where $l(\phi, \boldsymbol{\beta}^{(k+1)})$ is the log-likelihood function with $\boldsymbol{\beta}$ fixed at $\boldsymbol{\beta}^{(k+1)}$.
6. Repeat steps 2–5 until convergence of the parameter estimates.
7. Let $\hat{\boldsymbol{\beta}}$, $\hat{\phi}$ and $\boldsymbol{A}$ be the final estimates after convergence. The variances can be estimated by
$$\widehat{\text{Cov}}(\hat{\boldsymbol{\beta}}) = \widetilde{\boldsymbol{B}}\boldsymbol{A}^{-1}\widetilde{\boldsymbol{B}}, \qquad \widehat{\text{Var}}(\hat{\phi}) = \left[-\frac{\partial^2 l(\phi, \widehat{\boldsymbol{\beta}})}{\partial\phi^2}\right]^{-1}\Bigg|_{\phi=\hat{\phi}},$$
where $\widetilde{\boldsymbol{B}} = (\boldsymbol{X}^{\tau}\boldsymbol{W}\boldsymbol{A}\boldsymbol{X})^{-1}\boldsymbol{X}^{\tau}\boldsymbol{W}\boldsymbol{A}$.

Table 12.2 Expression of z_j and a_{jj} in the IRLS algorithm for selected distributions

Distribution	z_j	a_{jj}
$Normal(\mu, \sigma^2)$	y_j	1
$Binomial(n, p)$	$\eta_j + \frac{y_j/n_j - p_j}{p_j(1-p_j)}$	$n_j p_j(1 - p_j)$
$Poisson(\mu)$	$\eta_j + \frac{y_j - \mu_j}{\mu_j}$	μ_j
$NB(\mu, \alpha)$	$\eta_j + \frac{y_j - \mu_j}{\mu_j}$	$\frac{\mu_j r}{\mu_j + r}$

If the model does not involve an overdispersion parameter such as binomial and Poisson, step 5 is skipped. Table 12.2 gives z_j and a_{jj} (iteration index suppressed) for Gaussian, logistic, Poisson and negative binomial geographically weighted regression models. Note that the expressions of z_j and a_{jj} are based on Fisher information, i.e., the negative of the expectation of the second derivative of the log-likelihood with regard to η_j. They can be based on the observed Fisher information (without taking expectation) as well, as da Silva and Rodrigues (2014) did for the negative binomial model.

12.2.5 Colinearity and Remedies

Hereinafter, we assume each model has a total of p rather than $p + 1$ covariates, which may or may not include an intercept. This is because some of the regularized models require or recommend the response variable $\boldsymbol{Y}$ to be standardized which will eliminate the intercept. Typically, GWR fits models with $n \times p$ parameters, using only n observations. This overfitting is constrained by local weight matrices to yield valid inference, but probably at certain price. Wheeler and Tiefelsdorf (2005) took a close look at how the multicolinearity among predictors (covariates) might affect the correlation among GWR-estimated coefficients and their interpretability. The correlation between estimated coefficients is twofold. First, at any given location, the estimated local coefficients are correlated in terms that the estimated covariance between them are nontrivial. Second, and more importantly, the estimated coefficients for a given pair of covariates are correlated across all observation locations.

Wheeler and Tiefelsdorf (2005) first showed the possibility of local coefficient estimates contradicting the global regression results and scientific evidence by analyzing the bladder cancer mortality data from the Atlas of Cancer Mortality from the National Cancer Institute. Bladder cancer mortality was expected to be positively associated with population density (a proxy for urban vs. rural environment) and lung cancer mortality rate (a proxy for smoking prevalence), consistent with the global regression results. However, the GWR showed vast geographic heterogeneity, and the local coefficient estimates were negatively correlated. Counter-intuitive negative association with the outcome variable was found for population density in the West and Northeast and for lung cancer in the Midwest.

They then performed a series of simulation studies and found that the local coefficient estimates could be substantially correlated with each other, even when the corresponding covariates are not correlated globally. (Figs. 12.8and 12.9), adapted from Wheeler and Tiefelsdorf (2005), illustrates the correlation in the second sense. The two covariates, called exogenous variables, are generated for two scenarios according to

$$\text{Scenario A (dashed curve)}: \; x_1 = Evac_3, \quad x_2 = \sin(\theta)Evac_3 + \cos(\theta)Evac_1,$$

$$\text{Scenario B (solid curve)}: \; x_1 = Evac_4, \quad x_2 = \sin(\theta)Evac_4 + \cos(\theta)Evac1,$$

where $Evac_k$, $k = 1, \ldots, n$ are eigenvalues of the spatial adjacency matrix based on all the counties of the Georgia State in the U.S., after certain transformation and re-scaling. These eigenvalues capture orthogonal spatial characteristics. The parameter θ induces correlation between x_1 and x_2 via $\text{corr}(x_1, x_2) = \sin(\theta)$. Both scenarios indicate strong negative associations: the higher the correlation between the covariates, the lower the correlation between the coefficient estimates. Most surprisingly, zero correlation between the covariates is associated with a high level of negative correlation, -0.8, between the coefficient estimates for scenario B.

Wheeler and Tiefelsdorf (2005) speculated that when two covariates are highly positively correlated, the GWR model tends to explain the variation in the outcome by one coefficient, while pushing the other coefficient to the opposite direction. However, this speculation does not explain the strong positive correlation in coefficient estimates when the covariates are highly negatively correlated as seen in Fig. 12.4. In addition, although the negative correlation between coefficient estimates is obvious in their simulations even when the covariates are not correlated (Figs. 12.8 and 12.9 in Wheeler and Tiefelsdorf (2005)), it is not clear whether such negative correlation matters in practice because the coefficient estimates are mostly close to their global true values (statistical significance level was not given). When nontrivial multicolinearity among covariates is present, however, caution and diagnostic efforts need to be taken, like in global regressions, e.g., examining correlation in the coefficient estimates and the sensitivity of coefficient estimates to addition or deletion of other covariates.

Local Linear Estimation

The local linear estimation approach was proposed by Wang, Mei, and Yan (2008) to target reduction of bias in coefficient estimates of GWR, not to directly address the issue of multicolinearity. In particular, they were concerned about the boundary-effect problem, that is, the GWR estimates tend to be more biased at the boundaries than in the interior part of the study area. Nevertheless, multicolinearity could contribute to bias as evidenced by above discussion. Therefore, the local linear estimation approach can potentially alleviate the problem caused by multicolinearity, while being able to reduce bias from other sources. The idea of this approach is based on first-order Taylor expansion of local coefficients with regard to spatial points:

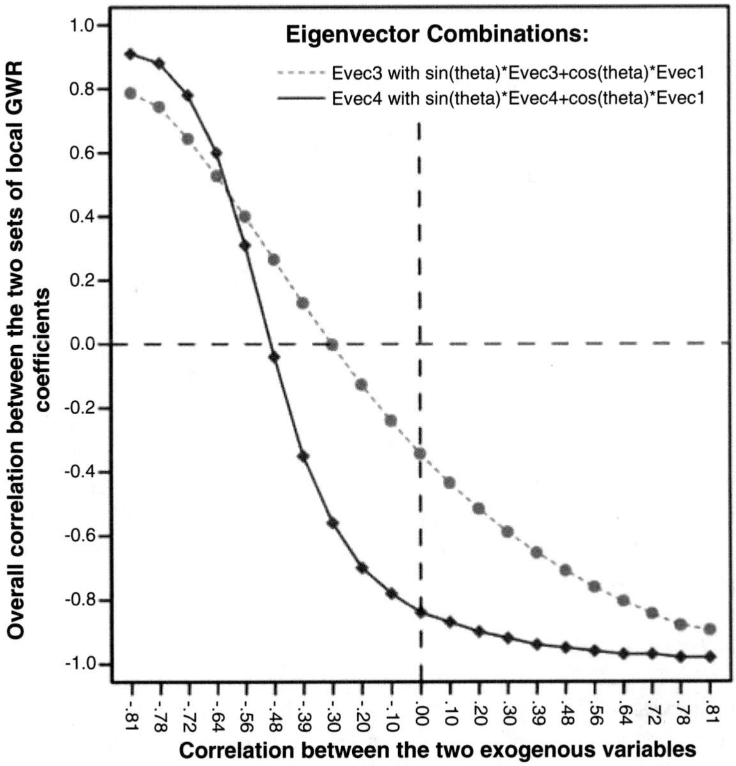

Fig. 12.4 Overall correlation between two coefficient estimates as a function of correlation between the two corresponding covariates, adapted from Wheeler and Tiefelsdorf (2005)

$$\beta_k(u, v) \approx \beta_k(u_i, v_i) + \beta_k^{(u)}(u_i, v_i)(u - u_i) + \beta_k^{(v)}(u_i, v_i)(v - v_i),$$

where $\beta_k^{(u)}(u_i, v_i)$ and $\beta_k^{(u)}(u_i, v_i)$ are partial derivatives of $\beta_k(u, v)$ with regard to u and v, respectively, evaluated at $s_j = (u_i, v_i)$. For each local regression centered at (u_i, v_i), it is no longer necessary to assume the same coefficients as at (u_i, v_i) for all other observation locations. Instead, the objective function becomes

$$\begin{aligned} L_i\big(\boldsymbol{\beta}(s_i)\big) &= \sum_{j=1}^{n} w_j(s_j)\Big\{y_j - \sum_{k=1}^{p} x_{jk}\big[\beta_k(u_i, v_i) + \beta_k^{(u)}(u_i, v_i)(u_j - u_i) \\ &\quad + \beta_k^{(v)}(u_i, v_i)(v_j - v_i)\big]\Big\}^2 \\ &= ||\boldsymbol{W}(s_i)^{1/2}(Y - \boldsymbol{X\beta}(s_i)||^2 \end{aligned} \tag{12.4}$$

The fitting of the model is as usual

$$\hat{\boldsymbol{\beta}}(s_i) = \left(\boldsymbol{X}(s_i)^\tau \boldsymbol{W}(s_i)\boldsymbol{X}(s_i)\right)^{-1}\boldsymbol{X}(s_i)^\tau \boldsymbol{W}(s_i)\boldsymbol{Y},$$

except that the coefficient vector and design matrix are of an extended form:

$$\boldsymbol{\beta}(s_i) = \left(\beta_1(s_i), \beta_1^{(u)}(s_i), \beta_1^{(v)}(s_i), \ldots, \beta_p(s_i), \beta_p^{(u)}(s_i), \beta_p^{(v)}(s_i)\right)^\tau$$

and

$$\boldsymbol{X}(s_i) = \begin{bmatrix} x_{11} & x_{11}(u_1-u_i) & x_{11}(v_1-v_i) & \cdots, & x_{1p} & x_{1p}(u_1-u_i) & x_{1p}(v_1-v_i) \\ x_{21} & x_{21}(u_2-u_i) & x_{21}(v_2-v_i) & \cdots, & x_{2p} & x_{2p}(u_2-u_i) & x_{2p}(v_2-v_i) \\ \vdots & \vdots & \vdots & \vdots & \vdots & \vdots & \vdots \\ x_{n1} & x_{n1}(u_n-u_i) & x_{n1}(v_n-v_i) & \cdots, & x_{np} & x_{np}(u_n-u_i) & x_{np}(v_n-v_i) \end{bmatrix}.$$

Note that $\boldsymbol{X}(s_i)$ depends on location s_i, different from the traditional GWR. In their simulation studies, Wang et al. (2008) generated two coefficients as nonlinear continuous functions of the spatial coordinates (Fig.12.5), and the local linear fitting approach (Fig. 12.6b, d) clearly demonstrated its bias reduction utility in comparison to the traditional GWR (Fig. 12.6a, c).

Regularized Fitting

Ridge Regression To further constrain the coefficient estimates which serves both purposes of reducing correlation in coefficient estimates and variable selection, Wheeler (2007) suggested the coupling of GWR with ridge regression (GWRR), i.e., adding a penalty term for the L_2 norm of the coefficients:

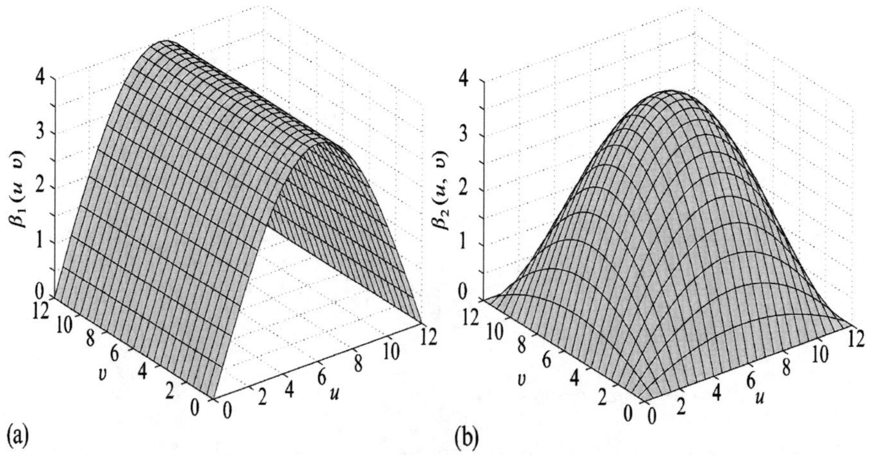

Fig. 12.5 True coefficient functions of geocoordinates in a simulation study in Wang et al. (2008): (**a**) coeficient $\beta_1(u, v)$ for predictor 1; (**b**) coeficient $\beta_2(u, v)$ for predictor 2

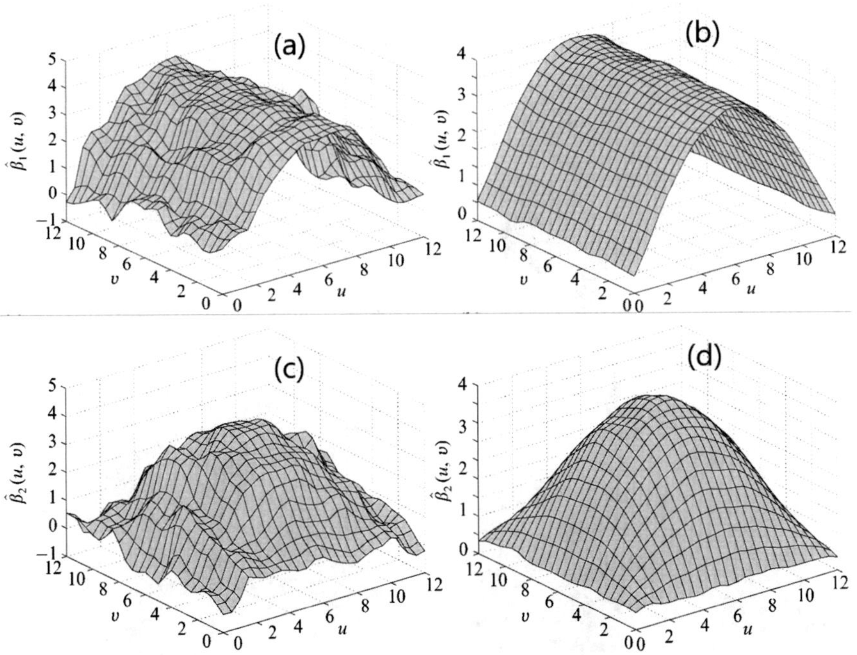

Fig. 12.6 Coefficient functions fitted by GWR (left) and local linear fitting (right) in a simulation study in Wang et al. (2008)

$$\hat{\boldsymbol{\beta}}(s_i) = \arg\min_{\boldsymbol{\beta}} \Big\{ \sum_{j=1}^{n} w_j(s_i) \big[\tilde{y}_j - \tilde{\boldsymbol{X}}_j^{\tau} \boldsymbol{\beta}(s_i) \big]^2 + \lambda \sum_{k=1}^{p} \beta_k^2(s_i) \Big\} \tag{12.5}$$

$$= \big[\tilde{\boldsymbol{X}}^{\tau} \boldsymbol{W}(s_i) \tilde{\boldsymbol{X}} + \lambda \boldsymbol{I} \big]^{-1} \tilde{\boldsymbol{X}}^{\tau} \boldsymbol{W}(s_i) \tilde{\boldsymbol{Y}}, \tag{12.6}$$

where $\tilde{\boldsymbol{X}}_j$ and $\tilde{y}_j$ are standardized covariates and response, $\tilde{\boldsymbol{X}}$ and $\tilde{\boldsymbol{Y}}$ are the standardized version of the covariate matrix and response vector, and λ is the global shrinkage parameter. Several standardization schemes were discussed by Wheeler (2007), but here we only introduce the most straightforward scheme:

$$\tilde{x}_{jk} = \frac{x_{jk} - \bar{x}_k\big(\boldsymbol{W}(s_i)\big)}{\hat{\sigma}_k^{(x)}}, \quad \tilde{y}_j = \frac{y_j - \bar{y}\big(\boldsymbol{W}(s_i)\big)}{\hat{\sigma}^{(y)}},$$

where

$$\bar{x}_k\big(\boldsymbol{W}(s_i)\big) = \sum_{i=1}^{n} \sqrt{w_j(s_i)} x_{jk} \Big/ \sum_{i=1}^{n} \sqrt{w_j(s_i)},$$

$$\bar{y}_k\big(\boldsymbol{W}(s_i)\big) = \sum_{i=1}^{n} \sqrt{w_j(s_i)} y_{jk} \Big/ \sum_{i=1}^{n} \sqrt{w_j(s_i)}$$

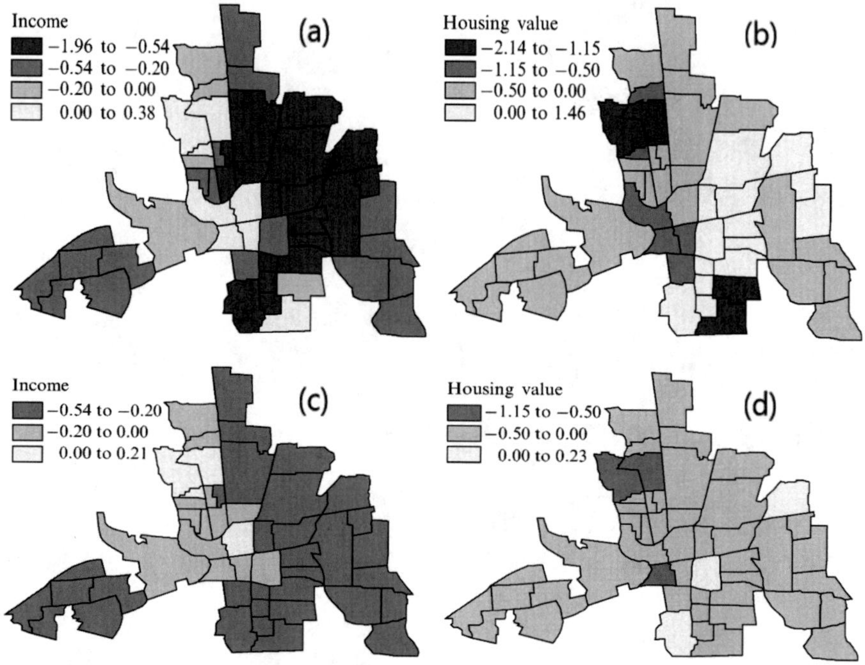

Fig. 12.7 Spatial distributions of coefficient estimates based on GWR and GWRR of crime rate on household income and housing value in Columbus, Ohio: (**a**) Household income, GWR; (**b**) Housing value, GWR; (**c**) Household income, GWRR; and (**d**) Housing value, GWRR (adapted from Wheeler (2007))

are the weighted means, and $\hat{\sigma}_k^{(x)}$ and $\hat{\sigma}^{(y)}$ are the unweighted sample standard deviations, of the kth covariate and the response. Standardization matters for ridge regression, because centering removes the intercept from the model, as ridge regression does not regulate intercept, and rescaling by sample standard deviation ensures fair shrinkage of the regression coefficients. Similar to the bandwidth h, the shrinkage parameter λ can be chosen by cross-validation, and Wheeler (2007) recommended tuning h and λ simultaneously. In his example of fitting crime rate on household income and housing value in Columbus, Ohio, Wheeler (2007) showed appreciable reduction in the correlation between coefficient estimates and more reasonable local coefficient estimates (Fig. 12.7) provided by the GWRR as compared to traditional GWR. Indeed, in Fig. 12.7, the negative association between the coefficient estimates by contrasting (c) with (d) for GWRR is much less obvious than that by contrasting (a) with (b). In addition, the counter-intuitive positive association between crime rate and housing value in East Columbus with GWR (b) become largely negative with GWRR (d).

GWGlasso Analogous to the ridge regression, Wang and Li (2017) proposed a method that couples GWR with adaptive group LASSO to identify model structure and select variables, and named it GWGlasso. The shrinkage of classic lasso is reached by using the L_1-norm penalty, $\lambda \sum_{k=1}^{p} |\beta_k(s_i)|$, instead of square of the L_2 norm, $\lambda \sum_{k=1}^{p} \beta_k^2(s_i)$. One major distinction between ridge regression and lasso is that the former tends to allow for small coefficients close to 0 whereas the latter shrinks small coefficients to 0 exactly (Wheeler 2007). Group lasso applies L_2 norm to the each group of coefficients, $\lambda \sum_{g=1}^{G} \sqrt{\sum_{k=1}^{p_g} \beta_k^2(s_i)}$, where G is the number of groups and p_g is the number of coefficients in group g. It reduces to classic lasso when $p_g = 1$ for all groups. Rather than shrinking each coefficient separately, group lasso shrinks the whole group of coefficients to 0, if shrinkage does occur. As a result, group lasso serves better as a model selector. Adaptive group lasso attaches a different tuning parameter to each group, $\sum_{g=1}^{G} \lambda_g \sqrt{\sum_{k=1}^{p_g} \beta_k^2(s_i)}$. Due to the adaptive feature, it is not necessary to remove the intercept by centering the responses and covariates.

To facilitate the description of GWGlasso, the following notation is defined. Let $\boldsymbol{a}$ be a $n \times p$ matrix with its element at ith row and kth column being $a_{ik} = \beta_k(s_i)$. We denote the columns and rows of $\boldsymbol{a}$ by $\boldsymbol{a}_{,k} = (\beta_k(s_1), \ldots, \beta_k(s_n))^\tau$, $k = 1, \ldots, p$, and $\boldsymbol{a}_{i,} = (\beta_1(s_i), \ldots, \beta_p(s_i))^\tau$, $i = 1, \ldots, n$, respectively. Note that both $\boldsymbol{a}_{,k}$ and $\boldsymbol{a}_{i,}$ are column vectors. Let $\boldsymbol{b}$ be a $2n \times p$ matrix with its element at ith row and kth column being

$$b_{ik} = \begin{cases} \beta_k^{(u)}(s_i), & 1 \le i \le n, \\ \beta_k^{(v)}(s_{i-n}), & n < i \le 2n \end{cases}.$$

Similarly, the columns of $\boldsymbol{b}$ are represented by $\boldsymbol{b}_{,k} = \left(\beta_k^{(u)}(s_1), \ldots, \beta_k^{(u)}(s_n), \beta_k^{(v)}(s_1), \ldots, \beta_k^{(v)}(s_n)\right)^\tau$, $k = 1, \ldots, p$. The rows of $\boldsymbol{b}$ are represented by $\boldsymbol{b}_{i,} = \left(\beta_1^{(u)}(s_i), \ldots, \beta_p^{(u)}(s_i)\right)^\tau$ for $1 \le i \le n$, and $\boldsymbol{b}_{i,} = \left(\beta_1^{(v)}(s_1), \ldots, \beta_p^{(v)}(s_i)\right)^\tau$ for $n < i \le 2n$. The objective function to be minimized is

$$L(\boldsymbol{a}, \boldsymbol{b}) = \sum_{i=1}^{n} L_i\big(\boldsymbol{\beta}(s_i)\big) + 2\lambda \sum_{k=1}^{p} \Big(\omega_{1k}||\boldsymbol{a}_{,k}||_2 + \omega_{2k}||\boldsymbol{b}_{,k}||_2\Big), \tag{12.7}$$

where $L_i\big((\boldsymbol{\beta}(s_i)$ is given in (12.4), $||\boldsymbol{a}_{,k}||_2 = \sqrt{\sum_{i=1}^{n}[\beta_k(s_i)]^2}$, and $||\boldsymbol{b}_{,k}||_2 = \sqrt{\sum_{i=1}^{n}[\beta_k^{(u)}(s_i)]^2 + [\beta_k^{(v)}(s_i)]^2}$. $||\cdot||_2$ is the L_2 norm (also called Euclidean norm). The weights, $\omega_{1k} = \sqrt{n}/||\hat{\boldsymbol{a}}_{,k}^{(0)}||_2$ and $\omega_{2k} = \sqrt{2n}/||\hat{\boldsymbol{b}}_{,k}^{(0)}||_2$, are used to account for the scales of the coefficient groups and turn multiple tuning parameters to a single one, where $\hat{\boldsymbol{a}}_{,k}^{(0)}$ and $\hat{\boldsymbol{b}}_{,k}^{(0)}$ are estimates of $\boldsymbol{a}_{,k}$ and $\boldsymbol{b}_{,k}$ without the penalty (Wang & Li, 2017). The objective function is not differentiable at the origin for the same reason that $f(x) = |x|$ is not. To circumvent this difficulty, a local quadratic approximation can be used (Wang & Li, 2017). For example, suppose the current estimate of $\boldsymbol{a}_{,k}$ is $\hat{\boldsymbol{a}}_{,k}^{(m)}$ at the mth iteration in an iterative evaluation procedure. Based on the first-order Taylor expansion of $f(y) = \sqrt{y}$, the approximation is

$$||\boldsymbol{a}_{,k}||_2 \approx ||\hat{\boldsymbol{a}}_{,k}^{(m)}||_2 + \frac{||\boldsymbol{a}_{,k}||_2{}^2 - ||\hat{\boldsymbol{a}}_{,k}^{(m)}||_2{}^2}{2||\hat{\boldsymbol{a}}_{,k}^{(m)}||_2}.$$

$||\boldsymbol{a}_k||_2{}^2$ is differentiable everywhere. The same approximation applies to $||\boldsymbol{b}_k||$ as well. With such approximations plugged in, the objective function becomes

$$L(\boldsymbol{a}, \boldsymbol{b}) \propto \sum_{i=1}^{n} \Big[L_i(\boldsymbol{\beta}(s_i)) + \lambda \big(\boldsymbol{a}_{i,}^{\tau} \boldsymbol{D}_1^{(m)} \boldsymbol{a}_{i,} + \boldsymbol{b}_{i,}^{\tau} \boldsymbol{D}_2^{(m)} \boldsymbol{b}_{i,} + \boldsymbol{b}_{n+i,}^{\tau} \boldsymbol{D}_2^{(m)} \boldsymbol{b}_{n+i,} \big) \Big],$$

where $\boldsymbol{D}_1^{(m)} = \text{diag}\big(\omega_{11}/||\boldsymbol{a}_{,1}^{(m)}||_2, \ldots, \omega_{1p}/||\boldsymbol{a}_{,p}^{(m)}||_2\big)$ and $\boldsymbol{D}_2^{(m)} = \text{diag}\big(\omega_{21p}/||\boldsymbol{b}_{,1}^{(m)}||_2, \ldots, \omega_{2p}/||\boldsymbol{b}_{,p}^{(m)}||_2\big)$.

Depending on whether the coefficient groups are shrunk to 0 or not, the model is naturally structured:

- When $\hat{\boldsymbol{a}}_{,k} = \hat{\boldsymbol{b}}_{,k} = \mathbf{0}$, then we conclude $\beta_k(s_i) = 0$ for all i, i.e., the kth covariate is not influential.
- When $\hat{\boldsymbol{b}}_{,k} = \mathbf{0}$ but $\hat{\boldsymbol{a}}_{,k} \neq \mathbf{0}$, then $\beta_k(s_i) = \beta_k$ for all i, i.e., there is no spatial heterogeneity in the effect of the kth covariate, and β_k is estimated by $\frac{1}{n}\sum_{i=1}^{n} \hat{\beta}_k(s_i)$, where $\hat{\beta}_k(s_i)$'s are elements of $\hat{\boldsymbol{a}}, k$.
- When $\hat{\boldsymbol{a}}_{,k} \neq \mathbf{0}$ and $\hat{\boldsymbol{b}}_{,k} \neq \mathbf{0}$, then there is spatial heterogeneity in the effect of the kth covariate, and $\beta_k(s_i)$ is estimated by $\hat{\beta}_k(s_i)$.

To alleviate computational overhead, Wang and Li (2017) suggested the optimal bandwidth, $h^{\star}$, be chosen using cross-validation based on the unpenalized local linear estimation approach. After fixing the bandwidth, the shrinkage parameter λ can be chosen to minimize the Bayesian information criteria,

$$BIC = \log\Big[\frac{1}{n^2}\sum_{i=1}^{n} L_i\big(\hat{\boldsymbol{\beta}}_{\lambda}(s_i)\big)\Big] + df_{\lambda}\frac{\log(nh)}{nh} + (p - df_{\lambda})\frac{\log(n)}{n},$$

where df_{λ} is the number of spatially-varying coefficients, $L_i\big(\hat{\boldsymbol{\beta}}_{\lambda}(s_i)\big)$ is given in (12.4), and $\hat{\boldsymbol{\beta}}_{\lambda}(s_i), i = 1, \ldots, n$, are the estimated coefficients in $\boldsymbol{a}$ and $\boldsymbol{b}$ under a given value of λ.

While GWGlasso is able to identify model structures, it is often desired to find sparse local coefficients within groups. Such desire entails the need for a method between lasso and group lasso, where the sparse group lasso fits (Simon et al. 2001). A possible extension of (12.7) is to incorporate sparse group lasso into GWGlasso is

$$L(\boldsymbol{a}, \boldsymbol{b}) = \sum_{i=1}^{n} L_i(\boldsymbol{\beta}(s_i)) + 2\lambda_1 \sum_{k=1}^{p} \Big(\omega_{1k}||\boldsymbol{a}_{,k}||_2 + \omega_{2k}||\boldsymbol{b}_{,k}||_2 \Big)$$
$$+ \lambda_2 \sum_{k=1}^{p} \Big(\omega_{1k}^{\star}||\boldsymbol{a}_{,k}||_1 + \omega_{2k}^{\star}||\boldsymbol{b}_{,k}||_1 \Big),$$

where $||\boldsymbol{a}_{,k}||_1 = \sum_{i=1}^{n} |a_{ik}|$ is the L_1 norm. Whether this is a valid extension, as well as what form should $\omega_{1k}^{\star}$ and $\omega_{2k}^{\star}$ take, are open questions.

GW Elastic Net lasso is able to identify influential covariates to form a parsimonious model, sacrificing the predictive power of the model to some level. On the other hand, ridge regression is able to reduce the impact of multicolinearity without compromising predictive performance, but it may retain non-predictive covariates. To find a balance between parsimony and predictive performance, a geographically weighted elastic net (GWEN) blends lasso and ridge penalties (Li & Lam, 2018):

$$L_i(\boldsymbol{\beta}(s_i)) = \sum_{j=1}^{n} w_j(s_i)\Big[y_j \quad \beta_0(s_i) \quad \sum_{k=1}^{p} \beta_k(s_i)x_{jk}\Big]^2 + \lambda \sum_{k=1}^{p} \big[(1-\alpha)\beta_k^2(s_i) + \alpha|\beta_k(s_i)|\big]$$

Similar to (12.5), one can center and rescale covariates and responses to remove the intercept:

$$L_i(\boldsymbol{\beta}(s_i)) = \sum_{j=1}^{n} w_j(s_i)\big[\tilde{y}_j - \tilde{\boldsymbol{X}}_j^{T}\boldsymbol{\beta}(s_i)\big]^2 + \lambda \sum_{k=1}^{p} \big[(1-\alpha)\beta_k^2(s_i) + \alpha|\beta_k(s_i)|\big]$$

where $\tilde{\boldsymbol{X}}_j$ and $\tilde{y}_j$, $j = 1, \ldots, n$, are standardized covariates and responses.

In an analysis of population size change from 2000 to 2010 regressed on thirty-five socio-environmental variables in the Lower Mississippi River Basin, Li and Lam (2018) compared the results between several GWR models as shown in Table 12.3. In this table, root MSE measures goodness of fit, mean VIF measures multicolinearity among covariates, and global Moran's I measures spatial assesses spatial autocorrelation among residuals. For all these quantities, the lower the better. GWEN resembles GWR-lasso in model parsimony and explaining spatial correlation, and is comparable to GWR-Ridge in terms of goodness-of-fit and multicolinearity. As expected, GWEN offers a reasonable trade-off between parsimony and goodness-of-fit.

Table 12.3 Comparison between various GWR models

Metrics	Classic GWR	GWR-Ridge	GWR-lasso	GWEN
Root MSE	0.42	0.51	0.59	0.55
Mean VIF	252.64	4.92	2.78	4.04
Average # of selected covariates	35.00	35.00	10.18	10.18
Global Moran's I	0.009	0.019	0.046	0.045

This table is adapted from Li and Lam (2018)

12.3 Software and Case Study

Currently, there are multiple choices of software tools implementing various versions of GWR. GWR4 is a standalone software package dedicated to GWR, implementing GWR for three distribution families (Gaussian, Poisson and Logistic), with useful features such as variable selection and simultaneously considering global and local regression coefficients (Nakaya, Fotheringham, Charlton, & Brunsdon, 2009). GWR has also been integrated into several commonly used GIS or spatial statistics software tools such as ArcGIS (Environmental Systems Resource Institute 2013), SpaceStat (BioMedware 2011), and SAM (Rangel, Diniz-Filho, & Bini, 2010). Both ArcGIS and SpaceStat are commercial software packages that are not free. We introduce three GWR-related R packages, spgwr, gwrr and GWmodel using a case study with a real data set, mainly for the free availability and versatility of R as a software platform for data manipulation, data presentation, and statistical analysis. To facilitate our description, we refer to the three regularized models (GW ridge regression, GWR with lasso and GWR with locally compensated ridge) available in packages gwrr and GWmodel as GWR-Ridge, GWR-LASSO and GWR-LCR. A brief comparison of features of the three packages is shown in Table 12.4. Clearly, these packages have some non-overlapping features, and it could be fruitful to use them in combination.

12.3.1 Data

For the case study we use the hand, foot and mouth disease (HFMD) surveillance data during 2009 in China, provided by the courtesy of Chinese Center for Disease Control and Prevention (CCDC). Epidemiological description and statistical analyses of these data can be found elsewhere (Tang, Yang, Yu, Liao, & Bliznyuk, 2019; Wang et al. 2011). Briefly, HFMD is a disease mainly among children under 6 years of age caused by a spectrum of enteroviruses. In China, mandated reporting of this disease was initiated by a large outbreak in 2008. The reporting became well established and relatively complete since 2009. As in Wang et al. (2011), we will analyze the data at the prefecture level, which is an administrative level between province and county. The dependent variable (outcome) of interest is disease incidence, i.e., number of cases per year and 100,000 people, after log-transformation. The independent variables (predictors) are log-transformed population density, (log-popden) temperature (temp), relative humidity (rh), and wind speed (ws), and all three climatic predictors are taken as annual averages. All predictors have been standardized to have 0 for sample means and 1 for sample variance. The spatial distributions of case numbers and incidences are shown in Fig. 12.8. High disease incidences are found in Guangxi, Guang and northern Hunan provinces. Moron's I statistic based on Euclidean distances as the weights is -0.056 with a p-value <0.001, indicating a pattern of more spatially dispersed than expected.

Table 12.4 Comparison of features between various GWR-related R packages, partially adapted from Gollini et al. (2015)

			Packages			
Model	Function	Option	spgwr	gwrr	GWmodel	McSpatial
All	Kernel[a]	Gaussian	Y	Y	Y	Y
		Bi-square	Y		Y	Y
		Tri-cube			Y	Y
		Exponential		Y	Y	
Classic GWR	Bandwidth Selection	CV	Y	Y	Y	Y
		AICc	Y		Y	
	Adaptive Bandwidth		Y		Y	
	Colinearity Diagnosis	VIF			Y	
		VDP		Y	Y	
		Condition number		Y	Y	
	Colinearity Solution	Global ridge		Y	Y[b]	
		Local ridge			Y[b]	
		LASSO		Y		
	Test global vs. local coefficients		Y		Y	
Generalized GWR	Distribution[c]	Poisson	Y		Y	
		Binomial	Y		Y	Y
		Multinomial				Y
		Quasi-Poisson	Y			
	Bandwidth Selection	CV	Y		Y	Y
		AICc			Y	
	Adaptive Bandwidth		Y		Y	

[a] GWmodel and McSpatial provide additional kernel functions
[b] GWmodel requires users to provide ridge parameters, i.e., no optimization
[c] spgwr offers additional distributions as specified in glm() function

12.3.2 *Data Analysis with R Packages*

We use R 3.3.0 for all the analyses (R Core Team 2013). The following packages are to be loaded.

```
Packages <- c("maptools", "shapefiles", "RColorBrewer", "rgdal", "spdep",
         "sp", "spgwr", "gwrr", "GWmodel", "lattice", "ape")
invisible(lapply(Packages, library, character.only = TRUE))
```

To load an individual package, e.g., gwrr, simply use "library(gwrr)". To load the data, use either of the following options:

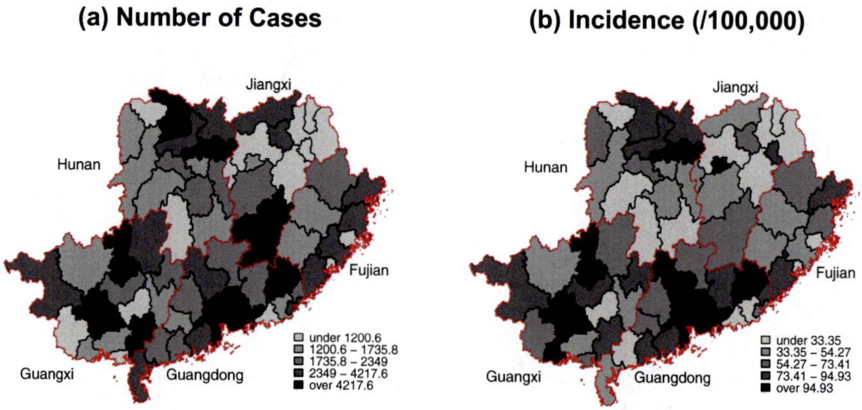

Fig. 12.8 Spatial distributions of (**a**) numbers of cases and (**b**) annual incidences at the prefecture level in five southern provinces of China during the 2009 epidemic of the hand, foot and mouth disease

```
# Option 1
setwd(path); load(case_study_gwr.RData)
# Option 2
load(paste(path, "case_study_gwr.RData", sep=''))
```

where *path* is the directory where your put the data, e.g., "C:/gwr/data/". Three data sets will be loaded, two spatial data objects (of type SpatialPolygonsDataFrame in R spatial statistics packages), named "south5.shp" and "`south5_province_line`", and one usual data frame, named "my.data", which contains the same data as in south5.shp but no polygon structures. "`south5_province_line`" is only for drawing provincial boundaries.

To assess Moran's I for disease incidence, use the code

```
centroids <- coordinates(south5.shp)
my.dMat <- gw.dist(centroids)
Moran.I(my.data$log_incidence, my.dMat)
```

We first examine the relationship between the outcome and the predictors to see if nonlinear trend exists. There appears to moderate levels of nonlinear trends for population density, temperature and wind speed (Fig. 12.9). However, for illustrative purpose, we move ahead with only linear terms. To select a bandwidth via cross-validation using the Gaussian kernel and to fit a classic GWR with the chosen bandwidth, one can use the following functions from the spgwr package:

```
bw.gwr<-gwr.sel(log_incidence~log_popden+rh+temp+ws, data=south5.shp,
                adapt=FALSE, gweight=gwr.Gauss, verbose=TRUE)
fit.gwr<-gwr(log_incidence~log_popden+rh+temp+ws, data=south5.shp,
             bandwidth=bw.gwr, gweight=gwr.Gauss, hatmatrix=TRUE)
```

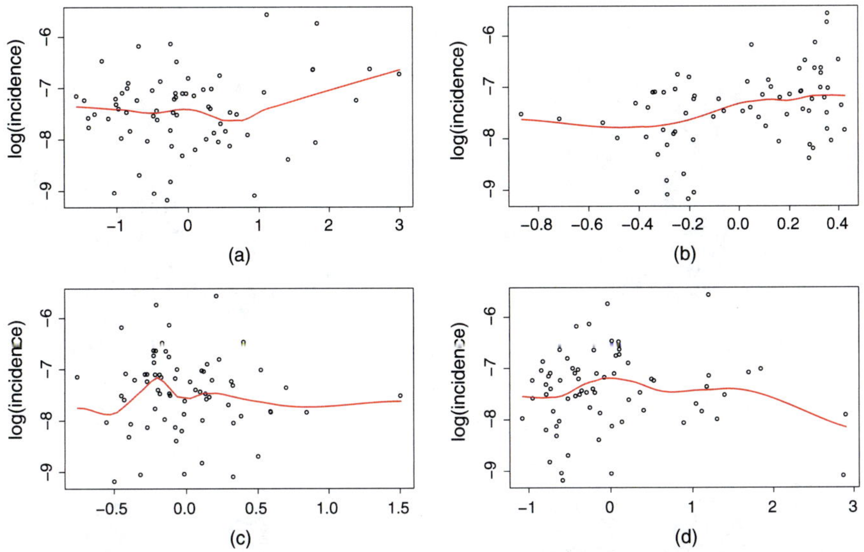

Fig. 12.9 Scatter plots of the outcome with (**a**) log(population density), (**b**) temperature, (**c**) relative humidity and (**d**) wind speed. The red solid curves represent loess smoothing

The option adapt=FALSE tells gwr.sel() that a fixed rather than adaptive bandwidth is desired. If adapt=TRUE, then a fraction is returned. For example, if the optimal fraction found by gwr.sel() is 0.8, then the nearest 80% of all data points will be included for analysis at each location. The option hatmatrix=TRUE specifies that the hat matrix is to be included in the returned object fit.gwr, in addition to other model outputs. The spatial distributions of the estimated coefficients, as shown in Fig. 12.9, are produced by

```
par(mfrow=c(2,2))
do.map(fit.gwr$SDF, fit.gwr$SDF$log_popden, '(a) log(Pop Density)')
do.map(fit.gwr$SDF, fit.gwr$SDF$temp, '(b) Temperature')
do.map(fit.gwr$SDF, fit.gwr$SDF$rh, '(c) Rel. Humidity')
do.map(fit.gwr$SDF, fit.gwr$SDF$ws, '(d) Wind Speed')
```

and the function *do.map()* can be found in the accompanying online code with this book. Figure 12.10 appears to indicate geographical clustering of different levels of regression coefficients for each predictor, particularly relative humidity and wind speed; nevertheless, such geographic heterogeneity may not be of practical importance. For example, the absolute value of the coefficient of variation is 0.23 for the estimated coefficients for temperature, much lower than 3.33 and 3.35 for relative humidity and wind speed, suggesting a lesser degree of spatial heterogeneity for temperature. The coefficient of variation is simply the ratio of standard deviation to mean and can be computed by `sd(fit.gwr$SDF$temp)/mean(fit.gwr$SDF$temp)`. Formal statistical tests can be used to test for spatial nonstationary in all or specific predictors:

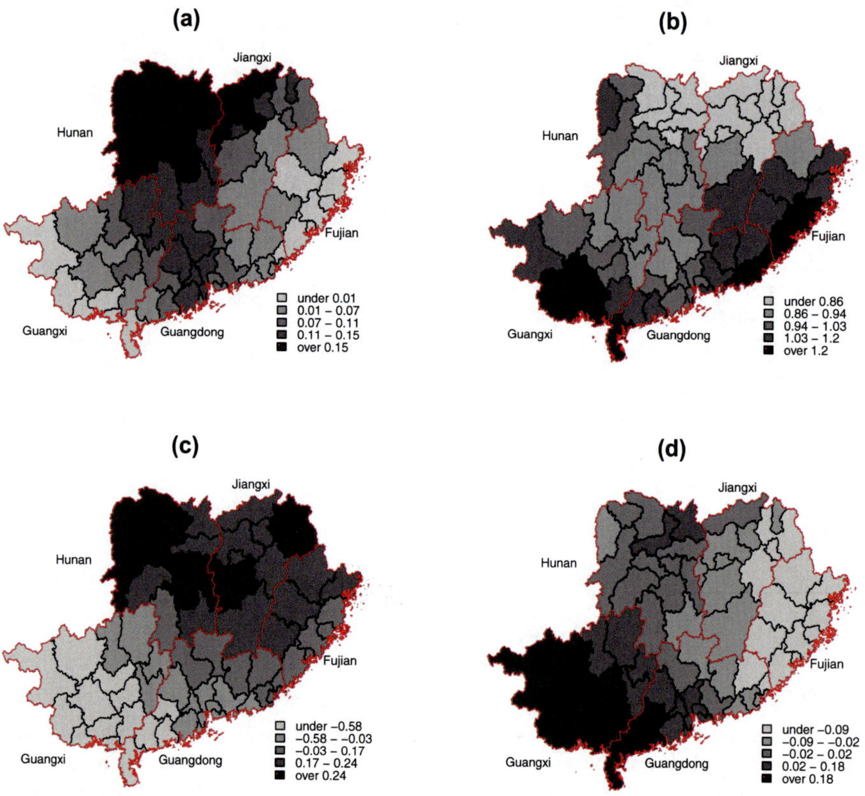

Fig. 12.10 Spatial distributions of local coefficients estimated by classic GWR with a fixed Gaussian kernel for (**a**) log(population density), (**b**) temperature, (**c**) relative humidity, and (**d**) wind speed

```
> BFC02.gwr.test(fit.gwr)$p.value
0.1932179
> LMZ.F1GWR.test(fit.gwr)$p.value
0.4162748
> LMZ.F2GWR.test(fit.gwr)$p.value
0.2315591
> LMZ.F3GWR.test(fit.gwr)
Leung et al. (2000) F(3) test

            F statistic  Numerator d.f.  Denominator d.f.      Pr(>)
(Intercept)     0.87779        34.29761            58.356    0.65434
log_popden      0.96944        23.37794            58.356    0.51567
rh              4.21961        31.52168            58.356  1.008e-06 ***
temp            0.57866        22.33473            58.356    0.92288
ws              1.71297        23.17358            58.356    0.05019 .
---
Signif. codes:  0 '***' 0.001 '**' 0.01 '*' 0.05 '.' 0.1 ' ' 1
```

BFC02.gwr refers to the resampling-based test (Brunsdon et al. 1996; Fotheringham et al. 2002), and LMZ.F1GWR and LMZ.F2GWR refer to the asymptotic test (Leung et al. 2000), for the global null (spatial stationarity in all coefficients). LMZ.F3GWR refers to the asymptotic tests for specific predictors (Leung et al. 2000). Spatial nonstationarity seems to be significant for relative humidity and marginally significant for wind speed. However, none of the global tests are significant. Statistically speaking, one should take the tests for specific predictors seriously only if the global test is significant.

To assess colinearity in predictors and its impact on GWR, we look at local weighted correlations among predictors' values (weights determined by the same distance matrix as in GWR) and correlations among GWR-estimated local coefficients of these predictors.

```
> var.list <- c('log_popden', 'temp', 'rh', 'ws')
> cov.gwr<-gw.cov(fit.gwr$SDF, vars=var.list,
+                 bw=bw.gwr, gweight=gwr.Gauss)
> mean.cor.gwr<-with(cov.gwr$SDF@data, apply(cbind(cor.log_popden.temp.,
+                    cor.log_popden.rh., cor.log_popden.ws., cor.temp.rh.,
+                    cor.temp.ws., cor.rh.ws.), 2, mean))
> b<-matrix(0, nrow=4, ncol=4, dimnames=list(var.list, var.list))
> b[lower.tri(b, diag=FALSE)] <- mean.cor.gwr
> t(b)
           log_popden       temp         rh          ws
log_popden          0 -0.6352849  0.3803019  0.01462292
temp                0  0.0000000 -0.4499036  0.16462085
rh                  0  0.0000000  0.0000000 -0.81590363
ws                  0  0.0000000  0.0000000  0.00000000
> with(fit.gwr$SDF@data, cor(cbind(log_popden, temp, rh, ws)))
           log_popden       temp         rh         ws
log_popden  1.0000000 -0.5994083  0.4320501 -0.1735663
temp       -0.5994083  1.0000000 -0.5898919  0.4249700
rh          0.4320501 -0.5898919  1.0000000 -0.9482771
ws         -0.1735663  0.4249700 -0.9482771  1.0000000
```

The local weighted correlations flagged alarming colinearity between population density and temperature, −0.63, as well as between relative humidity and wind speed, −0.82. The impact of colinearity of the latter pair on GWR is confirmed by the high negative correlation, −0.95, in local coefficients between relative humidity and wind speed. The colinearity associated with relative humidity and wind speed are visualized as the scatter plot of the estimated local coefficients (Fig. 12.11a) and the mapping of estimated local correlation based on Fisher information in the estimates of local coefficients (Fig. 12.11b). Unfortunately, the package spgwr does not provide means of addressing colinearity. It is probably worth mentioning that, for colinearity in the GWR setting, it could be misleading to only check the global correlations among the predictors, as the following code shows.

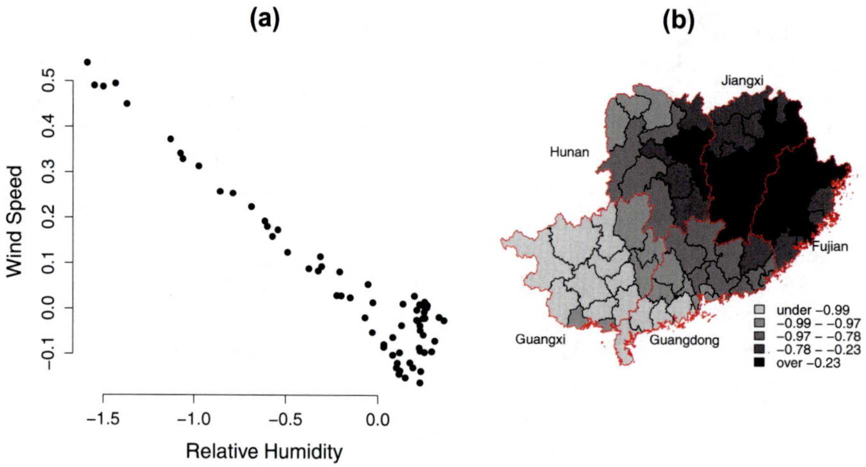

Fig. 12.11 Colinearity between relative humidity and wind speed is examined by (**a**) scatter plot of estimated local coefficients and (**b**) spatial distribution of estimated local correlation (using Fisher information) in the estimates of local coefficients

```
> with(my.data, cor(cbind(log_popden, temp, rh, ws)))
             log_popden        temp          rh         ws
log_popden  1.00000000  0.27318920 -0.05270545 0.44078059
temp        0.27318920  1.00000000 -0.11509446 0.04691729
rh         -0.05270545 -0.11509446  1.00000000 0.34480512
ws          0.44078059  0.04691729  0.34480512 1.00000000
```

The package spgwr does provide generalized GWR models, and the distribution families are as many wide as specified by glm(). The Poisson family is appropriate if we model the number of cases directly with population size as an offset.

```
bw.ggwr<-ggwr.sel(n_cases~log_popden+rh+temp+ws+offset(log(pop)),
                  data = south5.shp, family=poisson, adapt = FALSE,
                  gweight = gwr.Gauss, verbose = TRUE)
fit.ggwr<-ggwr(n_cases~log_popden+rh+temp+ws+offset(log(pop)),
               data = south5.shp, family=poisson,
               bandwidth=bw.ggwr, gweight=gwr.Gauss)
```

This Poisson GWR yields largely similar spatial patterns of local coefficient estimates (Fig. 12.12) as compared to the classic GWR (Fig. 12.10), except that large coefficients for temperature became more clustered in the southwest corner of the study region. However, spgwr does not offer predicted values of generalized models (mean rate in the Poisson case) or any measure for goodness-of-fit to the data.

Before exploring the ridge regression and LASSO facilities in the gwrr package, we first introduce the function vdp.gwr() in this package for diagnosing colinearity. Unlike spgwr, functions in gwrr do not handle spatial data structure (such as

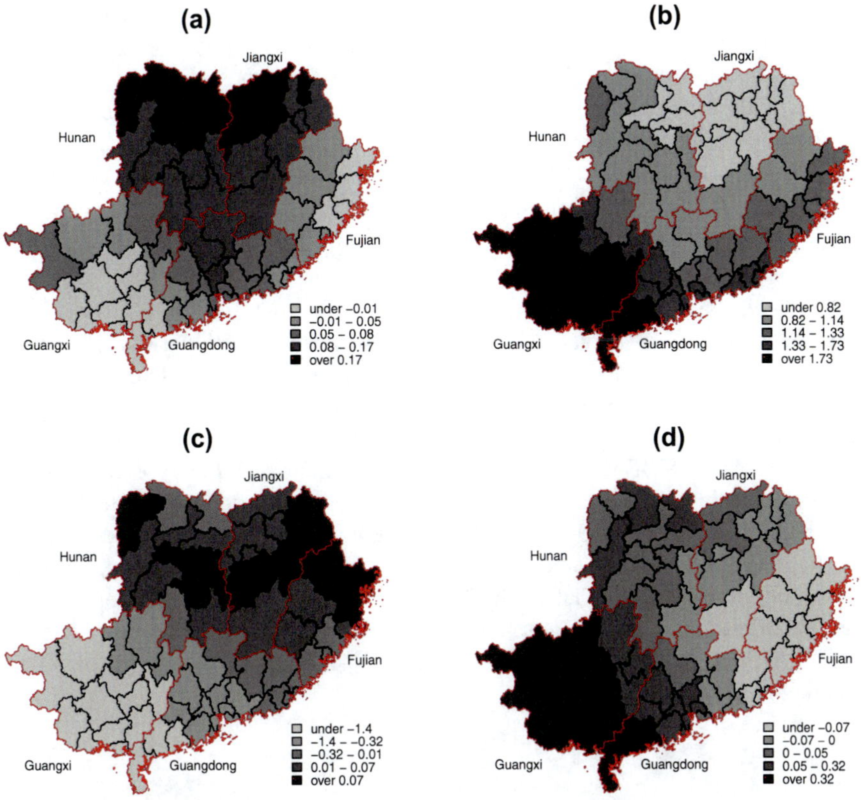

Fig. 12.12 Spatial distributions of local coefficients estimated by Poisson GWR with a fixed Gaussian kernel for (**a**) log(population density), (**b**) temperature, (**c**) relative humidity, and (**d**) wind speed

south5.shp used above) directly; instead, they require usual data frames with geo-coordinates as a separate argument.

```
bw.gwr.exp<-gwr.bw.est(log_incidence~log_popden+rh+temp+ws, data=my.data,
                        locs=centroids, kernel="exp")
vdp.gwr<-gwr.vdp(log_incidence~log_popden+rh+temp+ws, data=my.data,
                 locs=centroids, kernel="exp", phi=bw.gwr.exp$phi,
                 sel.ci = 30, sel.vdp = 0.5)
```

The first command optimizes the bandwidth via cross-validation, using the exponential kernel. Only two kernels are available in gwrr, Gaussian ("gauss") or exponential ("exp"). We got an numeric error by using the Gaussian kernel on the HFMD data, which leaves exponential as the only feasible option. Function gwr.bw.est() returns a structure rather than a value, and the selected bandwidth can be retrieved with `bw.gwr.exp$phi`. Function gwr.vdp() outputs both variance decomposition proportions (VDP) and condition numbers (CN), both derived from the weighted covariance matrix $\sqrt{\boldsymbol{W}(s_i)}\boldsymbol{X}$. According to Wheeler (2007), let the singular value decomposition of $\sqrt{\boldsymbol{W}(s_i)}\boldsymbol{X}$ be $\sqrt{\boldsymbol{W}(s_i)}\boldsymbol{X} = \boldsymbol{U}\boldsymbol{D}\boldsymbol{V}^{\tau}$, where $\boldsymbol{U}$ is a $n \times (p+1)$ matrix with orthogonal columns, $\boldsymbol{D}$ is a $(p+1) \times (p+1)$ diagonal matrix, and $\boldsymbol{V}$ is a $(p+1) \times (p+1)$ matrix with orthogonal columns. The diagonal elements $(d_1, \ldots, d_{p+1})$ of $\boldsymbol{D}$ are called singular values, and the columns of $\boldsymbol{V}$ are called (right) singular vectors. CNs are defined as $CN_j = \max(d_1, \ldots, d_{p+1})/d_j$ for $j = 1, \ldots, p+1$, and VDPs are defined as a matrix $\boldsymbol{\Phi} = \{\phi_{ij} = \frac{v_{ij}^2}{d_j^2}\}_{(p+1)\times(p+1)}$ rescaled by its row sums, i.e., $VDP_{ij} = \phi_{ij}/\phi_i$, where $\phi_i = \sum_{k=1}^{p+1} \phi_{ik}$. The rationale behind VDP is $\mathrm{Var}(\hat{\beta}_k(s_i)) = \sigma^2\phi_i$. However, function gwr.vdp() returns only a single value rather than a vector for CN and a vector rather than a matrix for VDP. After some investigation (see the online R code associated with this book), we found that the returned CN is the ratio of the largest to the smallest singular value, and the returned VDP vector is the column of the matrix $\{VDP_{ij}\}$ associated with the smallest singular value. This CN definition is analogous to (not exactly the same as) the one introduced in Gollini, Lu, Charlton, Brunsdon, and Harris (2015) for the package GWmodel. CN values > 30 or VDPs > 0.5 are thought to flag potential issues of colinearity, and that is why 30 and 0.5 are used for threshold options sel.ci and sel.vdp in the above code to indicate which locations have alarming RNs and VDPs. CN is also called condition index in Wheeler (2007), which explains the naming of the option sel.ci.

```
> summary(vdp.gwr$condition)
   Min. 1st Qu.  Median    Mean 3rd Qu.    Max.
  1.831   2.344   2.581   2.616   2.787   3.978
> apply(vdp.gwr$vdp, 2, summary)
              [,1]    [,2]      [,3]      [,4]    [,5]
Min.     6.206e-05 0.01967 2.764e-05 0.0001593 0.02339
1st Qu.  1.260e-02 0.23340 4.909e-02 0.3273000 0.16460
Median   2.410e-01 0.35770 1.298e-01 0.6547000 0.31700
Mean     2.994e-01 0.39300 2.208e-01 0.5513000 0.39120
3rd Qu.  5.281e-01 0.52170 4.188e-01 0.8028000 0.66820
Max.     8.384e-01 0.84120 6.724e-01 0.8949000 0.86160
```

For the HFMD data, none of the CNs are over the threshold, but a substantial amount of VDPs are exceeding 0.5, suggesting that a certain level of colinearity. The following code fits classic GWR and GWRs with ridge and LASSO penalties using functions in the gwrr package, where both bandwidth and shrinkage parameter are automatically chosen via cross-validation.

```
fit2.gwr<-gwr.est(log_incidence~log_popden+rh+temp+ws, data=my.data,
                  locs=centroids, kernel="exp", bw=bw.gwr.exp$phi)
fit.gwrr<-gwrr.est(log_incidence~log_popden+rh+temp+ws, data=my.data,
                   locs=centroids, kernel="exp", bw=TRUE, rd=TRUE)
fit.gwl<-gwl.est(log_incidence~log_popden+rh+temp+ws,
                 data=my.data, locs=centroids, kernel="exp")
```

We found that the ridge shrinkage parameter chosen by gwrr.est() for the HFMD data was 0, i.e., no shrinkage at all. For illustration, we fitted a GWR-Ridge model with a bandwidth equal to `bw.gwr.exp$phi` and an rather arbitrary shrinkage parameter of 0.01, and presented all results about GWR-Ridge based on this model.

```
> fit.gwrr<-gwrr.est(log_incidence~log_popden+rh+temp+ws,
+                    data=my.data, locs=centroids, kernel="exp",
+                    bw=bw.gwr.exp$phi, rd=0.01)
>  gof <-rbind(c(fit2.gwr$rsquare, fit.gwrr$rsquare, fit.gwl$rsquare),
+              c(fit2.gwr$RMSE, fit.gwrr$RMSE, fit.gwl$RMSE))
> dimnames(gof)<-list(c('R-square', 'RMSE'),
+                     c('Classic GWR', 'GWR-Ridge', 'GWR-LASSO'))
> gof
          Classic GWR GWR-Ridge GWR-LASSO
R-square    0.4584649 0.5085547 0.6956734
RMSE        0.5431182 0.5173908 0.4071468
```

The approximate R-squares of the regularized GWRs are larger, whereas the root mean square errors (RMSE) are smaller, than those of the classic GWR, indicating better goodness-of-fit to the data for the regularized regressions. Nonetheless, this does not necessarily imply better predictive power on new data. The scales and spatial distributions of local coefficients are shown in Fig. 12.13 for GWR-Ridge and in Fig. 12.14 for GWR-LASSO. Compared to classic GWR (Fig. 12.10), GWR-Ridge yielded more or less similar spatial patterns of coefficients except for temperature for which large coefficients in southern Guangxi province shifted to northern Hunan province. Shrinkage of coefficients towards zero is only noticeable for temperature. GWR-LASSO clearly shrank local coefficients towards 0 more aggressively, and led to more scattered spatial patterns of coefficients than the other two models.

Gollini et al. (2015) proposed a GWR approach with locally compensated ridge (GWR-LCR) parameters which is implemented in the R package GWmodel. However, the statistical presentation in the paper was a little loose, and we were not able to find further technical details elsewhere. As a result, we briefly summarize the rationale here, per our understanding of the paper. In a global regression setting, the standard solution to ridge regression is expressed as $\hat{\boldsymbol{\beta}} = (\boldsymbol{X}^{\tau}\boldsymbol{X} + \lambda\boldsymbol{I})^{-1}\boldsymbol{X}^{\tau}\boldsymbol{Y}$, where λ is the ridge penalty tuning parameter and $\boldsymbol{I}$ is the identity matrix. Let $\theta_1, \ldots, \theta_p$ be the eigenvalues of $\boldsymbol{X}^{\tau}\boldsymbol{X}$ in decreasing order, i.e., θ_1 and θ_p are the largest and smallest eigenvalues. Eigenvalues returned by R functions usually are also ordered decreasingly. Gollini et al. (2015) defined the condition number as θ_1/θ_p. The eigenvalues of the ridge-adjusted cross-product matrix $\boldsymbol{X}^{\tau}\boldsymbol{X} + \lambda\boldsymbol{I}$ is $\theta_1 + \lambda, \ldots, \theta_p + \lambda$, and the associated CN is $(\theta_1 + \lambda)/(\theta_p + \lambda)$. To have $CN \leq \kappa$ for some threshold κ, one can choose $\lambda \geq (\theta_1 - \kappa\theta_p)/(\kappa - 1)$. In a GWR-Ridge setting where a local ridge penalty is applied to each location, the local solution

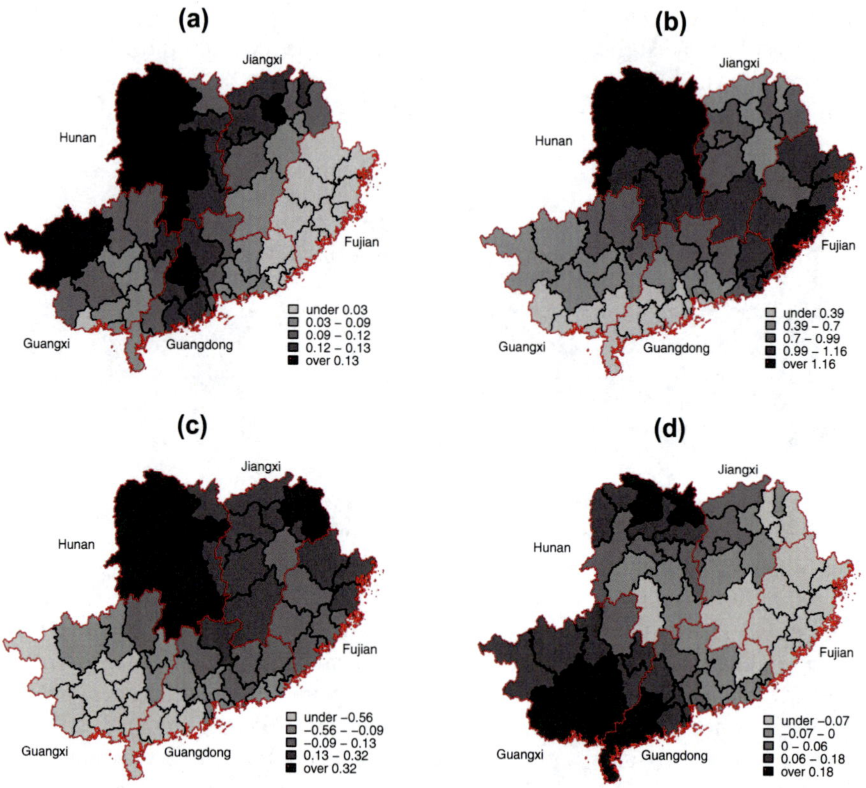

Fig. 12.13 Spatial distributions of local coefficients estimated by GWR-Ridge with an exponential kernel and a fixed bandwidth for (**a**) log(population density), (**b**) temperature, (**c**) relative humidity, and (**d**) wind speed

is given by $\hat{\boldsymbol{\beta}}(s_i) = (\boldsymbol{X}^\tau \boldsymbol{W}(s_i)\boldsymbol{X} + \lambda_i \boldsymbol{I})^{-1}\boldsymbol{X}^\tau \boldsymbol{W}(s_i)\boldsymbol{Y}$. The local ridge parameters λ_i's can be tuned separately to reach acceptable local CNs. This is in contrast to the usual GWR-Ridge where a global λ is tuned to minimize prediction error via cross-validation. Tuning of either fixed or adaptive bandwidth proceeds as usual, using either cross validation or AICc.

We want to point out that, the definition of CN differs from that in Wheeler (2007). The eigenvalues of $\boldsymbol{X}^\tau \boldsymbol{W}(s_i)\boldsymbol{X}$ and the singular values of $\sqrt{\boldsymbol{W}(s_i)}\boldsymbol{X}$ do not yield exactly the same CN because of their relationship $\theta_j = d_j^2$. If the definitions of CN are accurate in the two papers, we suspect that CNs produced by GWmodel are squares of those produced by gwrr. We compared the CNs produced by the two packages in Fig. 12.15, which was generated by the following code:

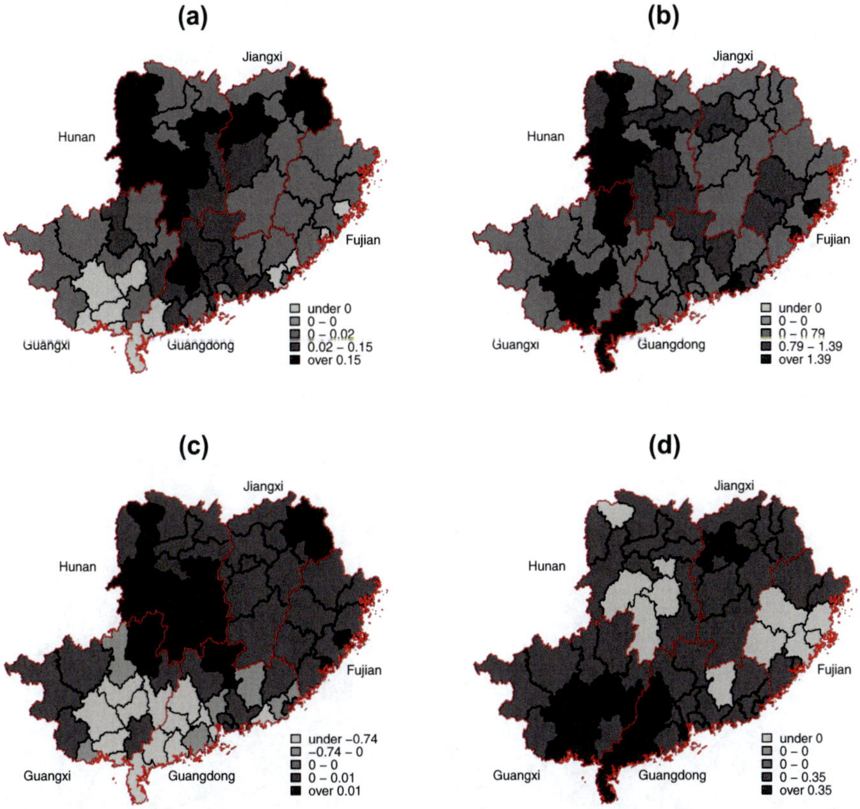

Fig. 12.14 Spatial distributions of local coefficients estimated by GWR-LASSO with an exponential kernel and a fixed bandwidth for (**a**) log(population density), (**b**) temperature, (**c**) relative humidity, and (**d**) wind speed

```
fit0<-gwr.lcr(log_incidence~log_popden+rh+temp+ws,
              data=south5.shp, kernel='exponential',
              bw=bw.gwr$phi, lambda=0, adaptive=FALSE, dMat=my.dMat)
bound<-max(c(fit0$SDF$Local_CN, vdp.gwr$condition))
plot(fit0$SDF$Local_CN, vdp.gwr$condition, xlim=c(0, bound),
     ylim=c(0,bound), xlab='GW-LCR', ylab='GWR', type='p',
     pch=19, main='Local condition indices')
points(sqrt(fit0$SDF$Local_CN), vdp.gwr$condition, pch=1, col='blue')
abline(coef = c(0,1))
```

The original CN outputs of the two packages are very different, shown by the black dots. The square roots of the CNs produced by GWmodel are close to the CNs produced by gwrr, but not exactly. We are not sure about the source of the subtle differences even after taking square root. Both packages recommended the same threshold (30) for flagging potentially problematic CNs.

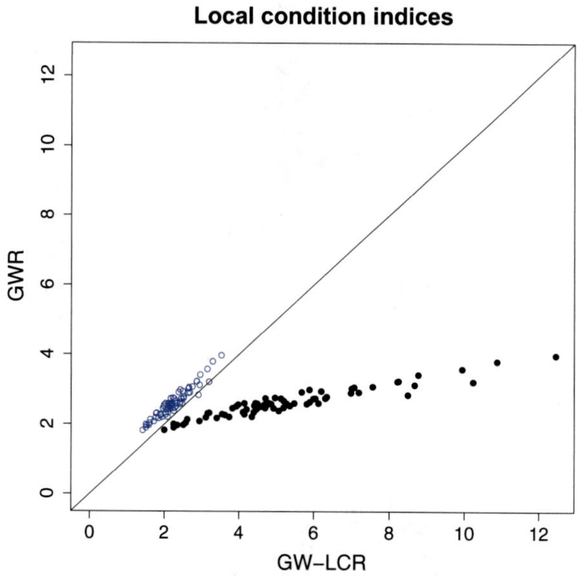

Fig. 12.15 Comparison between condition numbers produced by function gwr.vdp() in gwrr and those by function gwr.lcr() in GWmodel. Black solid dots are scatter plot of the CNs from the two functions. Blue circles are scatter plot after applying square root to the CNs produced by gwr.lcr()

The following code selects bandwidth for and fits the GWR-LCR model, using the exponential kernel and an adaptive bandwidth.

```
bw.lcr <- bw.gwr.lcr(log_incidence~log_popden + rh + temp + ws,
                     data=south5.shp, kernel='exponential',
                     adaptive=TRUE, lambda.adjust=TRUE, cn.thresh=30)
fit.lcr <- gwr.lcr(log_incidence~log_popden + rh + temp + ws,
                   data=south5.shp, kernel='exponential', bw=bw.lcr,
                   adaptive=TRUE, lambda.adjust=TRUE, cn. thresh=30)
```

The AIC, AICc and residual sum of squares obtained from GWR-LCR are 178, 191 and 24.4 respectively, compared to 137, 157 and 24.9 for the classic GWR. The less satisfactory AIC and AICc of GWR-LCR compared to the classic GWR could be due to the weak association of the predictors with the outcome and the substantially more parameters in the GWR-LCR model. The spatial patterns of local predictor coefficients fitted by GWR-LCR are shown in Fig. 12.16. The shrinkage effect of GWR-LCR is clear for relative humidity and wind speed. Interestingly, the spatial patterns are more comparable to the results of the classic GWR (Fig. 12.10) than to those of GWR-Ridge (Fig. 12.13), especially for temperature and population density.

The following code uses Moran's I to test spatial randomness of residuals for all four models. No special spatial patterns were found as all p-values are relatively large. This result suggests that, while the predictors did not show high predictive power overall, they indeed explain the spatial auto-correlation in the HFMD incidences.

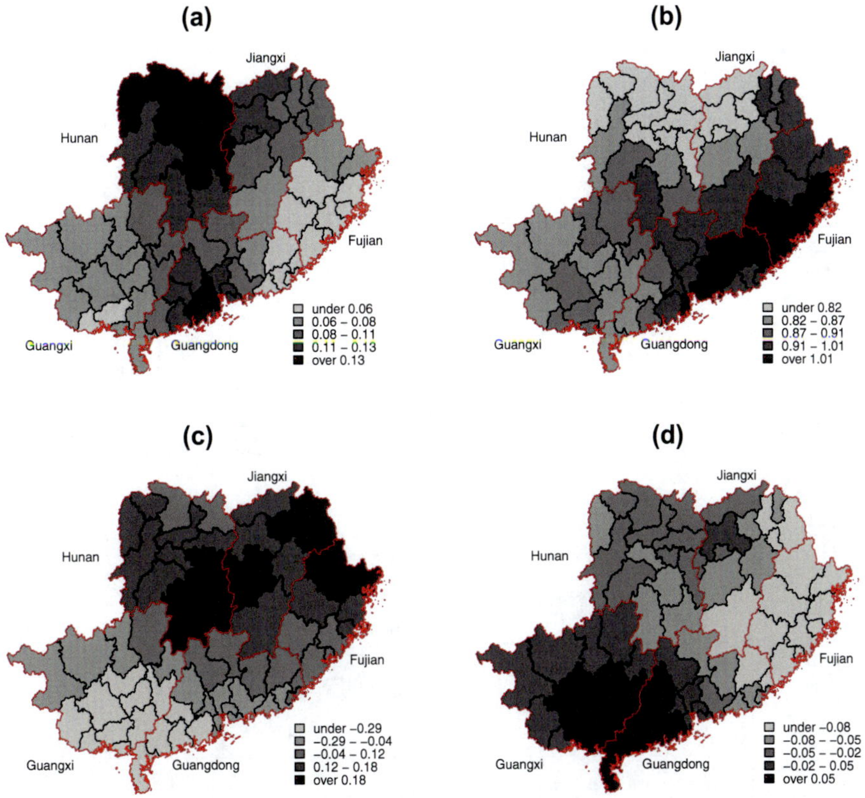

Fig. 12.16 Spatial distributions of local coefficients estimated by GWR-CLR with an exponential kernel and a adaptive bandwidth for (**a**) log(population density), (**b**) temperature, (**c**) relative humidity, and (**d**) wind speed

```
> res.gwr <- fit.gwr$SDF$pred - my.data$log_incidence
> res.gwrr <- fit.gwrr$yhat - my.data$log_incidence
> res.gwl <- fit.gwl$yhat - my.data$log_incidence
> res.lcr <- fit.lcr$SDF$yhat - my.data$log_incidence
> out<-rbind(Moran.I(my.data$log_incidence, my.dMat),
+       Moran.I(res.gwr, my.dMat), Moran.I(res.gwrr, my.dMat),
+       Moran.I(res.gwl, my.dMat), Moran.I(res.lcr, my.dMat))
> rownames(out) <- c('Raw Response', 'Residual:GWR',
+   'Residual:GWR-Ridge', 'Residual:GWR-LASSO', 'Residual:GWR-LCR')
> out
                    observed     expected    sd          p.value
Raw Response        -0.05610592  -0.01470588 0.008402828 8.353727e-07
Residual:GWR        -0.007730267 -0.01470588 0.008427097 0.4078063
Residual:GWR-Ridge  -0.008066695 -0.01470588 0.00844284  0.4316514
Residual:GWR-LASSO  -0.009189744 -0.01470588 0.008329576 0.5078205
Residual:GWR-LCR    -0.007598853 -0.01470588 0.008431426 0.3992724
```

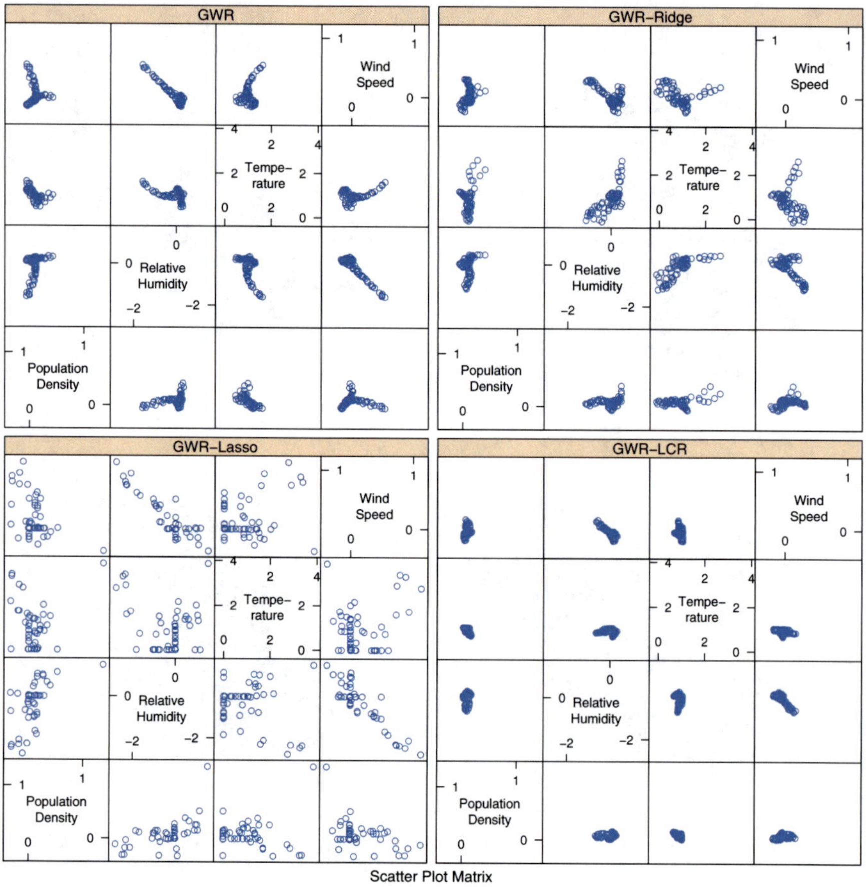

Fig. 12.17 Comparison of correlations among local regression coefficients for classic GWR (upper left), GWR-Ridge (upper right), GWR-LASSO (lower left) and GWR-LCR (lower right)

We further compared at colinearity in local coefficients of all four models, classic GWR, GWR-Ridge, GWR-LASSO and GWR-LCR in Fig. 12.17. The regularized models all reduced colinearity to some extent, and GWR-LASSO did a more satisfactory job. GWR-LCR shrank the ranges of coefficients for all parameters, particularly so for temperature and population density, but such shrinkage is not necessarily towards 0. Although the linear correlation in coefficients between relative humidity and wind speed still remains clear in the regularized models, it is generally not wise to increase the shrinkage level too much, as the price paid for less colinearity is bias in the estimated coefficients (Gollini et al. 2015).

12.3.3 Conclusion

We have introduced the theoretical background of the classic GWR and several regularized versions that impose different constraints on the magnitude of regression coefficients. We also touched the base of some diagnostic statistics such as VDP and condition number. In the case study, we reviewed the use of three R packages dedicated to GWR. We conclude this chapter with comments on future development of GWR and a brief introduction of a Bayesian GWR framework. Thus far, most applications of GWR are limited to cross-sectional data, despite valuable information such as seasonality contained in longitudinal data. There seems to be no theoretical obstacle to the application of GWR to longitudinal data, as long as a reasonable distance can be defined in space-time. However, there is no consensus or guideline on such definitions. One possibility is to introduce an extra tuning parameter for the importance of time relative to space in the construction of distance, and let data guide the choice of this parameter, e.g., via cross-validation. Through the case study, we have seen the difficulties in real data analysis. The existing software packages may not offer the desired tools or output for diagnosis or inference. Documentation of most packages is far from sufficient. For instance, we had to do our own investigation to find out how VDP and condition number are calculated in some packages, and yet did not succeed in such investigation for other packages. Better documentation and literature support will greatly increase the popularity of GWR methods. Finally, there appears to be a gap in the GWR literature about how to handle missing data.

All the methods formally introduced in this chapter are likelihood- or frequentist-oriented. The Bayesian approach is known to be able to incorporate prior knowledge about parameters, which is useful when data are inadequate to support inference about some parameters. Another advantage of the Bayesian approach is its convenience in handling complex likelihood with latent or missing data, when the inference is performed by Markov chain Monte Carlo (MCMC), e.g., using either Gibb's sampler or the Metropolis-Hasting's algorithm (Gelman, Carlin, Stern, & Rubin, 1995; Gilks, Richardson, & Spiegelhalter, 1996). A promising direction that has been researched in the past two decades is the Bayesian spatially varying coefficient (SVC) models (Banerjee, Carlin, & Gelfand, 2004; Finley 2011; Gelfand, Kim, Sirmans, & Banerjee, 2003; Wheeler & Calder, 2007; Wheeler & Waller, 2009). The basic hierarchical structure of the Bayesian SVC model is

$$
\begin{aligned}
\boldsymbol{Y} &= \boldsymbol{X}^{\star}\boldsymbol{\beta} + \boldsymbol{\epsilon} \\
\boldsymbol{\epsilon} &\sim \mathcal{N}(\mathbf{0}, \sigma_{\epsilon}^{2}\boldsymbol{I}) \\
\boldsymbol{\beta} &\sim \mathcal{N}(\mathbf{1}_{n\times 1} \otimes \boldsymbol{\mu}, \boldsymbol{H}(\phi) \otimes \boldsymbol{T}) \\
\boldsymbol{\mu} &\sim \mathcal{N}(\boldsymbol{\eta}, \sigma_{\mu}^{2}\boldsymbol{I}) \\
\boldsymbol{T} &\sim InverseWishart_{\nu}(\boldsymbol{\Omega}^{-1}) \\
\phi &\sim gamma(a_{\phi}, b_{\phi}) \\
\sigma_{\epsilon}^{2} &\sim InverseGamma(a_{\tau}, b_{\tau})
\end{aligned}
\tag{12.8}
$$

where $\boldsymbol{Y}$ is the outcome vector of length n, $\boldsymbol{\beta}$ is a vector of length $n \times p$ stacking regression coefficients at all locations together, $\boldsymbol{X}^{\star}$ is a $n \times np$ block diagonal matrix with $\boldsymbol{X}_i$ (ith row of $\boldsymbol{X}$) as each diagonal block ad 0 elsewhere, and $\boldsymbol{\epsilon}$ is the vector of *i.i.d.* normal errors. The prior distribution of $\boldsymbol{\beta}$ is the essence of the Bayesian SVC model. The notation $\boldsymbol{A} \otimes \boldsymbol{B}$ denotes the Kronecker product which multiplies every element of matrix $\boldsymbol{A}$ with matrix B and yields a block matrix of dimensions as the products of corresponding dimensions of $\boldsymbol{A}$ and $\boldsymbol{B}$. For example, the mean of $\boldsymbol{\beta}$, $\mathbf{1}_{n\times 1} \otimes \boldsymbol{\mu}$, gives a column vector with n $\boldsymbol{\mu}$'s stacked together, where $\mathbf{1}_{n\times 1}$ is a column vector of n 1's. The covariance matrix of $\boldsymbol{\beta}$ is the Kronecker product of a $n \times n$ correlation matrix $\boldsymbol{H}(\phi)$ and a $p \times p$ covariance matrix $\boldsymbol{T}$. $\boldsymbol{H}(\phi)$ captures spatial correlation between study locations and is assumed to depend only on distance and a decay parameter ϕ, e.g., the (i, j)th element being $h_{ij} = \exp(-d_{ij}/\phi)$, where d_{ij} is the distance between locations i and j. $\boldsymbol{T}$ is the covariance among regression coefficient at any location. This Kronecker product structure ensures $\boldsymbol{\Sigma}$ is positive definite and hence a valid covariance matrix. The last four expressions in (12.8) specify prior distributions of $\boldsymbol{\mu}$, $\boldsymbol{T}$, ϕ and σ_{ϵ} with known hyper-parameters. The inference of model was implemented via MCMC in Wheeler and Calder (2007). Due to the high-dimension nature of GWR (number of coefficients increases with locations), the computational burden of this model can be heavy. There are two R packages, spBayes (Finley 2011; Finley & Banerjee, 2019) and spTDyn (Bakar, Kokic, & Jin, 2016), implementing Bayesian SVC models. In particular, parallel computing via openMP is available in spBayes to expedite computation. As computer engineering continues to advance at a fast pace, we can see that Bayesian approach will become more computationally affordable and popular.

References

Bakar, K., Kokic, P., & Jin, H. (2016). Hierarchical spatially varying coefficient and temporal dynamic process models using spTDyn. *Journal of Statistical Computation and Simulation, 86*, 820–840.

Banerjee, S., Carlin, B., & Gelfand, A. (2004). *Hierarchical modeling and analysis for spatial data*. Boca Raton, FL: Chapman & Hall/CRC.

BioMedware. (2011). *Spacestat user manual, version 2.2.* http://www.biomedware.com/

Brunsdon, C., Fotheringham, A., & Charlton, M. (1996). Geographically weighted regression: A method for exploring spatial nonstationarity. *Geographical Analysis, 28*(4), 281–298.

Casetti, E. (1972). Generating models by the expansion method: Applications to geographic research. *Geographical Analysis, 4*, 81–91.

da Silva, A., & Rodrigues, T. (2014). Geographically weighted negative binomial regression–incorporating overdispersion. *Statistics and Computing, 24*, 769–783.

Environmental Systems Resource Institute. (2013). ArcGIS Resource Center, version 10.2. http://www.arcgis.com/

Finley, A. (2011). Comparing spatially-varying coefficients models for analysis of ecological data with non-stationary and anisotropic residual dependence. *Methods in Ecology and Evolution, 2*, 143–154.

Finley, A., & Banerjee, S. (2019). Bayesian spatially varying coefficient models in the spBayes R package. arXiv:1903.03028v1. https://arxiv.org/pdf/1903.03028

Fotheringham, A., Brunsdon, C., & Charlton, M. (2002). *Geographically weighted regression: The analysis of spatially varying relationships*. West Sussex, UK: Wiley.

Fotheringham, A., Charlton, M., & Brunsdon, C. (1998). Geographically weighted regression: A natural evolution of the expansion method for spatial data analysis. *Environment and Planning A, 30*, 1905–1927.

Gelfand, A., Kim, H., Sirmans, C., & Banerjee, S. (2003). Spatial modelling with spatially varying coefficient processes. *Journal of American Statistical Association, 98*, 387–396.

Gelman, A., Carlin, J., Stern, H., & Rubin, D. (1995). *Bayesian data analysis*. London, UK: Chapman & Hall.

Gilks, W., Richardson, S., & Spiegelhalter, D. J. (1996). *Markov chain Monte Carlo in practice*. Boca Raton, FL: Chapman & Hall/CRC.

Gollini, I., Lu, B., Charlton, M., Brunsdon, C., & Harris, P. (2015). Gwmodel: An r package for exploring spatial heterogeneity using geographically weighted models. *Journal of Statistical Software, 63*(17), 1–50.

Jones, K. (1992). Specifying and estimating multilevel models for geographical research. *Transactions of the Institute of British Geographers, 16*, 148–159.

Leung, Y., Mei, C., & Zhang, W. (2000). Statistical tests for spatial nonstationarity based on the geographically weighted regression model. *Environment and Planning A, 32*, 9–32.

Li, K., & Lam, N. (2018). Geographically weighted elastic net: A variable-selection and modeling method under the spatially nonstationary condition. *Annals of the American Association of Geographers, 108*, 1582–1600.

Mei, C.-L., Wang, N., & Zhang, W.-X. (2006). Testing the importance of the explanatory variables in a mixed geographically weighted regression model. *Environment and Planning A, 38*(14), 587–598.

Nakaya, T., Fotheringham, A., Brunsdon, C., & Charlton, M. (2005). Geographically weighted Poisson regression for disease association mapping. *Statistics in Medicine, 24*, 2695–2717.

Nakaya, T., Fotheringham, A., Charlton, M., & Brunsdon, C. (2009). Semiparametric geographically weighted generalised linear modelling in GWR 4.0. In *10th International Conference on GeoComputation*, Sydney, Australia. Available at http://mural.maynoothuniversity.ie/4846/

Nelder, J., & Wedderburn, R. (1972). Generalized linear models. *Journal of the Royal Statistical Society, 135*, 370–384.

R Core Team. (2013). *R: A language and environment for statistical computing*. Vienna, Austria: R Foundation for Statistical Computing. http://www.R-project.org/

Rangel, T., Diniz-Filho, J. A. F., & Bini, L. M. (2010). Sam: A comprehensive application for spatial analysis in macroecology. *Ecography, 33*, 46–50.

Shoff, C., & Yang, T.-C. (2012). Spatially varying predictors of teenage birth rates among counties in the United States. *Demographic Research, 27*(14), 377–418.

Simon, N., Friedman, J., Hastie, T., & Tibshirani, R. (2001). A sparse-group lasso. *Journal of Computational and Graphical Statistics, 22*(2), 231–245.

Tang, X.-Y., Yang, Y., Yu, H.-J., Liao, Q.-H., & Bliznyuk, N. (2019). A spatio-temporal modeling framework for surveillance data of multiple infectious pathogens with small laboratory validation sets. *Journal of the American Statistical Association, 114*(528), 1561–1573.

Wakefield, J. (2008). Ecologic studies revisited. *Annu Review of Public Health, 29*, 75–90.

Wang, N., Mei, C.-L., & Yan, X.-D. (2008). Local linear estimation of spatially varying coefficient models: An improvement on the geographically weighted regression technique. *Environment and Planning A, 40*, 986–1005.

Wang, W., & Li, D. (2017). Structure identification and variable selection in geographically weighted regression models. *Journal of Statistical Computation and Simulation, 87*(10), 2050–2068.

Wang, Y., Feng, Z., Yang, Y., Self, S., Gao, Y., Wakefield, J., . . . , Yang, W. (2011). Hand, foot and mouth disease in China: Patterns of spread during 2008–2009. *Epidemiology, 22*, 781–792.

Wheeler, D. (2007). Diagnostic tools and a remedial method for collinearity in geographically weighted regression. *Environment and Planning A, 39*, 2464–2481.
Wheeler, D., & Calder, C. (2007). An assessment of coefficient accuracy in linear regression models with spatially varying coefficients. *Journal of Geographical Systems, 9*, 145–166.
Wheeler, D., & Tiefelsdorf, M. (2005). Multicollinearity and correlation among local regression coefficients in geographically weighted regression. *Journal of Geographical Systems, 7*, 161–187.
Wheeler, D., & Waller, L. (2009). Comparing spatially varying coefficient models: A case study examining violent crime rates and their relationships to alcohol outlets and illegal drug arrests. *Journal of Geographical Systems, 11*, 1–22.
Zhang, C., & Murayama, Y. (2000). Testing local spatial autocorrelation using k-order neighbors. *International Journal of Geographical Information Science, 14*, 681–692.
Zhou, Y., Wang, Q., Yang, M., Gong, Y., Yang, Y., Nie, S. J., . . . , Jiang, Q. (2016). Geographical variations of risk factors associated with HCV infection in drug users in southwestern China. *Epidemiology and Infection, 144*, 1291–1300.

Part III
Advanced Statistical Methods

Chapter 13
Bayesian Spatial-Temporal Disease Modeling with Application to Malaria

Ropo Ebenezer Ogunsakin and (Din) Ding-Geng Chen

Abstract *Background*: Malaria remains a major public health challenge in Nigeria. Considerable effort has been made to reduce the prevalence and impact of the disease. The National Malaria Control Programme conducted a nationally representative Malaria Indicator Survey (MIS) within the malaria peak transmission season in 2008, 2010, 2013 and 2015 which comprises of all the six region of Nigeria. In this study, the spatial and temporal modeling of malaria risk within each region of Nigeria were studied using the MIS survey data. *Methods*: This study used data obtained from the Nigeria demographic health survey (NDHS) database to assess models; data were collected in 37 states between 2008, 2010, 2013 and 2015. We examine associations between malaria risk and socio-demographic factors using 16 Bayesian Poisson spatial-temporal models that incorporate spatial and temporal autocorrelations. The optimum model selected according to the deviance information criterion and effective number of parameters in the Bayesian paradigm. The models were implemented in R-INLA package. *Results*: The model included spatially uncorrelated heterogeneity, temporally correlated random-walk autocorrelation, and spatial temporal interaction model had small deviance information criteria. This model was the best in examining the association between malaria risk and socio-demographic factors using NDHS. The relationship between malaria risk and socio-demographic factor is statistically significant. *Conclusion*: The spatial-temporal interaction was statistically meaningful and the prevalence of malaria was influenced by the time and space interaction effect. Wealth index and place of residence have influence on malaria. To further reduce malaria burden, current tools should be supplemented by socio-demographic development.

The original version of this chapter was revised: An appendix has been added at the end of this chapter and page numbers in the subsequent chapters were corrected. The correction to this chapter is available at https://doi.org/10.1007/978-3-030-35260-8_17

R. E. Ogunsakin (✉)
University of Pretoria, Pretoria, South Africa

(Din) D.-G. Chen
School of Social Work, University of North Carolina, Chapel Hill, NC, USA
e-mail: dinchen@email.unc.edu

X. Chen, (Din) D.-G. Chen (eds.), *Statistical Methods for Global Health and Epidemiology*, ICSA Book Series in Statistics,
https://doi.org/10.1007/978-3-030-35260-8_13

13.1 Introduction

Malaria is endemic in Nigeria and remains a major public health burdens affecting the world despite the remarkable accomplishment made towards its control and prevention. Most of the burden of malaria is concentrated in Sub-Saharan Africa (SSA) (Israel et al. 2018). Estimates in 2016 affirmed that 90% and 92% of the global proportion of malaria cases and death were recorded in this region (Awuah et al. 2018; Israel et al. 2018; Odugbemi et al. 2018; World Health Organization 2015) and Nigeria accounts for about 29% of this burden. Malaria is the third leading cause of death among under five children globally and accounts for almost one out of every five deaths in under five children (Abah & Temple 2015; Israel et al. 2018; Singh, Musa, Singh, & Ebere 2014). In Nigeria, it is estimated that about 110 million clinically diagnosed cases of malaria and nearly 300,000 malaria-related childhood deaths occur each year (Israel et al. 2018; Kyu, Georgiades, Shannon, & Boyle 2013). Evidence shows that the disease contributes to about 60% of all outpatients visits, 30% of hospitalizations and 11% of maternal mortality in the country (Bennett et al. 2017; Kassegne et al. 2017).

Considerable effort has been made to reduce the prevalence and impact of the disease, however, the last decade of malaria control has witnessed increased support by government and its partners in the areas of insecticide-treated nets (ITNs), intermittent preventive treatment (IPT), indoor residual spraying (IRS), integrated programme (IVM) and environmental management (EM), long-lasting insecticidal net (LLIN) campaigns, replacement campaigns, intermittent preventive treatment (IPT), and a massive scale up in malaria case management. The National Malaria Control Programme (NMCP) in collaboration with Roll Back Malaria (RBM) also keying into these global strategies plan (2009–2013) (Kilian, Boulay, Koenker, & Lynch 2010). In 2010, more than 24 million long lasting impregnated net (LLIN) were distributed across 14 states of Nigeria through a campaign supported by the partners (Adigun, Gajere, Oresanya, & Vounatsou 2015). Preceding this time, one of the state in South-South Nigeria have received more than 600,000 LLINs between 2008 and part of 2009 through the help of United State Agency for International Development (USAID) (Kyu et al. 2013) for children under the age of five. These efforts resulted into about 425 of households having at least one ITN (Adigun et al. 2015).

In addition, more than 70 million rapid diagnostic tests (RDTs) were distributed among all the health facilities in the country between 2008 and 2010 which could be freely used in malaria diagnosis and to provide immediate treatment based on the results (World Health Organization 2015). It was further reported that 5% of malaria cases were screened with RDTs in 2008. But in 2010, the number of pregnant women who received preventive therapy during their routine antenatal care reached 13% which is an indication of low turnout for health care seeking behavior. In view of the aforementioned, the effective malaria control strategies suggest a better and comprehensive map of the spatial distribution of malaria prevalence. This can help in efficient resource allocation for planning and intervention implementation as well as the evaluation of their impact (Gemperli et al. 2006; Giardina et al. 2012;

Gosoniu, Msengwa, Lengeler, & Vounatsou 2012; Hay & Snow 2006; Riedel et al. 2010). It is essential to identify the association between malaria risk and socio-demographic factors. Such a study of the identification of the socio-demographic risk factors is helpful in identifying region who have a critical need for intervention. In Nigeria, previous studies have concluded that malaria risk are associated with environmental and climatic factors (Adigun et al. 2015; World Health Organization 2017). In particular it was noted that intervention appear not to have important effect on malaria risk. Nevertheless the spatial distribution of malaria was not investigated (Adigun et al. 2015). However, the modeling of malaria risk in each of the region in Nigeria has to be explored. Meanwhile, the spatial pattern of malaria risk is known to vary, its temporal evolution has yet to be evaluated. Therefore, the objective of this study was to determine the spatial-temporal modeling of malaria risk in Nigeria taking into consideration socio-demographic factors.

In this research, we introduce Bayesian spatial-temporal modeling that incorporate spatial information in such a way that not only reflect the influences of space and time but also reflect the interaction of space time on the preferred variable of interest. In doing so, we use 16 Bayesian Poisson spatial-temporal techniques in estimating model parameters.

13.2 Spatial-Temporal Data in Nigeria

13.2.1 Study Area

Nigeria is the most populous country in the continent of Africa, which is located in the west sub region of Africa. The country is divided into 37 states grouped into six (13.6) regions and covers an area of about 923,768 km^2. Nigeria has the largest population in Africa and the seventh largest in the world. The current population is estimated at 177.1 million based on an annual growth rate of 3.2% (National Population Commission [NPopC] 2016). Nigeria's population is young, with persons age 0–24 accounting for more than 62% of the country's residents (National Population Commission 2010). According to the World Bank's definition, Nigeria is a lower middle income country. The country has tropical climate with two rainfall seasons in a year (wet and dry season) which is accompanied with the movement of two dominant winds: the rain bearing south westerly winds, and the cold, dry and dusty north easterly wind generally referred to as the Harmattan. The wet season occurs from April to September, and the dry season from October to March. The annual rainfall ranges between 550 mm in some part of the north mainly in the fringes of Sahara desert to 4000 mm in the coastal region around Niger delta area in the south. The temperature in Nigeria ranges between 25 and 40 °C . The geographic location of Nigeria makes suitable climate for malaria transmission throughout the country and it is all year round in most part of the country (Adigun et al. 2015). Plasmodium falciparum is the most prevalent malaria parasite species in Nigeria (Mouzin et al. 2012; National Population Commission 2012). Malaria transmission intensity, and seasonality vary among the country's five ecological strata that extend from south to north (National Population Commission 2012). Considering population density and distribution of risk areas, an estimated 3%, 67% and 30% live in very low to low, moderate, and high to very high transmission intensities area, respectively (Mouzin et al. 2012). The transmission season increases from north to south in terms of duration, in the space of 3 months in the north area bordering Chad to perennial in the most southern part (Mouzin et al. 2012).

13.2.2 Country Profile

The data were collecteds using the standard malaria indicator questionnaires developed by the RBM and the demographic health surveillance programme. The dataset consists of information such as, demographic characteristics and socio-economic status which is on a nationally representative sample of around 6000 households from about 240 clusters. Detail description of the sampling strategies is reported in the final report of NMIS 2010 (National Population Commission 2012). The blood samples were taken from 239 clusters due to some security challenges in one of the clusters in northern part of Nigeria (National Population Commission 2012). The prevalence from two diagnostic methods: RDT and microscopy was recorded in the data (Wongsrichanalai, Barcus, Muth, Sutamihardja, & Wernsdorfer 2007). In 2015, malaria testing was done through both rapid diagnostic testing (RDT) as well as blood smear microscopy. Of the 6316 eligible children, 95% provided blood for RDT and 91% for malaria microscopy. The 2015 NMIS shows a malaria prevalence of 45% by RDT and 27% by microscopy. The geographical representation of the clusters involved and observed prevalence in the NMIS is displayed in Fig. 13.1. Figure 13.1 shows the map of Nigeria divided into various regions.

13.2.3 Ethical Approval

This study was based on the analysis of existing survey data-sets in the public domain that are available free online. The first author obtained permission for the download and usage of the NDHS dataset from http://www.dhsprogram.com/data/dataset_admin/login_main.cfm.

13.2.4 Predictor Variables

The transmission of malaria is known to be influenced by several factors such as socioeconomic, demographic factors and environmental/climatic. Demographic

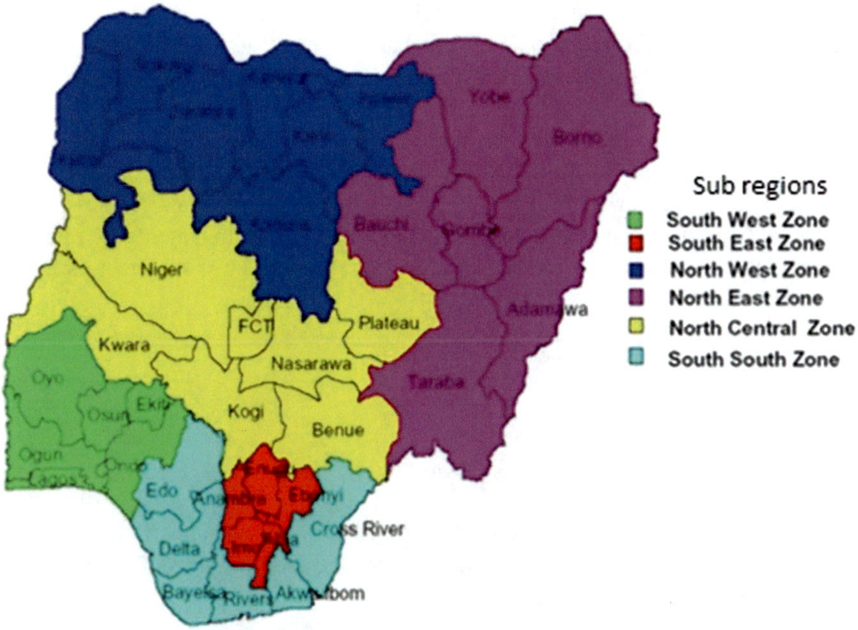

Fig. 13.1 Map of Nigeria showing the 37 states with six Geo-political region

variables were captured on survey tools, which include area type of the household, age, and mother's educational level. Information on socioeconomic status was measured by a wealth index. It was calculated as a weighted sum of household assets using principal component analysis.

13.3 Statistical Methodology

13.3.1 Malaria Spatial-Temporal Modeling

Spatial-temporal disease mapping has become an important tool in passive surveillance of diseases. Understanding how disease risks and prevalence and/or incidence vary over time may provide information that may be of great epidemiological significance. Spatial-temporal models are extensions of the basic spatial models by simply including a linear or a non-parametric trend in time, time space, time covariate and time-space-covariate interactions. When using spatial-temporal data to study occurrences such as diseases, researchers are often interested in both the spatial and temporal aspects of these data. For instance, researchers might want to investigate disease location and time of diagnosis along with the disease counts. This goal could be achieved by modeling the disease counts as a Poisson process while concurrently incorporating the space and time data with all other risk covariates. Because of the spatial-temporal autocorrelations, spatial-temporal disease data are typically modeled as multivariate with correlated observations of Poisson disease counts at a fixed spatial location that evolves over time.

In this study, our focus is on malaria data collected over a 4-year period (2–4) from 37 States in Nigeria. Suppose we let i represent the spatial location i = 1,. . . . . ., K (=37) states and t = 1,. . . . . .,T(=4) years, the number of malaria cases, y_{it}, is modeled as a Poisson spatial-temporal model with the expected incidence rates E_{it}, and the associated risk θ_{it}. The standard Besag-York-Mollie spatial analytic model is represented as follows:

Data Distribution

$$y_{it} \sim Pois(E_{it} \times \theta_{it}) \tag{13.1}$$

where y_i counts in area i are independently identically Poisson distributed and have an expectation in area i of E_i, the expected count, times θ_i, the risk for area i

Spatial-Temporal Mixed-Effects Regression Model

$$log(\theta_{it}) = \beta_o + \beta_1 x_{1it} + \cdots + \beta_j x_{jit} + S_i + T_t + ST_{it} \tag{13.2}$$

where S represent the random spatial term, T is the random temporal term, and ST is the random space-time interaction. Meanwhile, the fixed-effects component is $\beta_o + \beta_1 x_{1it} + \cdots + \beta_j x_{jit}$ where $x_{1it}, \ldots, x_{jit}$ are the risk factors to be modeled with the disease risk θ_{it}. In the present study, the two covariates included is wealth index (WI), and area type (AT). Hence, the model (13.2) is simplified as

$$log(\theta_{it}) = \beta_o + \beta_1 WI_{1it} + \beta_2 AT_{1it} + S_i + T_t + ST_{it} \tag{13.3}$$

From model (13.1), E_{it} represent the expected incidence rates and its values can be estimated by several approaches. The simplest overall average for the expected counts is given by:

$$E_{it} = p_{it} \times \frac{\sum_{i=1}^{K} \sum_{t=1}^{T} y_{it}}{\sum_{i=1}^{k} \sum_{t=1}^{T} p_{it}} \tag{13.4}$$

where p_{it} is the population at ith location (i.e., state) and tth time point (i.e., year) in this malaria data.

Specifically, eight models were constructed by considering the spatial effect, and the interaction between time and space (see Table 13.2). To evaluate the regional effects, the spatial-temporal model in expression (13.3) is built to include the six Nigeria region (Region) as:

$$log(\theta_{it}) = \beta_o + \beta_1 WI_{1it} + \beta_2 AT_{1it} + \beta_4 Region_{it} + S_i + T_t + ST_{it} \tag{13.5}$$

Hence, additional of eight spatial-temporal models are included, yielding a total of 16 fitted spatial-temporal models. These eight models comprises of different combinations of spatial random effect (UH), spatially structured heterogeneity, linear time trend, identically independent distributed time variable, random walk as well as spatial-temporal interactions (see Table 13.2 for the description of those models).

13.4 Bayesian Spatial-Temporal Models with INLA

In this section, we introduce how Bayesian spatial-temporal model can be implemented using R-INLA. Spatio-temporal disease mapping models are a well-known tool to explain the pattern of disease counts. Model of this kind is usually formulated within a Bayesian framework (Banerjee, Carlin, & Gelfand 2004) and computationally expensive Markov Chain Monte Carlo (MCMC) are needed to obtain the respective parameter estimates. Also, in order to get a reliable estimate for a complex spatial and spatio-temporal models, a specific block-sampling algorithms have to be applied. Furthermore, Bayesian spatial-temporal disease mapping via MCMC methods involve computationally and time intensive simulations to obtain the posterior distribution for the parameters. An approximate technique for parameter estimation in latent Gaussian models was proposed by Banerjee et al. (2004). This technique uses Integrated Nested Laplace Approximation (INLA). The advantage of INLA method is that it does not use iterative computation techniques like MCMC and it returns precise parameter estimates. The posterior approximation is achieved by applying numerical integrations for fixed effects and Laplace integral approximation to the random effects (Chen, Wakefield, & Lumely 2014). Primarily, INLA is designed for latent Gaussian models, a very wide and flexible class of models like spatial and spatio-temporal models, making INLA to be used widely in a great variety of applications (Spiegelhalter, Best, Carlin, & van der Linde 2003). In addition, the deviance information criterion (DIC) is provided by INLA for Bayesian model choice. For our analysis, INLA was implemented in the R package “INLA” (R-INLA). We used R for data management and R package , maptools for reading the shapefile.

13.4.1 Goodness of Fit Statistics

Modeling was done in R using the R-INLA package. The model were compared using the Deviance Information Criterion (DIC) as recommended by Khana, Rossen, Hedegaard, and Warner (2018) and Spiegelhalter, Best, Carlin, and Van Der Linde (2002). The ability to fit complex multilevel models using Markov Chain Monte Carlo (MCMC) techniques presents a need for methods to compare alternative models. The standard model comparison techniques such as AIC and BIC require the specification of the number of parameters in each model. For multilevel models which contain random effects, the number of parameters is not generally obvious and as such an alternative technique of comparison is demanded. The most widely used of such alternative technique is the Deviance information Criteria (DIC) as suggested by Spiegelhalter et al. (2002). The DIC statistic is a generalization of the AIC, and is based on the posterior mean of the deviance, which is also a measure of model complexity and fit. The deviance is defined as

$$D(\theta) = -2\log f(y|\theta).$$

since DIC is a measure of model complexity, it considers a measure of the effective number of parameters in a model, and is defined by

$$pD = \bar{D}(\theta) - (\breve{\theta}).$$

where $\bar{D}(\theta)$ is the posterior expectation of the deviance, given by

$$\bar{D}(\theta) = -2E\Big[\log f(y|\theta)|y\Big].$$

and $(\breve{\theta})$ is the deviance evaluated at some estimate $\breve{\theta}$ of θ. Therefore, we now define the deviance information criteria (DIC) by

$$DIC = \bar{D}(\theta) + pD = 2\bar{D}(\theta) - \hat{\theta}. \tag{13.6}$$

where $\bar{D}$ is the posterior mean of the deviance that measures the goodness of fit, and pD represent the effective number of parameters in the model. In the case of the Bayesian and bootstrapping models, low values of $\bar{D}$ imply a better fit, while small values of pD imply a parsimonious model. pD is higher for a more complex model, and DIC appears to select the correct model. The best fitting model is one with the smallest DIC, as suggested by Lesaffre and Lawson (2012) and Spiegelhalter et al. (2002). When comparing different models, how big the difference between the DIC value of the models need to be revealed so as to declare that one model is better than the other. Previous studies have shown that a difference of 3 in DIC between two models cannot be distinguished while a difference of between 3 and 7 can be weakly differentiated (Kazembe, Chirwa, Simbeye, & Namangale 2008; Spiegelhalter, Best, Carlin, & Linde 2014). For context, a DIC difference 3 to 5 is considered significant.

13.5 Results

To illustrate how the 16 Bayesian Poisson spatial-temporal models can be applied to real life data, we used the data on malaria risk from 37 states of Nigeria (see Fig. 13.1). In Table 13.1, we grouped the 37 states into six regions (i.e., North central, North east, North west, South east, South south and South west) to investigate regional differences. We extracted the malaria prevalence rate for the 4-year period. To obtain the malaria incidence rates, we merged these data to calculate the associated malaria incidences rates y_{it} and the expected incidence rates E_{it} to be used in Eqs. (13.1) and (13.4). As mentioned previously, malaria can be related to many risk factors. From the epidemiological perspective, malaria risk factors includes environmental/ climatic, socioeconomic status and socio-demographic and so on. The DHS database consists an extensive list of risk covariates that could be used to model the predictability of these risk factors to malaria prevalence rates; meanwhile, most of the covariates have a higher percentage of missing data (>90%). Hence, for demonstration purposes the current study utilizes wealth index, and area type as a possible covariates.

Meanwhile all the spatial-temporal data from 37 states collected for 4 years period were incorporated for a unified Bayesian spatial-temporal modeling. Table 13.2 presents series of spatial-temporal models fitted with the R-INLA package. Comparison results among different models affirmed that the DIC values of the two models with only spatial heterogeneity effect were: 1358.55 and 1358.36 respectively while the DIC values for models incorporating temporal heterogeneity were: 1338.26, 1336.49, 1339.86, and 1336.59, respectively. The last sets of two models considered assesses the spatial-temporal interaction. DIC values of the two UH random effect and convolution model with interaction term were: 1126.44 and 1125.92 respectively. Among the two interaction models, model taking the spatially temporally uncorrelated heterogeneity + UH, temporally correlated random walk autocorrelation, and spatial temporal interaction effect into consideration was the best fitting one with a smallest DIC as well as pD value. It should be acknowledged that the DIC values from the models 1–8 space-time interaction do not exhibit extreme differences. This can be attributed to all models taking the form shown in Eq. (13.3). Between the eight models fitted, model 7 and 8 has larger pD values which indicate that the two models are more complex, apparently because it incorporates a spatio-temporal interaction effect that is not part of model 1–6. Although, model 7 and 8 is weakly indistinguishable because of the differences between the DIC value is lesser than 3. Therefore, the higher complexity was beneficial as it led to lower DIC values in model 8 which indicates a better fit model to the data. Therefore, the best fitting DICs are seen with the interaction models.

With model 8 as the best fitting model, the estimated coefficients of place of residence (rural) and wealth index (poorer), (middle), (richer) and (richest) were: 0.04525, 0.01380, 0.11115, 0.000180 and 0.05793 respectively. Moreover, the estimated β for these socio-demographic variables were 1.04629(95% BCI: 0.905–1.209), 1.01389 (95% BCI: 0.887–1.158), 1.11797 (95% BCI: 0.966–1.292), 1.0001

Table 13.1 List of 37 Nigeria states and associated state code

RegionNum	RegionName	StateName	StateCode	RegionCode
1	North West	Sokoto	YYB	1.YYB
1	North West	Zamfara	ZAM	1.ZAM
1	North West	Katsina	KAT	1.KAT
1	North West	Jigawa	DTI	1.DTI
1	North West	Kano	KAN	1.KAN
1	North West	Kaduna	KAD	1.KAD
1	North West	Kebbi	KEB	1.KEB
2	North East	Yobe	DTR	2.DTR
2	North East	Borno	BOR	2.BOR
2	North East	Adamawa	YOL	2.YOL
2	North East	Gombe	GME	2.GME
2	North East	Bauchi	BAU	2.BAU
2	North East	Taraba	TAR	2.TAR
3	North Central	Niger	KNT	3.KNT
3	North Central	Abuja	FCT	3.FCT
3	North Central	Nasarawa	NAS	3.NAS
3	North Central	Plateau	JOS	3.JOS
3	North Central	Benue	BEN	3.BEN
3	North Central	Kogi	LOK	3.LOK
3	North Central	Kwara	ILO	3.ILO
4	South West	Oyo	OYD	4.OYD
4	South West	Osun	SGB	4.SGB
4	South West	Ekiti	ADK	4.ADK
4	South West	Ondo	ODK	4.ODK
4	South West	Lagos	KJA	4.KJA
4	South West	Ogun	ABG	4.ABG
5	South South	Edo	BED	5.BED
5	South South	Cross River	CAL	5.CAL
5	South South	Akwa Ibom	AKI	5.AKI
5	South South	Rivers	PHC	5.PHC
5	South South	Bayelsa	YEN	5.YEN
5	South South	Delta	WAR	5.WAR
6	South East	Anambra	ANA	6.ANA
6	South East	Enugu	ENU	6.ENU
6	South East	Ebonyi	EBO	6.EBO
6	South East	Abia	ABI	6.ABI
6	South East	Imo	WER	6.WER

Note: These 37 states are grouped into 6 regions ("RegionNum") under the region names ("RegionName"). For ease of representation in Figs. 13.1 and 13.2, we created the RegionCode abbreviation that combines the RegionNum and the StateCode

Table 13.2 Specific spatial-temporal models and associated fit statistics

Model	Details	DIC	n.eff
1	Spatial Only (UH)	1358.55	33.633
2	Spatial Only (UH+CH)	1358.36	33.664
3	Spatial(UH+CH) +Temporal trend	1338.26	34.364
4	Spatial(UH+CH) +Temporal(UH)	1336.49	36.358
5	Spatial(UH+CH)+Temporal(CH)	1339.86	42.938
6	Spatial(UH+CH)+Temporal(UH+CH)	1336.59	36.056
7	Spatial(UH)+Temporal(CH)+ST	1126.44	109.213
8	Spatial(UH+CH)+Temporal(CH)+ST	1125.92	108.740

Abbreviations: Spatial—UH: uncorrelated effect model; CH: correlated effect model. Temporal—UH: uncorrelated heterogeneity, CH: random walk; spatial-temporal interaction. ST: spatial-temporal. DIC: deviance information criterion, n.eff: effective number of parameters

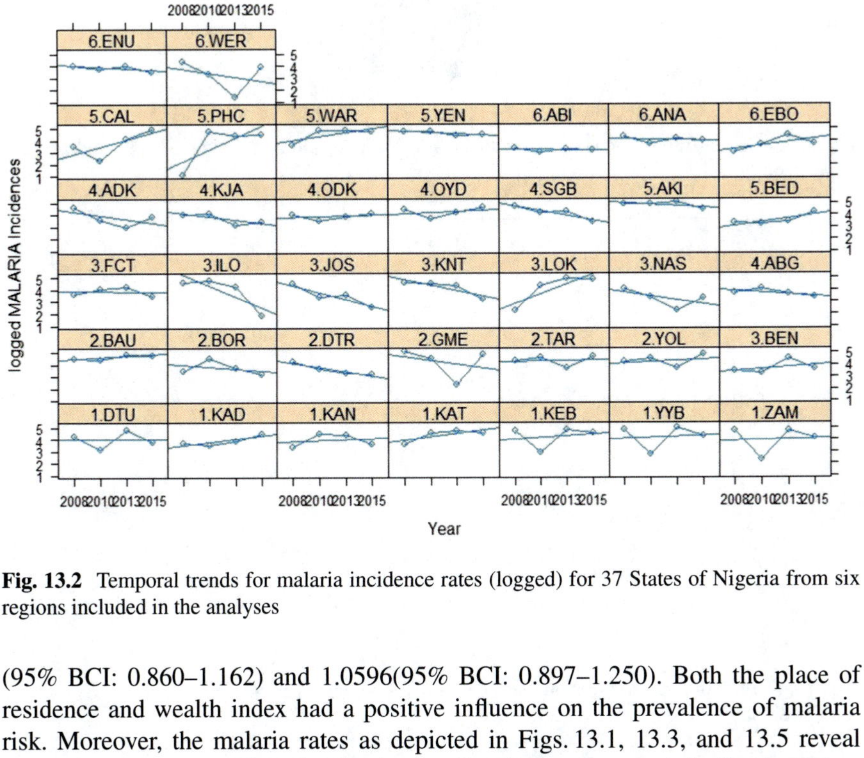

Fig. 13.2 Temporal trends for malaria incidence rates (logged) for 37 States of Nigeria from six regions included in the analyses

(95% BCI: 0.860–1.162) and 1.0596(95% BCI: 0.897–1.250). Both the place of residence and wealth index had a positive influence on the prevalence of malaria risk. Moreover, the malaria rates as depicted in Figs. 13.1, 13.3, and 13.5 reveal some signs of spatial trends despite the fact that there are no statistically significant spatial patterns. As shown in Fig. 13.2, reported cases of malaria prevalence in Nigeria declined year by year across the 37 states over the 4-year period.

Also, the map depicted in Fig. 13.3 shows the estimated overall pattern in the spatial random-residual effects revealing spatial autocorrelation as represented by S_i in expression (13.3). The implication of the map is that all the six regions in the country have had a mix of high and low malaria prevalence over time, which is

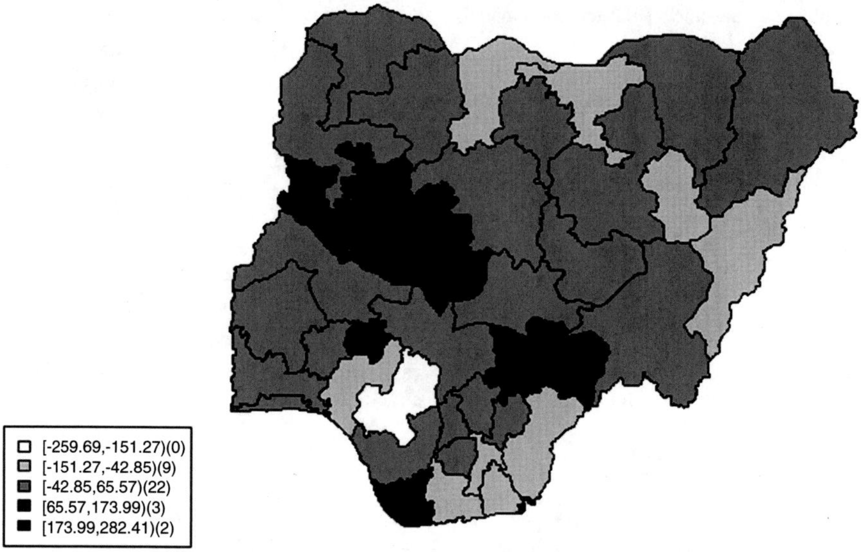

Fig. 13.3 Spatial random-residual effects showing spatial autocorrelation as indicated by S_i in expression (13.3)

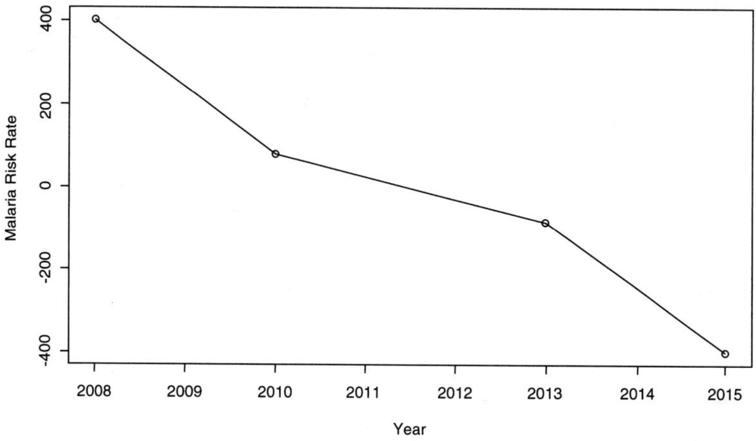

Fig. 13.4 Temporal random-residual effects showing temporal autocorrelation as indicated by T_t in expression (13.3)

indicated by the random effects S_i and fixed effects presented in expression (13.3). Figure 13.4 depicts only the overall temporal pattern of the malaria risk prevalence as reported by T_t in expression (13.3); the map indicates that Nigeria experienced uneven risk of malaria infection without giving much knowledge about differences across the geopolitical zone of the country. Hence, both the spatial-only patterns in Fig. 13.3 and temporal-only trends in Fig. 13.4 should be interpreted simultaneously.

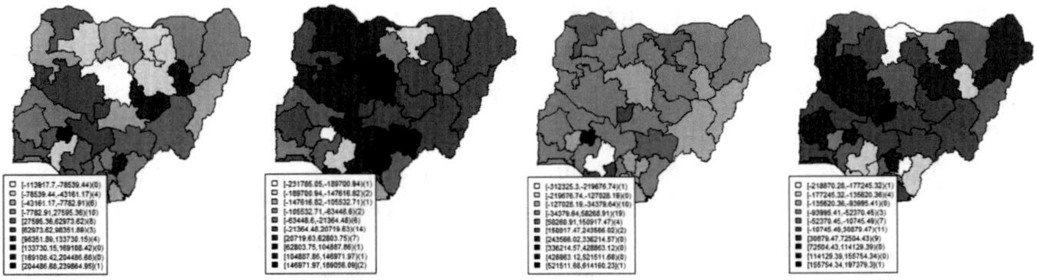

Fig. 13.5 Spatial and temporal random-residual effects showing spatial and temporal autocorrelation as indicated by ST_it in expression (13.3)

Table 13.3 Bayesian spatial-temporal models with regional effect

Model	Details	DIC	n.eff
9	Spatial Only (UH)	1359.45	35.221
10	Spatial Only (UH+CH)	1359.31	35.162
11	Spatial(UH+CH) +Temporal trend	1339.11	35.778
12	Spatial(UH+CH) +Temporal(UH)	1337.05	37.694
13	Spatial(UH+CH)+Temporal(CH)	1339.39	42.581
14	Spatial((UH+CH)+Temporal(UH+CH)	1337.21	37.427
15	Spatial(UH)+Temporal(CH)+ST	1126.34	112.183
16	Spatial(UH+CH)+Temporal(CH)+ST	1125.58	109.873

In addition, the interaction of spatial and temporal factors during 4 year period suggests the presence of convoluted spatial and temporal autocorrelation as indicated by ST_{it} in expression (13.3). Figure 13.5 also indicated some considerable differences in the relative risk of malaria across the six regions of Nigeria.

Moreover, in order to account for the remaining eight (8) models of our 16 Bayesian spatial-temporal model, we fitted a model accounting for the regional effects. The findings affirmed that the regional effects were statistically significant and the result is presented in Table 13.3. The results presented in Figs. 13.2, 13.3, 13.4 and 13.5 are for the first eight (8) models without the regional effect.

13.6 Conclusion and Summary of Findings

In this study, different models were compared for modeling and mapping of malaria risk in Nigeria. In particular, we considered series of Bayesian spatial-temporal models to examine the association or effects of socio-demographic on the malaria risk across the 37 states of Nigeria. This relationship is important to enable an effective policies as well as tools to tackle the menace of malaria transmission in Nigeria. These models were fitted to NDHS malaria prevalence data for 4-year period. Among the different spatial-temporal models examined, the model with spatial-temporal interaction fit the data well but model 8 appears better than model 7. The findings indicate that model with spatially uncorrelated heterogeneity, temporally correlated random-walk autocorrelation, and spatial temporal interaction was the best model for goodness of fit for modeling malaria risk. The finding is similar with previous studies (Abellan, Richardson, & Best 2008; Popoff 2014) which found potential use of spatial and temporal terms in the model. Although our study did not use the Bayesian hierarchical but previous studies that used Bayesian hierarchical framework for diseases mapping as well as ecological studies of health environment association (Ehlers & Zevallos 2015; Popoff 2014) affirmed that if data are collected over space and time, spatial and temporal terms in the model becomes necessary. The reason for this could be due to the complex dependence patterns over space and over time of the occurrence of malaria deaths. The study findings indicated an estimated positive association between socio-demographic factors and malaria risk. This finding confirms previous results that showed that malaria risk is positively associated with socio-economic status (Adigun et al. 2015; Giardina et al. 2012; Gosoniu et al. 2012; Gosoniu, Veta, & Vounatsou 2010). Moreover, we observed that the overall malaria risk among the 37 states was spatially uncorrelated when viewed from a historical point for the 4 years period. Estimations from model 8 affirmed that wealth index could be an influential factor on the prevalence of malaria. Specifically, with one unit increase of wealth index (poorer), the risk of new malaria case increased by 1.0139 times. This finding is similar to what the previous findings on Bayesian geostatistical modeling of malaria from Nigeria (Adigun et al. 2015). Therefore, the results of this study provide evidence on the spatial-temporal distribution of socio-demographic risk factors in the occurrence of malaria. Hence, the utilization of socio-demographic data on malaria rapid diagnosis test (RDT), clarifies the association of these factors. From the study it was affirmed that those people living in the North Central region were found to be more at risk of malaria compared to those living in the South West.

Meanwhile, the malaria map produced in this study affirms considerable shrinkage in malaria burden in comparison to results from the first MIS survey of 2010 that showed a high burden of malaria in the entire country. There are some limitations to consider when interpreting the findings of this study. Foremost, the current study relied on malaria test results from RDT. Secondly, one can think of the limitation of the current study in line with the data used which may contain spatially correlated malaria prevalence trends across the local government or towns that are not noticeable at the state level. Hence, for future study it is advisable to perform a sensitivity analysis in case of a study utilizing Bayesian spatial temporal modeling to check whether the results vary at different geographical scales. Thus, this will help the researchers to discuss the research policy in case the results differ. Moreover, in obtaining the incidence rates when using Bayesian spatial-temporal approaches, decisions as to whether to calculate the incidence rate as population-based, geographical area-based, or combination of both should be put into consideration. In case of the current study, the incidence rate in Eq. (13.4) is obtained using the population-based. As pointed out by Lesaffre (Lawson 2013; Lesaffre and Lawson 2012), that is the most commonly used incidence rate in spatial-temporal disease mapping. An important aspect that needs to be highlighted regarding this study is that the regional effects is statistically significant which requires the attention of the health policies makers in controlling the prevalence of malaria. Therefore, adequate effort should be targeted further in order to uncover factors that is responsible for the transmission so as to allow for the development of better malaria control measures.

A.1 Appendix 1: R Program Codes for Analysis.

```
StateList = rep(State,each=T)
CodeList = rep(Code, each=T)
region<-rep(1:m,each=T)
region2<-region
ind2<-rep(1:(m*T))
data<-data.frame(Mal,E,year,Year,region,region2,CodeList,
    StateList,ind2,Res, Weat)
data
####1. Spatial-temporal data are pre-processed and load them in

source("dataMALARIA.R")
# check the data
print(data)
summary(data)
subregion = read.csv("subregionMALARIApaper.csv", header=T)
data = merge(data,subregion)


#calculation of the population
ff = mean(data$Mal/data$E)
data$pop = data$Mal/ff


#create a new variable for plotting since the State names are
    to long
data$NewRegion = paste(data$subregion1,".",data$CodeList, sep
    ="")
# order the data by the new var
data= data[order(data$NewRegion),]
head(data)


#make table 1
d1 = data.frame(StateList=unique(data$StateList),Code=unique(
    data$CodeList),Region= unique(data$NewRegion))
d2 =merge(d1, subregion)
d3 = data.frame(RegionNum = d2$subregion1, RegionName =
    d2$subregion, RegionCode=d2$Region,StateName= d2$StateList,
     StateCode = d2$Code)
d3
```

```
###2. pre-analysis for to identify the relationship for
    modelling

library(lattice)
# incidence time series
xyplot(log(Mal)~Year|as.factor(NewRegion),type=c("b","r"), data
    , xlab="Year", ylab="logged MALARIA Incidences")

xyplot(log(Mal)~Year|as.factor(NewRegion),layout = c(7, 6),type
    =c("b","r"), data, xlab="Year", ylab="logged MALARIA
    Incidences")


### 3. Now Spatial-temporal modelling
#
# R libraries
# load neccessary packages and download the map shapefile and
    therefater, read it into R  \\

library(maptools)
# get INLA
library(INLA)
inla.setOption(scale.model.default=FALSE)
require(splancs)
require(sp)
require(fields)
require(maptools)
require(abind)
library(rgdal)

 ## Meaning###
## The R tools maptools::readShapePoly() will read shapefiles
    into R, and spdep::poly2nb() followed by INLA::nb2INLA()
    are used to create the adjacency matrix neighbor structures
     for use with a CAR model. To map results, you can use sp::
    spplot()

source("Malaria3.R")

 # model 1: spatial only UH
model1 = Mal~1+as.factor(Res)+as.factor(Weat)+subregion+f(
    region,model="iid")
result1  = inla(model1,family="poisson",data=data,E=E,control.
    compute=list(dic=TRUE,cpo=TRUE))
UH<-result1$summary.random$region[,2]
summary(model1)

## where:

 # Mal is the disease count or outcome from your dataset.
## 1 forces an intercept onto the model.
## f() specify the spatial region and how it should be modeled.
```

```
## In the case of our study, spatial region is modeled as "iid"
     which is a random effects term. One of the advantage of
    this function is that it is useful when invoking any
    spatial model, especially the geograhically weighted
    regressions.
## Also, f() functions can be added to each other in order to
    build up models.
## model1 refers to and invokes the previously defined model.
## family = specifies the likelihood.
## data = specifies the data.

## control.compute specifies options like DICand DCO.
## Note: CPO is the conditional predictive ordinate, a cross
    validation tool that predicts an area value using all the
    data except that area and compare that value to the actual
    value.
## E = specifies the offset variable required for a Poisson
    likelihood


# model 2: UH and CH effects
model2<-Mal~1+as.factor(Res)+as.factor(Weat)+subregion+f(region
    ,model="iid")+f(region2,model="bym",graph="
    nga_admbnda_adm1_osgof_20161215.graph")
result2<-inla(model2,family="poisson",data=data,E=E,control.
    compute=list(dic=TRUE))
summary(result2)


# model 3: spatial + time trend   (model 1a)
model3<-Mal~1+as.factor(Res)+as.factor(Weat)+year+subregion+f(
    region,model="iid")+f(region2,model="bym",graph="
    nga_admbnda_adm1_osgof_20161215.graph")
result3 = inla(model3,family="poisson",data=data,E=E,control.
    compute=list(dic=TRUE,cpo=TRUE))
summary(result3)


# model 4: UH + CH + year IID
model4<-Mal~1+as.factor(Res)+as.factor(Weat)+subregion+f(region
    ,model="iid")+f(region2,model="bym",graph="
    nga_admbnda_adm1_osgof_20161215.graph")+f(year,model="iid")
result4<-inla(model4,family="poisson",data=data,E=E,control.
    compute=list(dic=TRUE,cpo=TRUE))
summary(result4)

 # model 5: UH + CH + year RW1   (model 1b)
model5<-Mal~1+as.factor(Res)+as.factor(Weat)+subregion+f(region
    ,model="iid",param=c(2,1))+f(region2,model="bym",graph="
    nga_admbnda_adm1_osgof_20161215.graph")+f(year,model="rw1",
    param=c(1,0.01))
result5<-inla(model5,family="poisson",data=data,E=E,control.
    compute=list(dic=TRUE,cpo=TRUE))
summary(result5)
```

```
UH<-result4$summary.random\$region[,2]
yearR<-result4$summary.random\$year[,2]


# model 6:  UH +CH +year UH +CH    (model 2)
year2<-year
model6<-Mal~1+as.factor(Res)+as.factor(Weat)+subregion+f(region
    ,model="iid")+f(region2,model="bym",graph="
    nga_admbnda_adm1_osgof_20161215.graph")+f(year,model="rw1")
    +f(year2,model="iid")
result6<-inla(model6,family="poisson",data=data,E=E,control.
    compute=list(dic=TRUE,cpo=TRUE))

# modle 7: UH+ year RW1 +INT  IID
model7<-Mal~1+as.factor(Res)+as.factor(Weat)+subregion+f(region
    ,model="iid")+f(year,model="rw1")+f(ind2,model="iid")
result7<-inla(model7,family="poisson",data=data,E=E,control.
    compute=list(dic=TRUE,cpo=TRUE))


# model 8: UH +CH + year RW1 + INT IID  (model 3)
model8<-Mal~1+as.factor(Res)+as.factor(Weat)+subregion+f(region
    ,model="iid")+f(region2,model="bym",graph="
    nga_admbnda_adm1_osgof_20161215.graph")+f(year,model="rw1")
    +f(ind2,model="iid")
result8<-inla(model8,family="poisson",data=data,E=E,control.
    compute=list(dic=TRUE,cpo=TRUE))


result1$dic$dic;result1$dic$p.eff
result2$dic$dic;result2$dic$p.eff
result3$dic$dic;result3$dic$p.eff
result4$dic$dic;result4$dic$p.eff
result5$dic$dic;result5$dic$p.eff
result6$dic$dic;result6$dic$p.eff
result7$dic$dic;result7$dic$p.eff
result8$dic$dic;result8$dic$p.eff

##The best model is model 8
#
# summary of the model 8
summary(result8)
# fixed effects
betas = result8$summary.fixed
betas

exp(betas)

## results for model 8

# get the shape file
library(maptools)
```

```
cities <- readOGR(dsn=dsn,layer="
    nga_admbnda_adm1_osgof_20161215")
plot(cities)
names(cities)
# extract the data
UH = result7$summary.random$region[,2]*100000
yearR<-result7$summary.random$year[,2]*100000
STint<-result7$summary.random$ind2[,2]*100000

# plot risk rate by state
fillmap(cities,"Spatial Pattern for Nigeria Malaria Prevalence
    Risk ",UH,n.col=10)
fillmap(cities,"",UH,n.col=5)

plot(cities)
fillmap(cities,"",UH,n.col=5)

# plot risk rate by year
time<- c("2008", "2010","2013","2015")
plot(time,yearR, xlab="Year", ylab = " Risk Rates",main="
    Temporal Pattern for Malaria Risk Rates")
plot(time,yearR, xlab="Year", ylab = " Malaria Risk Rate")
lines(time,yearR)

# the S-T interaction
STest<-matrix(STint,ncol=4, byrow=T)

 ST1<-STest[,1]
ST2<-STest[,2]

par(mfrow=c(1,2), mai=c(0,0,0.3,0),mar=c(2,1,1,1))
for(i in 1:4){
  #x11()
  fillmap(cities,paste("Spatial-Temporal in Year",2008+i,sep="
      "),STest[,i]*5,n.col=10)
  }
x11()
for(i in 3:4){
  fillmap(cities,paste("Spatial-Temporal in Year",2008+i,sep="
      "),STest[,i]*10,n.col=10)
  }

STest<-matrix(0,nrow = 88, ncol=10)

for(i in 1:4){i=ceiling(i/10) j=i-10*(k-1) STest[i,j]<-STint[i]
     }
```

References

Abah, A., & Temple, B. (2015). Prevalence of malaria parasite among asymptomatic primary school children in Angiama Community, Bayelsa State, Nigeria. *Tropical Medicine & Surgery, 4*, 203–207.

Abellan, J. J., Richardson, S., & Best, N. (2008). Use of space–time models to investigate the stability of patterns of disease. *Environmental Health Perspectives, 116*(8), 1111.

Adigun, A. B., Gajere, E. N., Oresanya, O., & Vounatsou, P. (2015). Malaria risk in Nigeria: Bayesian geostatistical modelling of 2010 malaria indicator survey data. *Malaria Journal, 14*(1), 156.

Awuah, R. B., Asante, P. Y., Sakyi, L., Biney, A. A., Kushitor, M. K., Agyei, F., & Aikins, A. d.-G. (2018). Factors associated with treatment-seeking for malaria in urban poor communities in Accra, Ghana. *Malaria Journal, 17*(1), 168.

Banerjee, S., Carlin, B. P., & Gelfand, A. E. (2004). *Hierarchical modeling and analysis for spatial data*. New York, NY: Chapman and Hall/CRC.

Bennett, A., Bisanzio, D., Yukich, J. O., Mappin, B., Fergus, C. A., Lynch, M., ..., Eisele, T. P. (2017). Population coverage of Artemisinin-based combination treatment in children younger than 5 years with fever and Plasmodium falciparum infection in Africa, 2003–2015: A modelling study using data from national surveys. *The Lancet Global Health, 5*(4), e418–e427.

Chen, C., Wakefield, J., & Lumely, T. (2014). The use of sampling weights in Bayesian hierarchical models for small area estimation. *Spatial and Spatio-Temporal Epidemiology, 11*, 33–43.

Ehlers, R., & Zevallos, M. (2015). Bayesian estimation and prediction of stochastic volatility models via INLA. *Communications in Statistics-Simulation and Computation, 44*(3), 683–693.

Gemperli, A., Sogoba, N., Fondjo, E., Mabaso, M., Bagayoko, M., Briët, O. J., ..., Vounatsou, P. (2006). Mapping malaria transmission in West and Central Africa. *Tropical Medicine & International Health, 11*(7), 1032–1046.

Giardina, F., Gosoniu, L., Konate, L., Diouf, M. B., Perry, R., Gaye, O., ..., Vounatsou, P. (2012). Estimating the burden of malaria in Senegal: Bayesian zero-inflated binomial geostatistical modeling of the MIS 2008 data. *PLoS One, 7*(3), e32625.

Gosoniu, L., Msengwa, A., Lengeler, C., & Vounatsou, P. (2012). Spatially explicit burden estimates of malaria in Tanzania: Bayesian geostatistical modeling of the malaria indicator survey data. *PloS One, 7*(5), e23966.

Gosoniu, L., Veta, A. M., & Vounatsou, P. (2010). Bayesian geostatistical modeling of malaria indicator survey data in Angola. *PloS One, 5*(3), e9322.

Hay, S. I., & Snow, R. W. (2006). The malaria atlas project: Developing global maps of malaria risk. *PLoS Medicine, 3*(12), e473.

Israel, O. K., Fawole, O. I., Adebowale, A. S., Ajayi, I. O., Yusuf, O. B., Oladimeji, A., & Ajumobi, O. (2018). Caregivers' knowledge and utilization of long-lasting insecticidal nets among under-five children in Osun State, Southwest, Nigeria. *Malaria Journal, 17*(1), 231.

Kassegne, K., Zhang, T., Chen, S.-B., Xu, B., Dang, Z.-S., Deng, W.-P., ..., Zhou, X.-N. (2017). Study roadmap for high-throughput development of easy to use and affordable biomarkers as diagnostics for tropical diseases: A focus on malaria and schistosomiasis. *Infectious Diseases of Poverty, 6*(1), 130.

Kazembe, L. N., Chirwa, T. F., Simbeye, J. S., & Namangale, J. J. (2008). Applications of bayesian approach in modelling risk of malaria-related hospital mortality. *BMC Medical Research Methodology, 8*(1), 6.

Khana, D., Rossen, L. M., Hedegaard, H., & Warner, M. (2018). A Bayesian spatial and temporal modeling approach to mapping geographic variation in mortality rates for subnational areas with R-INLA. *Journal of Data Science, 16*(1), 147.

Kilian, A., Boulay, M., Koenker, H., & Lynch, M. (2010). How many mosquito nets are needed to achieve universal coverage? recommendations for the quantification and allocation of long-lasting insecticidal nets for mass campaigns. *Malaria Journal, 9*(1), 330.

Kyu, H. H., Georgiades, K., Shannon, H. S., & Boyle, M. H. (2013). Evaluation of the association between long-lasting insecticidal nets mass distribution campaigns and child malaria in Nigeria. *Malaria Journal, 12*(1), 14.

Lawson, A. B. (2013). *Bayesian disease mapping: Hierarchical modeling in spatial epidemiology*. Boca Raton, FL: Chapman and Hall/CRC.

Lesaffre, E., & Lawson, A. B. (2012). *Bayesian biostatistics*. New York, NY: Wiley.

Mouzin, E. (2012). *Focus on Nigeria*. https://apps.who.int/iris/bitstream/handle/10665/87100/9789241503310_eng.pdf. Accessed 10 Jan 2020.

National Population Commission. (2010). Population and housing census of the Federal Republic of Nigeria 2006.

National Population Commission. (2012). Nigeria malaria indicator survey 2010.

National Population Commission. (2016). *Nigeria population projections by age and sex from 2006 to 2017*. Abuja: National Population Commission.

Odugbemi, B., Ezeudu, C., Ekanem, A., Kolawole, M., Akanmu, I., Olawole, A., . . . , Babatunde, S. (2018). Private sector malaria RDT initiative in Nigeria: Lessons from an end-of-project stakeholder engagement meeting. *Malaria Journal, 17*, 70.

Popoff, E. (2014). *An approximate spatio-temporal Bayesian model for Alberta wheat yield*. PhD thesis, University of British Columbia.

Riedel, N., Vounatsou, P., Miller, J. M., Gosoniu, L., Chizema-Kawesha, E., Mukonka, V., & Steketee, R. W. (2010). Geographical patterns and predictors of malaria risk in Zambia: Bayesian geostatistical modelling of the 2006 Zambia National Malaria Indicator Survey (ZMIS). *Malaria Journal, 9*(1), 37.

Singh, R., Musa, J., Singh, S., & Ebere, U. V. (2014). Knowledge, attitude and practices on malaria among the rural communities in Aliero, Northern Nigeria. *Journal of Family Medicine and Primary Care, 3*(1), 39.

Spiegelhalter, D., Best, N. G., Carlin, B. P., & van der Linde, A. (2003). Bayesian measures of model complexity and fit. *Quality Control and Applied Statistics, 48*(4), 431–432.

Spiegelhalter, D. J., Best, N. G., Carlin, B. P., & Linde, A. (2014). The deviance information criterion: 12 years on. *Journal of the Royal Statistical Society: Series B (Statistical Methodology), 76*(3), 485–493.

Spiegelhalter, D. J., Best, N. G., Carlin, B. P., & Van Der Linde, A. (2002). Bayesian measures of model complexity and fit. *Journal of the Royal Statistical Society: Series B (Statistical Methodology), 64*(4), 583–639.

Wongsrichanalai, C., Barcus, M. J., Muth, S., Sutamihardja, A., & Wernsdorfer, W. H. (2007). A review of malaria diagnostic tools: Microscopy and rapid diagnostic test (RDT). *The American Journal of Tropical Medicine and Hygiene, 77*(6_Suppl.), 119–127.

World Health Organization. (2015). *World malaria report 2014*. World Health Organization.

World Health Organization. (2017). *Global hepatitis report 2017*. World Health Organization.

Chapter 14
BCEWMA: A New and Effective Biosurveillance System for Disease Outbreak Detection

Kai Yang and Peihua Qiu

Abstract Disease outbreaks need to be detected in a timely manner for effective disease control. For disease surveillance, conventional statistical process control charts are often included in public health surveillance systems, without taking into account the complicated structure of the disease incidence data and/or additional covariate information. This chapter presents a novel prospective disease surveillance system, named BCEWMA (Biosurveillance via Covariate-Assisted Exponentially Weighted Moving Average Control Chart), which can accommodate seasonality and arbitrary distribution of disease incidence data. Methodologically, BCEWMA is based on the widely used exponentially weighted moving average control chart, incorporating useful information in covariates. This new surveillance system is applied to two real disease incidence datasets: one regarding the hand, foot and mouth disease in Sichuan province of China and the other about the influenza-like-illness in Florida. These real-data examples show the reliability and effectiveness of BCEWMA in disease outbreak detection.

Keywords Control chart; Covariates; Disease surveillance; Exponentially weighted moving average; Semiparametric regression; Statistical process control.

14.1 Introduction

Prospective disease surveillance, also referred to as *biosurveillance*, aims to monitor disease incidence data sequentially and detect disease outbreaks or other unusual disease patterns in a timely manner, so that effective disease control and prevention measures can be implemented promptly. In recent years, numerous statistical and epidemiological methods concerning prospective disease outbreak detection have been developed. A recent review paper by Unkel, Farrington, and Garthwaite

K. Yang (✉) · P. Qiu
Department of Biostatistics, University of Florida, Gainesville, FL, USA
e-mail: yklmy1994121@ufl.edu

X. Chen, (Din) D.-G. Chen (eds.), *Statistical Methods for Global Health and Epidemiology*, ICSA Book Series in Statistics,
https://doi.org/10.1007/978-3-030-35260-8_14

(2012) classifies existing biosurveillance methods into five categories, including regression techniques, time series methods, statistical process control (SPC) charts, surveillance methods using spatial information, and multivariate outbreak detection methods. This paper aims to develop a new and effective biosurveillance method using SPC.

Among all existing biosurveillance methods, SPC charts has a long history of application to public health surveillance problems. To monitor disease incidence data, Dong, Hedayat, and Sinha (2008) suggested an exponentially weighted moving average (EWMA) control chart based on the assumption that the disease incidence rates are normally distributed. Instead of using normality assumption, Zhou and Lawson (2008) assumed that the observed number of disease cases was Poisson-distributed, and then they proposed a likelihood-ratio-based control chart to detect possible disease outbreaks. Based on the assumption that disease incidence is either Bernoulli or Poisson distributed, Kulldorff (1997) suggested a spatial scan statistic to analyze disease incidence data. The generalized versions of this scan statistic have also been developed for analyzing ordinal data (Jung, Kulldorff, & Klassen 2007) or continuous data (Kulldorff, Huang, & Konty 2009). Based on the scan statistic, Sonesson (2007) established a cumulative sum (CUSUM) control chart to detect unusual disease clusters in space-time setting. In the literature, there are some other control charts for prospective disease surveillance, including the CUSUM chart using a local Knox statistic to detect unusual space-time disease interactions (Marshall, Spitzner, & Woodall 2007) and the Shewhart chart that can accommodate the day-of-week variation (Zhao et al. 2011).

Conventional SPC charts were originally designed for detecting defective products in industrial production processes. Recently, they are used in many biosurveillance applications. This is because the detection of disease outbreaks has a similar nature to the detection of defective products. However, conventional SPC charts are usually based on the assumptions that process observations are independent and identically distributed (i.i.d.) and they follow a parametric distribution (e.g., normal or Poisson distribution), which are often invalid in biosurveillance applications. For instance, seasonality is common in disease incidence, and their distribution is often too complicated to be described by a parametric form. Furthermore, conventional SPC charts use the observed disease incidence data only. In practice, disease incidence is often associated with covariates like humidity, temperature and other weather or environmental factors. Information in these covariates should be incorporated to improve model performance in detecting disease outbreaks. Recently, Yang and Qiu (2020) suggested an exponentially weighted moving average (EWMA) control chart for online process monitoring, and this method can utilize information in covariates. However, this method assumes a steady in-control (IC) process distribution. In this chapter, we generalize the EWMA chart in Yang and Qiu (2020) to cases when the IC process distribution changes over time to accommodate seasonality and other IC longitudinal patterns. The generalized method can accommodate arbitrary data distribution as well.

The rest of the chapter is organized as follows. In Sect. 14.2, we will introduce some basic SPC concepts and control charts. In Sect. 14.3, our approach BCEWMA will be described in detail. In Sect. 14.4, BCEWMA will be tested with two real datasets as examples. Finally, some remarks conclude the chapter in Sect. 14.5.

14.2 Some Basic SPC Concepts and Methods

Since the first control chart introduced by Shewhart (1931), SPC charts have become a major statistical tool for monitoring production processes in manufacturing industries to ensure the stability of the processes over time. The main objective of SPC is to distinguish any *special cause variation* from the *common cause variation* in a production process of interest. A common cause variation is the variation due to random noise, and is considered to be an inherent part of the production process. It cannot be changed without changing the process itself (cf., Qiu 2014). In cases when only common cause variation is present, the production process is considered to be *in-control (IC)*. When some components of the process (e.g., raw materials) become out-of-order, the product quality would have a systematic shift, and the resulting variation is referred to as special cause variation. When a special cause variation occurs in a production process, the process is considered to be *out-of-control (OC)*. SPC charts are designed to detect possible special cause variation and give a signal as soon as it occurs. In the SPC literature, there are four main types of control charts, including Shewhart, CUSUM, EWMA and change-point detection (CPD) charts, each of which will be briefly discussed below.

The first control chart by Shewhart (1931) is called Shewhart chart nowadays, where the observed quality variable at the n-th time point, denoted as Y_n, is assumed to be normally distributed when the process is IC, i.e., $Y_n \sim N(\mu_0, \sigma^2)$. The two IC parameters μ_0 and σ^2 are assumed to be known or can be estimated from an IC dataset. Then, if

$$\frac{|Y_n - \mu_0|}{\sigma} > Z_{1-\alpha/2}, \tag{14.1}$$

the chart will give a signal of process mean shift, where $Z_{1-\alpha/2}$ is the $(1 - \alpha/2)$-quantile of the standard normal distribution and α is a significance level. In (14.1), if a batch of m observations are available at each time, then Y_n should be replaced by the sample mean of the observations in the batch and σ should be replaced by $\sigma/\sqrt{m}$ accordingly. In some real-world applications, including disease surveillance, we are only concerned about upward mean shifts. In such cases, we can compare $(Y_n - \mu_0)/\sigma$ with $Z_{1-\alpha}$, and the chart will give a signal of upward mean shift if $(Y_n - \mu_0)/\sigma > Z_{1-\alpha}$.

To evaluate the performance of a control chart, we usually use the IC average run length (ARL), denoted as ARL_0, which is defined to be the average number of time points from the beginning of process monitoring to the signal time when the process is IC, and the OC ARL, denoted as ARL_1, which is the average number of time points from the occurrence of a shift to the signal time after the process becomes

OC. Usually, ARL_0 is specified at a specific level, and the chart performs better if its ARL_1 value is smaller for detecting a given shift.

From Eq. (14.1), it is clear that the Shewhart chart only uses the observed data at the current time when making a decision whether or not the process is IC. All past observations $\{Y_1, Y_2, \ldots, Y_{n-1}\}$ are ignored. To overcome this limitation, Page (1954) suggested the following CUSUM chart:

$$C_n^+ = \max\{0, C_{n-1}^+ + \frac{Y_n - \mu_0}{\sigma} - k\}, \quad \text{for } n \geq 1, \tag{14.2}$$

where $C_0^+ = 0$ and $k > 0$ is an allowance constant. This chart gives a signal of upward mean shift if $C_n^+ > \rho$, where $\rho > 0$ is a control limit. From (14.2), it is obvious that past observations have been used in the charting statistic C_n^+. In the CUSUM chart (14.2), the allowance constant k is often specified in advance, and it has been well studied in the SPC literature that small k values are ideal for detecting relatively small mean shifts and large k values are ideal for detecting relatively large mean shifts. After k is specified, the control limit ρ can be chosen to achieve a given ARL_0 value. For the CUSUM charting statistics C_n^+ defined in (14.2), it is obvious that C_n^+ is reset to 0 each time when $C_{n-1}^+ + (Y_n - \mu_0)/\sigma \leq k$. This is the so-called re-starting mechanism of CUSUM chart, and under some regularity conditions, Moustakides (1986) showed that the CUSUM chart had some good theoretical properties.

Although the CUSUM chart (14.2) has certain good theoretical properties, it is difficult to follow for many users, partly due to the re-starting mechanism. To overcome this difficulty, Roberts (1959) proposed the EWMA control chart:

$$E_n = \lambda \frac{Y_n - \mu_0}{\sigma} + (1 - \lambda) E_{n-1} = \lambda \sum_{i=1}^{n} (1 - \lambda)^{n-i} \frac{Y_n - \mu_0}{\sigma}, \quad \text{for } n \geq 1, \tag{14.3}$$

where $E_0 = 0$ and $\lambda \in (0, 1]$ is a weighting parameter. The EWMA chart gives a signal of upward mean shift if $E_n > \rho$, where $\rho > 0$ is a control limit. From (14.3), it is clear that E_n is a weighted average of $(Y_1 - \mu_0)/\sigma, (Y_2 - \mu_0)/\sigma, \ldots, (Y_n - \mu_0)/\sigma$, and the weight $(1 - \lambda)^{n-i}$ decreases exponentially fast when i moves away from n. For the EWMA chart, the weighting parameter λ is often pre-specified, and small λ values are ideal for detecting relatively small mean shifts and large λ values are ideal for detecting relatively large mean shifts. Similar to the CUSUM chart, after the weighting parameter λ is given, the control limit ρ can be chosen to achieve a given ARL_0 value. In the SPC literature, it has been well discussed that CUSUM and EWMA charts are more effective to detect small and persistent shifts in a process, compared with the Shewhart chart (cf., Qiu 2014).

For the Shewhart, CUSUM and EWMA charts, they require the IC parameters μ_0 and σ^2 to be known in advance or they can be estimated from an IC dataset, which makes them inconvenient to use in some applications. To overcome this difficulty, a

CPD chart was suggested by Hawkins, Qiu, and Kang (2003). Assume that process observations $\{Y_1, Y_2, \ldots, Y_n\}$ by the current time point n follow the change-point model

$$\begin{aligned} Y_i &\sim N(\mu_0, \sigma^2), \ \text{ for } i = 1, 2, \ldots, \tau; \\ Y_i &\sim N(\mu_1, \sigma^2), \ \text{ for } i = \tau + 1, \ldots, n, \end{aligned} \tag{14.4}$$

where τ is an unknown change-point, $\mu_0 < \mu_1$ are the process means before and after the change-point τ, and σ^2 is the process variance. So, in the above change-point model (14.4), it is assumed that the process mean has an upward shift at τ and the process variance does not change. To test the existence of the change-point, the related likelihood ratio test (LRT) statistic is defined as

$$T_{\max,n} = \max_{1 \le j \le n-1} \sqrt{\frac{j(n-j)}{n}} \left(\frac{\overline{Y}^*_{jn} - \overline{Y}_{jn}}{\widehat{\sigma}_{jn}} \right), \tag{14.5}$$

where $\overline{Y}_{jn}$ and $\overline{Y}^*_{jn}$ are the sample means of $\{Y_i, i = 1, \ldots, j\}$ and $\{Y_i, i = j + 1, \ldots, n\}$, respectively, and $\widehat{\sigma}_{jn} = \sum_{i=1}^{j} (Y_i - \overline{Y}_{jn})^2 + \sum_{i=j+1}^{n} (Y_i - \overline{Y}^*_{jn})^2$. The CPD chart gives a signal of upward mean shift when

$$T_{\max,n} > \rho_n, \tag{14.6}$$

where $\rho_n > 0$ is a control limit chosen to achieve a given ARL_0 value. After a signal is given by the CPD chart defined above, the change-point τ can be estimated immediately by

$$\widehat{\tau} = \arg \max_{1 \le j \le n-1} \sqrt{\frac{j(n-j)}{n}} \left(\frac{\overline{Y}^*_{jn} - \overline{Y}_{jn}}{\widehat{\sigma}_{jn}} \right). \tag{14.7}$$

From the description above, the CPD chart does not require the parameters μ_0, μ_1 and σ^2 to be known in advance, and it can report a shift position immediately after a signal is given. However, the computational burden to calculate the time-varying control limit ρ_n and the charting statistic $T_{\max,n}$ is quite heavy. Also, a shift could be left undetected if it cannot be detected early by the chart. See Chapter 6 in Qiu (2014) for a more detailed discussion.

The SPC control charts discussed above are mainly for detecting upward mean shifts when the quality variable is univariate and continuous. Other cases, including the ones when we are interested in detecting downward or arbitrary mean shifts or when the quality variable is multivariate and/or discrete, can be discussed similarly. There are also control charts designed for detecting variance shifts or shifts in other parameters of the process distribution. See Qiu (2014) for a related discussion on all these topics.

14.3 A New Biosurveillance System

In this section, the newly proposed biosurveillance system BCEWMA is discussed in detail. BCEWMA is a generalization of the EWMA chart discussed in Yang and Qiu (2020), and it consists of three main steps: (i) estimation of a semiparametric baseline model to describe regular disease incidence pattern for cases when no disease outbreaks are present, (ii) extraction of useful information from covariates by applying an EWMA chart on the covariates, and (iii) detection of unusual disease incidence pattern (or disease outbreak) by another EWMA chart, in which the weighting parameter is determined by the extracted covariate information. All the details of these three steps are described below.

14.3.1 A Baseline Model and Its Estimation

Recall that, when no special cause variation is present in a process, the process is considered to be IC, and a dataset collected in cases when the process is in IC is referred to as an IC dataset. For disease surveillance, IC data refer to observations collected in time periods when no disease outbreaks are present. In the first step of BCEWMA, we aim to describe the IC longitudinal disease incidence pattern by a baseline model, and then this baseline model can be estimated from an IC dataset.

Let $[0, T]$ be the basic time interval of the baseline model. In practice, this time interval $[0, T]$ is often chosen to be a whole year. For any $t \in [0, T]$, let $N(t; dt)$ be the number of disease cases in the time interval $[t, t + dt]$, and $M(t)$ be the population size at time t. Then, $Y(t) = N(t; dt)/[M(t)dt]$ is defined to be the disease incidence rate. This is a commonly used definition in the epidemiological literature. See, for instance, Last (2001) for a related discussion. Assume that $\{Y(t_i), i = 1, 2, \ldots, n\}$ is an observed IC disease incidence dataset, and $\mathbf{X}(t_i) = \left(X_1(t_i), X_2(t_i), \ldots, X_p(t_i)\right)^T$ is a measurement of a p-dimensional covariate vector $\mathbf{X}$ at the time point $t_i \in [0, T]$, for $1 \le i \le n$. In cases when no disease outbreaks are present, the observed IC incidence rates are assumed to follow the semiparametric baseline model

$$Y(t_i) = f(t_i) + \mathbf{X}(t_i)^T \boldsymbol{\beta} + \varepsilon(t_i), \qquad \text{for } i = 1, 2, \ldots, n, \tag{14.8}$$

where $f(t)$ is an unknown smooth function used to describe the temporal variation (e.g., seasonality) of the disease incidence rate, $\boldsymbol{\beta} = (\beta_1, \beta_2, \ldots, \beta_p)^T$ are the regression coefficients, and $\{\varepsilon(t_i), i = 1, 2, \ldots n\}$ are the zero-mean random errors. Furthermore, for $i = 1, 2, \ldots, n$, denote

$$E(\mathbf{X}(t_i)) = \boldsymbol{\mu}_{\mathbf{X}}(t_i), \;\; \text{Var}(\mathbf{X}(t_i)) = \boldsymbol{\Sigma}_{\mathbf{X}}(t_i), \tag{14.9}$$

and

$$\text{Var}(Y(t_i)) = \sigma_Y^2(t_i), \tag{14.10}$$

where $\boldsymbol{\mu}_{\mathbf{X}}(t_i)$ is a vector with length p, $\boldsymbol{\Sigma}_{\mathbf{X}}(t_i)$ is a $p \times p$ matrix, and $\sigma_Y^2(t_i) \geq 0$ is the variance of the observed incidence rate $Y(t_i)$. In Eqs. (14.8)–(14.10), no parametric assumptions are imposed on $f(t)$, $\boldsymbol{\mu}_{\mathbf{X}}(t)$, $\boldsymbol{\Sigma}_{\mathbf{X}}(t)$, $\sigma_Y^2(t)$, and the distributions of $\mathbf{X}(t)$ and $\varepsilon(t)$, to ensure high flexibility and generalizability.

The $\boldsymbol{\beta}$ and $f(t)$ in Eq. (14.8) can be estimated in the following four steps: (i) provide an initial estimate of $f(t)$, (ii) estimate the parametric part $\boldsymbol{\beta}$, (iii) estimate the nonparametric part $f(t)$, and (iv) iterate steps (ii) and (iii) until convergence. Next, we will describe these four steps in detail.

In step one, an initial estimate of $f(t)$ is needed. To this end, $\boldsymbol{\beta}$ is assumed to be $\mathbf{0}$, and the following local linear kernel smoothing (LLKS) procedure is used to estimate $f(t)$:

$$\underset{\boldsymbol{\alpha}\in\mathbb{R}^2}{\arg\min} \sum_{i=1}^{n}\sum_{j=1}^{m_i} \left[Y(t_i) - \alpha_0 - \alpha_1(t_i - t)\right]^2 K_h(t_i - t), \tag{14.11}$$

where $\boldsymbol{\alpha} = (\alpha_0, \alpha_1)^T$, $K_h(t_i - t) = K((t_i - t)/h)$, $h > 0$ is a bandwidth and $K(\cdot)$ is a kernel function. Let $\mathbf{G}_i = (1, (t_i - t))^T$, for $i = 1, 2, \ldots, n$, then the solution of (14.11) to α_0 is the LLKS estimate of $f(t)$, which can be expressed as

$$\widehat{f}(t) = \boldsymbol{e}_1^T \left(\mathbf{G}^T\mathbf{W}\mathbf{G}\right)^{-1} \mathbf{G}^T\mathbf{W}\mathbf{Y}, \tag{14.12}$$

where $\boldsymbol{e}_1 = (1, 0)^T$, $\mathbf{G} = (\mathbf{G}_1, \ldots, \mathbf{G}_n)^T$, $\mathbf{W} = \text{diag}\{K_h(t_i - t), \ldots, K_h(t_n - t)\}$, and $\mathbf{Y} = (Y(t_1), \ldots, Y(t_n))^T$. The estimate $\widehat{f}(t)$ is actually a weighted average of all observations in a neighborhood of t, with the weights controlled by $K(u)$ and the neighborhood size controlled by h.

To ensure that the LLKS procedure works well, the kernel function $K(u)$ and the bandwidth h should be chosen properly. For the kernel function, since the Epanechnikov kernel function $K_e(u) = [3(1 - u^2)/4]I(|u| \leq 1)$ has some good theoretical properties, it is chosen for $K(u)$. Regarding the choice of the bandwidth h, note that disease incidence rates at different observation times are often correlated, and it has been well discussed in the literature that conventional bandwidth selection approaches like the leave-one-out cross-validation (CV) would not perform well when the observations are correlated, because these conventional bandwidth selection procedures cannot properly distinguish the data correlation structure from the data mean function. See, for instance, Altman (1990) and Opsomer, Wang, and Yang (2001). To overcome this difficulty, Brabanter, Brabanter, Suykens, and De Moor (2011) suggested a modified CV (MCV) procedure to handle the correlated data. According to their suggestion, we can choose the bandwidth h by minimizing the following MCV score:

$$\mathrm{MCV}(h) = \frac{1}{n}\sum_{i=1}^{n}\left[\widehat{f}_{-(i)}(t_i) - Y(t_i)\right]^2, \tag{14.13}$$

where $\widehat{f}_{-(i)}(t_i)$ is the leave-one-out estimate of $f(t_i)$ by (14.11) when the observation $Y(t_i)$ is left out and when the kernel function is chosen to be the following bimodal kernel

$$\widetilde{K}_\epsilon(u) = \frac{4}{4-3\epsilon-\epsilon^3}\begin{cases} \frac{3}{4}(1-u^2)I(|u|\le 1), & \text{if } |u| \ge \epsilon; \\ \frac{3(1-\epsilon^2)}{4\epsilon}|u|, & \text{if } |u| < \epsilon, \end{cases} \tag{14.14}$$

and $\epsilon \in (0, 1)$ is a constant. By using this bimodal kernel function, observations around t_i are down-weighted when computing $\widehat{f}_{-(i)}(t_i)$ in (14.13) to reduce the impact of data correlation on bandwidth selection. Based on a large simulation study, Brabanter et al. (2011) suggested choosing ϵ to be 0.1, and this suggestion is adopted throughout this chapter.

In step two of model estimation, we estimate the parametric component $\boldsymbol{\beta}$. Denote $\mathbf{X} = (\mathbf{X}(t_1), \ldots, \mathbf{X}(t_n))^T$, $Z(t_i) = Y(t_i) - \widehat{f}(t_i)$, and $\mathbf{Z} = (Z(t_1), \ldots, Z(t_n))^T$. In order to estimate the parametric part $\boldsymbol{\beta}$, the following ordinary least square procedure can be considered:

$$\widehat{\boldsymbol{\beta}} = \left(\mathbf{X}^T\mathbf{X}\right)^{-1}\mathbf{X}^T\mathbf{Z}. \tag{14.15}$$

In step three, we can specify $\boldsymbol{\beta}$ to be $\widehat{\boldsymbol{\beta}}$, and update the estimate of the nonparametric part $f(t)$ by the LLKS procedure (14.12), with $Y(t_i)$ replaced by $\widetilde{Y}(t_i) = Y(t_i) - \mathbf{X}(t_i)^T\widehat{\boldsymbol{\beta}}$. In this step, for simplicity, the same bandwidth as in calculating the initial estimate of $f(t)$ is recommended for use.

As last step of model estimation, we can iterate between the second and the third steps described above to obtain the final estimates of $\boldsymbol{\beta}$ and $f(t)$, after certain convergence criteria are met. Suppose the estimate of $\boldsymbol{\beta}$ at the k-th iteration is $\widehat{\boldsymbol{\beta}}_{(k)}$, the iterative procedure will stop at the k-th iteration if the following criterion is satisfied:

$$||\widehat{\boldsymbol{\beta}}_{(k)} - \widehat{\boldsymbol{\beta}}_{(k-1)}||_1 / ||\widehat{\boldsymbol{\beta}}_{(k-1)}||_1 \le err,$$

where $err > 0$ is a pre-specified small number (we use $err = 10^{-6}$ in real data examples), and $||\cdot||_1$ is the summation of the absolute values of all the elements in a vector.

For $\boldsymbol{\mu}_{\mathbf{X}}(t)$ and $\boldsymbol{\Sigma}_{\mathbf{X}}(t)$ defined in (14.9), they can be estimated from the observed covariate vectors $\{\mathbf{X}(t_i) : i = 1, 2, \ldots, n\}$ directly. More specifically, $\boldsymbol{\mu}_{\mathbf{X}}(t)$ can be estimated by

$$\widehat{\boldsymbol{\mu}}_{\mathbf{X}}(t) = \frac{\sum_{i=1}^{n} K_h(t_i - t)\mathbf{X}(t_i)}{\sum_{i=1}^{n} K_h(t_i - t)}, \tag{14.16}$$

and we can estimate $\mathbf{\Sigma_X}(t)$ by

$$\widehat{\mathbf{\Sigma}}_{\mathbf{X}}(t) = \frac{\sum_{i=1}^{n} K_h(t_i - t)\,(\mathbf{X}(t_i) - \widehat{\boldsymbol{\mu}}_{\mathbf{X}}(t_i))\,(\mathbf{X}(t_i) - \widehat{\boldsymbol{\mu}}_{\mathbf{X}}(t_i))^T}{\sum_{i=1}^{n} K_h(t_i - t)}. \tag{14.17}$$

From (14.8), it is clear that the mean of $Y(t)$ is $\mu_Y(t) = f(t) + \boldsymbol{\mu}_{\mathbf{X}}(t)^T \boldsymbol{\beta}$. After obtaining the estimates $\widehat{\boldsymbol{\beta}}$, $\widehat{f}(t)$ and $\widehat{\boldsymbol{\mu}}_{\mathbf{X}}(t)$, we can define $\widehat{\mu}_Y(t) = \widehat{f}(t) + \widehat{\boldsymbol{\mu}}_{\mathbf{X}}(t)^T \widehat{\boldsymbol{\beta}}$ to be the estimate of $\mu_Y(t)$. Then, let $\widehat{e}(t_i) = Y(t_i) - \widehat{\mu}_Y(t_i)$. For $t \in [0, T]$, the variance function of $Y(t)$ can be estimated by

$$\widehat{\sigma}_Y^2(t) = \frac{\sum_{i=1}^{n} K_h(t_i - t)\widehat{e}^2(t_i)}{\sum_{i=1}^{n} K_h(t_i - t)}. \tag{14.18}$$

So far, we have discussed the estimation of $\boldsymbol{\mu}_{\mathbf{X}}(t)$, $\mathbf{\Sigma}_{\mathbf{X}}(t)$, $\mu_Y(t)$, and $\sigma_Y^2(t)$ in (14.16)–(14.18) for cases when $t \in [0, T]$. With the assumption that these functions are periodic in time with a period of T, these estimates can be extended to the entire time interval $[0, \infty)$.

14.3.2 Sequential Monitoring of Disease Incidence Rates

In the EWMA chart proposed by Yang and Qiu (2020), the IC distributions (including the means and the variances) of $Y(t)$ and $\mathbf{X}(t)$ are assumed to be time-independent. In biosurveillance applications, however, these IC distributions are usually time-varying, as discussed in Sect. 14.1. In the previous subsection, estimation of the means, variances and other related IC quantities of $Y(t)$ and $\mathbf{X}(t)$ has been discussed. More specifically, the estimates $\widehat{f}(t)$, $\widehat{\boldsymbol{\mu}}_{\mathbf{X}}(t)$, $\widehat{\mathbf{\Sigma}}_{\mathbf{X}}(t)$, $\widehat{\boldsymbol{\beta}}$, $\widehat{\mu}_Y(t)$ and $\widehat{\sigma}_Y^2(t)$ have been obtained from an IC dataset. These estimates can thus be used to describe IC longitudinal patterns of disease incidence rates and the corresponding covariates for online sequential monitoring. A unique notion of the generalized EWMA chart proposed in this chapter is that the estimated IC quantities of $Y(t)$ and $\mathbf{X}(t)$ can be used to standardize the future observations of $Y(t)$ and $\mathbf{X}(t)$, and then the chart in Yang and Qiu (2020) can be applied to the standardized future observations. Detailed description of the generalized EWMA chart is provided below.

Suppose the incidence rates for a disease to be monitored are observed at times $\{t_i^* : i = 1, 2, \ldots\}$, and let the observed incidence rates and the corresponding covariates be $\{Y(t_i^*), i = 1, 2, \ldots\}$ and $\{\mathbf{X}(t_i^*), i = 1, 2, \ldots\}$, respectively. From the equation in (14.8), we know that the p-dimensional covariate vector $\mathbf{X}(t)$ can affect $Y(t)$ through a linear combination $\mathbf{X}(t)^T \boldsymbol{\beta}$ such that changes in $\mathbf{X}(t)^T \boldsymbol{\beta}$ result in a mean shift in $Y(t)$. So, the covariates could contain information about disease incidence. In BCEWMA, the covariate information can be extracted by using the following EWMA charting statistic

$$E_{\mathbf{X},i} = \lambda \left[\frac{(\mathbf{X}(t_i^*) - \widehat{\boldsymbol{\mu}}_{\mathbf{X}}(t_i^*))^T \widehat{\boldsymbol{\beta}}}{\sqrt{\widehat{\boldsymbol{\beta}}^T \widehat{\boldsymbol{\Sigma}}_{\mathbf{X}}(t_i^*) \widehat{\boldsymbol{\beta}}}} \right] + (1-\lambda) E_{\mathbf{X},i-1}, \text{ for } i \geq 1, \tag{14.19}$$

where $E_{\mathbf{X},0} = 0$, and $\lambda \in (0, 1]$ is a weighting parameter.

Note that a large absolute value of $E_{\mathbf{X},i}$ implies that it is likely to have a shift in the mean of $\mathbf{X}(t)^T \boldsymbol{\beta}$. Therefore, $E_{\mathbf{X},i}$ can be used for measuring the possibility of a mean shift in $\mathbf{X}(t)^T \boldsymbol{\beta}$. For disease outbreak detection, usually only upward shifts in the disease incidence rate $Y(t)$ are of interest. Thus, we focus on upward shifts in $\mathbf{X}(t)^T \boldsymbol{\beta}$ as well, because of the relationship between $\mathbf{X}(t)^T \boldsymbol{\beta}$ and $Y(t)$ described in (14.8). For the EWMA chart (14.19), it would give a signal of an upward shift in $\mathbf{X}(t)^T \boldsymbol{\beta}$ if

$$E_{\mathbf{X},i} > \rho_{\mathbf{X}}, \tag{14.20}$$

where $\rho_{\mathbf{X}} > 0$ is a control limit chosen to achieve a pre-specified value of ARL_0, denoted as $ARL_{\mathbf{X},0}$.

Given the value of $ARL_{\mathbf{X},0}$ and λ, $\rho_{\mathbf{X}}$ can be computed by a resampling approach from an IC dataset (cf., Chatterjee & Qiu 2009). Because the observed covariate vectors at different time points are often correlated, we suggest using a block bootstrap procedure that is described below. Suppose the IC dataset used to search for the control limit $\rho_{\mathbf{X}}$ is $\{(\mathbf{X}(t_i^{**}), Y(t_i^{**})), i = 1, 2 \ldots, \widetilde{n}\}$. Then, the block bootstrap procedure with block length l can be described as follows:

1. Calculate $\widetilde{Q}(t_i^{**}) = \frac{(\mathbf{X}(t_i^{**}) - \widehat{\boldsymbol{\mu}}_{\mathbf{X}}(t_i^{**}))^T \widehat{\boldsymbol{\beta}}}{\sqrt{\widehat{\boldsymbol{\beta}}^T \widehat{\boldsymbol{\Sigma}}_{\mathbf{X}}(t_i^{**}) \widehat{\boldsymbol{\beta}}}}$, for $i = 1, 2, \ldots, \widetilde{n}$. Then, there are $\widetilde{n} - l + 1$ possible blocks of length l, with the k-th block being $\{\widetilde{Q}(t_i^{**}), k \leq i \leq k + l - 1\}$, for $k = 1, 2 \ldots, \widetilde{n} - l + 1$;
2. Randomly select a sequence of blocks from all $\widetilde{n} - l + 1$ possible blocks with replacement. The selected blocks are placed one after another according to the selection order, and they form a bootstrap sample, denoted as $\{\widetilde{Q}_i^* : i = 1, 2 \ldots\}$;
3. Compute the EWMA charting statistic $E_i = \lambda \widetilde{Q}_i^* + (1-\lambda) E_{i-1}$, for $i \geq 1$, where $E_0 = 0$. For a given control limit $\rho_{\mathbf{X}}$, define $RL_0(\rho_{\mathbf{X}}) = \min\{i : E_i > \rho_{\mathbf{X}}\}$;
4. Repeat the second and third steps for B times, and define $ARL_0(\rho_{\mathbf{X}})$ to be the average of B $RL_0(\rho_{\mathbf{X}})$ values obtained from the B replications;
5. Use the bisection search method to search for $\rho_{\mathbf{X}}$ such that $ARL_0(\rho_{\mathbf{X}})$ equal to the pre-specified $ARL_{0,\mathbf{X}}$ level.

To detect a disease outbreak using $E_{\mathbf{X},i}$, we propose to use the following EWMA chart:

$$E_{Y,i} = \phi(E_{\mathbf{X},i}; \lambda, \rho_{\mathbf{X}}) \left(\frac{Y(t_i^*) - \widehat{\mu}_Y(t_i^*)}{\widehat{\sigma}_Y(t_i^*)} \right) + \left(1 - \phi(E_{\mathbf{X},i}; \lambda, \rho_{\mathbf{X}})\right) E_{Y,i-1}, \text{ for } i \geq 1, \tag{14.21}$$

where $E_{Y,0} = 0$, and $\phi(E_{\mathbf{X},i}; \lambda, \rho_{\mathbf{X}}) \in (0, 1]$ is a weight that depends on $E_{\mathbf{X},i}$ and $(\lambda, \rho_{\mathbf{X}})$. This chart will trigger a signal of a disease outbreak if

$$E_{Y,i} > \rho_Y, \tag{14.22}$$

where $\rho_Y > 0$ is a control limit chosen to achieve a pre-specified value of ARL_0, denoted as $ARL_{Y,0}$. The weighting function $\phi(E_{\mathbf{X},i}; \lambda, \rho_{\mathbf{X}})$ and the value of $ARL_{Y,0}$ need to be chosen in advance, then ρ_Y can be determined by the block bootstrap procedure from the IC dataset, similar to the determination of the control limit $\rho_{\mathbf{X}}$ in (14.20).

As mentioned previously, the weighting function $\phi(E_{\mathbf{X},i}; \lambda, \rho_{\mathbf{X}})$ must be specified and used in the chart (14.21)–(14.22). It is obvious that more weight should be put on the current observation $Y(t_i^*)$ when we calculate the charting statistic $E_{Y,i}$ if the possibility of an upward shift in $\mathbf{X}(t)^T\boldsymbol{\beta}$ is larger at time t_i^*. So, $\phi(E_{\mathbf{X},i}; \lambda, \rho_{\mathbf{X}})$ should be chosen as a nondecreasing function of $E_{\mathbf{X},i}$. In this chapter, we suggest using the following weighting function:

$$\phi_H(x; \lambda, \rho_{\mathbf{X}}) = \begin{cases} 1 - (1-\lambda)\,/(x/\rho_{\mathbf{X}})\,, & \text{if } x > \rho_{\mathbf{X}}, \\ \lambda, & \text{otherwise}; \end{cases} \tag{14.23}$$

The function $\phi_H(x; \lambda, \rho_{\mathbf{X}})$ in (14.23) is inspired by the Huber's function (Huber 1981), and the resulting disease surveillance system is denoted as BCEWMA-H, where the last letter "H" denotes the fact that $\phi_H(x; \lambda, \rho_{\mathbf{X}})$ is used as the weighting function. From (14.23), it is obvious that $\rho_{\mathbf{X}}$ is a scale parameter of $E_{\mathbf{X},i}$ when we calculate the weight $\phi_H(E_{\mathbf{X},i}; \lambda, \rho_{\mathbf{X}})$.

14.4 Real Data Examples

In this section, we apply the new biosurveillance system BCEWMA to monitor the incidence rates of hand, foot, and mouth disease (HFMD) in China and the influenza-like-illness (ILI) in Florida. Besides the proposed approach using the weighting function $\phi_H(x; \lambda, \rho_{\mathbf{X}})$ (denoted as BCEWMA-H), we also consider the following three alternative methods:

- the proposed control chart with the weighting parameter to be a constant λ, denoted as BCEWMA-C,
- the EWMA chart for detecting upward mean shifts suggested by Dong et al. (2008), denoted as EWMA, and
- the Shewhart chart for detecting upward mean shifts, denoted as Shewhart.

For the alternative chart BCEWMA-C, the weighting parameter is chosen to be a constant. So, the covariate information is totally ignored by this chart. To investigate the benefit of using covariate information, we can compare the performance of

BCEWMA-H with that of BCEWMA-C. In the EWMA chart by Dong et al. (2008), the observed disease incidence rate is assumed to be normally distributed and this chart cannot handle the seasonality and other time-varying IC patterns. Besides the limitations of the EWMA by Dong et al. (2008), the Shewhart chart has another major disadvantage that it is ineffective in detecting small shifts.

14.4.1 The Hand, Foot and Mouth Disease Data

Hand, foot and mouth disease (HFMD) is a common infectious disease that often occurs in children under 5 years of age. During 2008–2015, the number of HFMD patients reported in China is about 13 millions, including 123,261 severe cases and 3322 deaths (c.f., Huang et al. 2018). Due to its high death rate, an effective biosurveillance system is needed to detect the disease outbreaks at an early stage, so that some disease control measures can be taken in a timely fashion to minimize its damage. In a HFMD dataset obtained from Chinese Center for Disease Control (CDC), we have the weekly disease incidence rates in Sichuan province of China during years 2012–2014. For HFMD, it has been well studied that it is closely associated with certain weather conditions like air temperature. See, for example, Wang et al. (2011). On the webpage of the National Oceanic and Atmospheric Administration (NOAA) of the United States, we can download the weekly average of temperature of Sichuan province during years 2012–2014. The observed weekly HFMD incidence rates and temperature levels are presented in Fig. 14.1. From Fig. 14.1, it is clear that the observed incidence rates in years 2012 and 2013 are quite stable, and we use these observations as IC data. The IC dataset is then divided into two parts. The observations in year 2013 are used to estimate the regular disease pattern, while the IC data in year 2012 is used to determine the control limits $\rho_{\mathbf{X}}$ and ρ_Y of the proposed method BCEWMA-H, by the block bootstrap

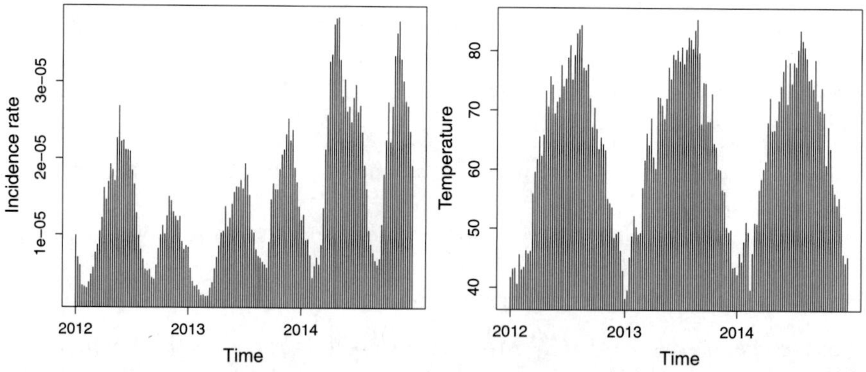

Fig. 14.1 Observed HFMD incidence rates and air temperatures in Sichuan province during years 2012–2014

procedure after the weighting function is chosen to be $\phi_H(x; \lambda, \rho_{\mathbf{X}})$, $\lambda = 0.3$ and $ARL_{\mathbf{X},0} = ARL_{Y,0} = 50$.

Then, we sequentially monitor the disease incidence rates from the beginning of year 2014, and this chart is presented in Fig. 14.2a. For comparison, the results of the BCEWMA-C chart with the weighting parameter $\lambda = 0.3$, the EWMA chart with $\lambda = 0.3$, and the Shewhart chart are presented in Fig. 14.2b–d. When we implement the four control charts in this example, all the control limits are chosen by the block bootstrap procedure with the bootstrap sample size $B = 10{,}000$ and the block size $l = 5$, using the IC data in year 2012. For the BCEWMA-C, EWMA and Shewhart charts, their ARL_0 values are also fixed at 50. From Fig. 14.3, we find that these four charts give signals of disease outbreak at the 11th, 12th, 14th, and 14th week, respectively. Next, the observed disease incidence rates in year 2014 is compared with their predicted values using the estimated regular pattern. In Fig. 14.3, the dark points denote the observed HFMD incidence rates in 2014, the solid curve denotes the predicted incidence rates using the estimated regular pattern obtained from the IC data, and the vertical dashed line denotes the signal

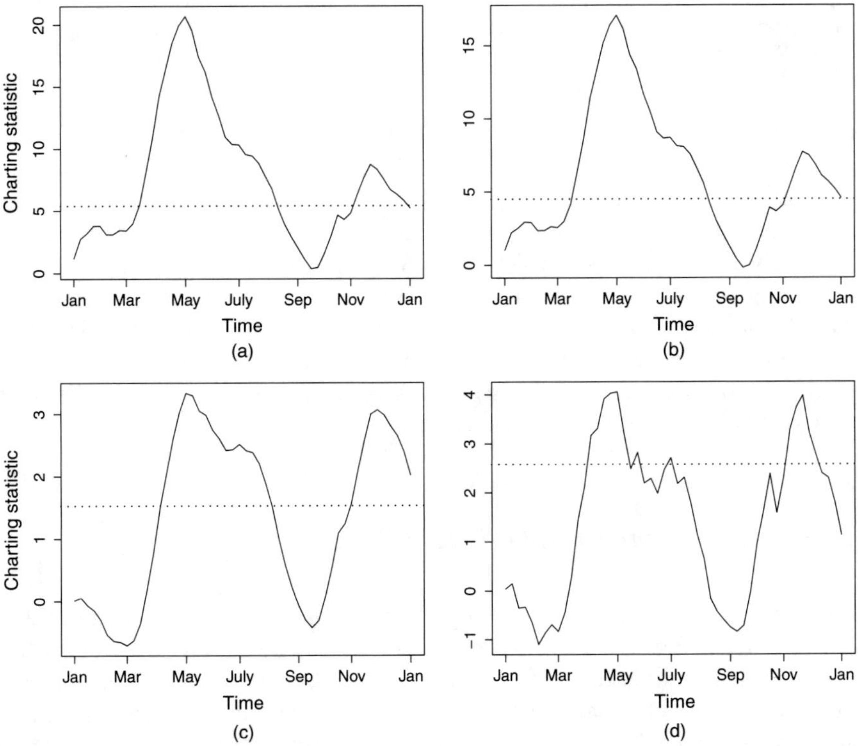

Fig. 14.2 The (**a**) BCEWMA-H, (**b**) BCEWMA-C, (**c**) EWMA and (**d**) Shewhart charts for monitoring the weekly HFMD disease incidence rates in year 2014, where the horizontal lines denote the control limits for the corresponding control charts

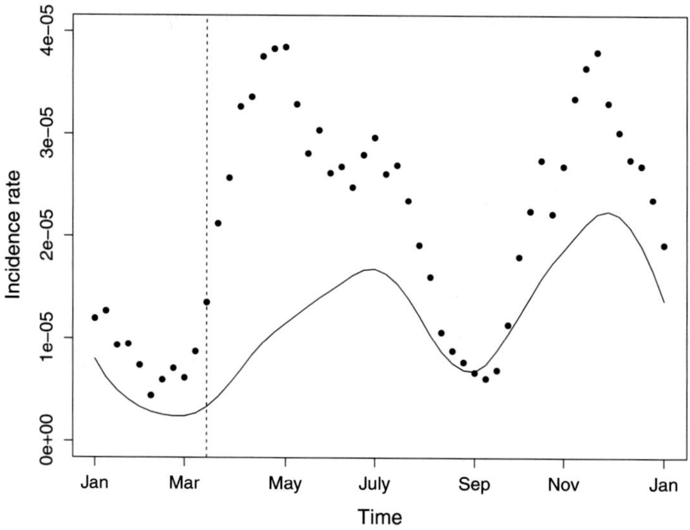

Fig. 14.3 Observed weekly HFMD incidence rates in year 2014 (little dots) and their predicted values from the estimated baseline model (solid curve). The vertical dashed line is the signal time of BCEWMA-H

time from BCEWMA-H. It can be seen that the observed HFMD incidence rates are indeed much higher than their predicted values, and BCEWMA-H catches this shift quite promptly. To investigate whether this shift is associated with temperature, we calculate the average temperature during years 2012–2013, and compare it with the yearly average temperature in 2014. We find that the average temperature in the year 2014 is 63.9 °F, which is a little bit lower than the average temperature of 64.1 °F during the years 2012 and 2013. So, the temperature during 2014 is indeed colder than that in 2012–2013, which might contribute to the higher incidence rates of HFMD in 2014. As a result, BCEWMA-H gives a signal 1 week earlier than BCEWMA-C, after using the temperature information.

14.4.2 The Influenza-Like-Illness Data

The second example is about the Florida influenza-like-illness (ILI) data. ILI is a severe respiratory infection that can cause serious illness and even death (Hu et al. 2018). Thus, it is critically important to provide an effective real-time disease monitoring such that its damage can be minimized. The ILI disease surveillance data are provided by the Florida Department of Health (FDOH), covering the years of 2012–2014 in Florida state. Due to the fact that ILI is highly associated with weather conditions such as temperature (cf., Noort, Aguas, Ballesteros, & Gomes 2012), we included the Florida temperature data obtained from the NOAA of the United

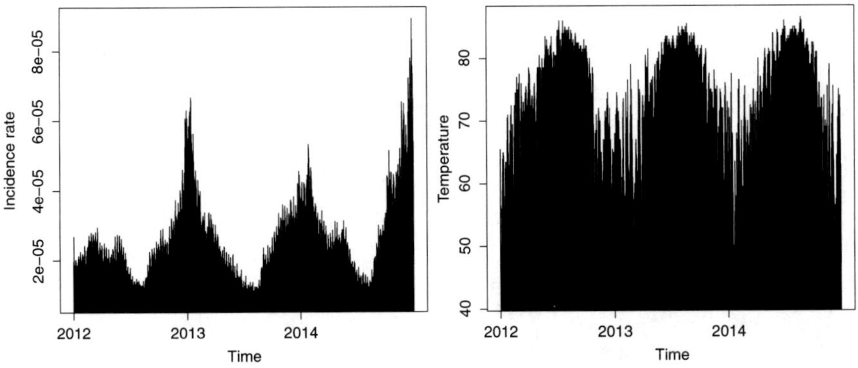

Fig. 14.4 Observed daily ILI incidence rates and air temperature data in Florida during years 2012–2014

States in our disease monitoring so that the helpful temperature information can be properly used to improve the disease outbreak detection. The observed Florida ILI incidence rates are presented in Fig. 14.4, together with the temperature data. From the figure, we can see that the observation disease incidence rates in years 2012 and 2013 are more stable, compared to those in year 2014. So, the observed data in these 2 years are used as the IC data. Based on the IC data, we can estimate the regular disease longitudinal pattern and determine the control limits used in our proposed chart as well. To this end, the data in year 2013 are used for estimating the baseline model and those in 2012 are used for determining the control limits of the chart BCEWMA-H by the block bootstrap approach.

Then, we apply the related control charts to the observed data in 2014 for online disease monitoring. In BCEWMA-H, both $ARL_{\mathbf{X},0}$ and $ARL_{Y,0}$ are fixed at 500. For the three competitive charts BCEWMA-C, EWMA and Shewhart, their ARL_0 values are also specified to be 500. In all the charts, λ is chosen to be 0.3, and their control limits are determined by the block bootstrap procedure with $B = 10{,}000$ and $l = 5$. The four charts are presented in Fig. 14.5, where the dotted horizontal lines denote the related control limits. From the plots in the figure, the BCEWMA-H, BCEWMA-C, EWMA and Shewhart charts give signals on Oct 7th, Oct 19th, Nov 13th, and Nov 13th, respectively. Therefore, the signal from of BCEWMA-H is about 2-week earlier than that of BCEWMA-C, and the signals from EWMA and Shewhart are more than 1-month later. To better perceive the observed disease incidence rates in year 2014, we present the observed data in that year and the corresponding predicted values from the estimated baseline model in Fig. 14.6 by the dark points and the solid curve, respectively. From the plot, it can be seen that major difference between the observed data and their predicted values starts in early September and the difference becomes more significant later on. The vertical dashed line in the plot denotes the signal time from BCEWMA-H. It can be seen that BCEWMA-H can detect such difference in a quite timely manner. In this study, we also compare the average temperature in year 2014 with that of years 2012 and

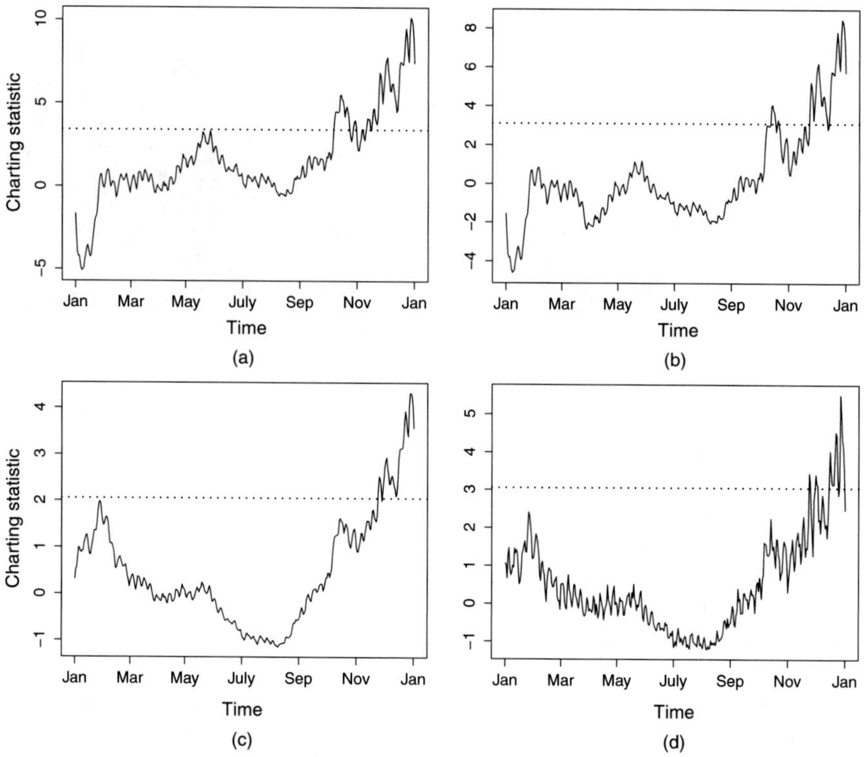

Fig. 14.5 The (**a**) BCEWMA-H, (**b**) BCEWMA-C, (**c**) EWMA and (**d**) Shewhart charts for monitoring the daily ILI disease incidence rates in year 2014. The horizontal lines denote the control limits of the related control charts

2013. Because the major difference between the observed and predicted incidence rates starts at the beginning of September, we only take average of the temperatures during 09/01 and 12/31. By some simple calculations, the average temperature during this time period in 2014 is 71.5 °F, which is 1.5 degrees lower than that in the previous 2 years. Therefore, temperature information should be helpful to predict the occurrence of unusual disease incidence patterns. This might explain the reason why the BCEWMA-H chart can detect the disease outbreak earlier than the other three charts.

14.5 Concluding Remarks

In this paper, we have proposed a new biosurveillance system BCEWMA for monitoring disease incidence data. The new biosurveillance system is a generalization of the online monitoring approach that was originally discussed in

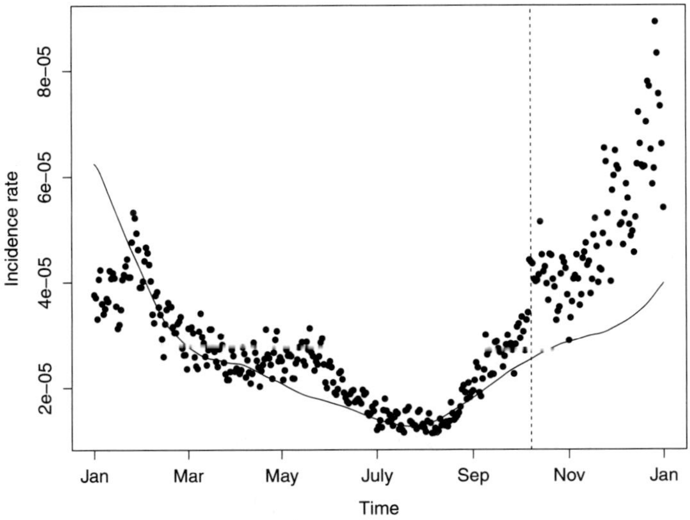

Fig. 14.6 Observed daily ILI incidence rates in year 2014 (little dots) and their predicted values from the estimated baseline model (solid curve). The vertical dashed line is the signal time of BCEWMA-H

Yang and Qiu (2020) for sequential monitoring of processes with time-independent IC distributions. The generalized method can accommodate helpful information from covariates, time-varying longitudinal pattern of the process observations (e.g., seasonality), and arbitrary data distribution. BCEWMA is applied to two real-data examples, and the results indicate that it works well in practice. In addition to disease surveillance, BCEWMA should also be useful for many other applications, including sequential monitoring of some environmental indexes like PM2.5 concentration levels. However, there are still some issues regarding BCEWMA that need to addressed in the future work. For instance, in practice, there could be a lot of covariates that might be relevant to the incidence rates of a disease in concern. In such cases, only those covariates that are strongly related to the disease incidence rates would be helpful for disease surveillance and thus should be included in the proposed surveillance system. Therefore, we need to decide which covariates should be included in the system in advance. To address this issue, an effective and reliable variable selection procedure should be developed, which will be studied in our future research.

References

Altman, N. S. (1990). Kernel smoothing of data with correlated errors. *Journal of the American Statistical Association, 85*, 749–758.

Brabanter, K. D., Brabanter, J. D., Suykens, J. A. K., & De Moor, B. (2011). Kernel regression in the presence of correlated errors. *Journal of Machine Learning Research, 12*, 1955–1976.

Chatterjee, S., & Qiu, P. (2009). Distribution-free cumulative sum control charts using bootstrap-based control limits. *The Annals of Applied Statistics, 3*, 349–369.
Dong, Y., Hedayat, A. S., & Sinha, B. K. (2008). Surveillance strategies for detecting changepoint in incidence rate based on exponentially weighted moving average methods. *Journal of the American Statistical Association, 103*, 843–853.
Hawkins, D., Qiu, P., & Kang, C. W. (2003). The changepoint model for statistical process control. *Journal of Quality Technology, 35*, 355–366.
Hu, H., Wang, H., Wang, F., Langley, D., Avram, A., & Liu, M. (2018). Prediction of influenza-like illness based on the improved artificial tree algorithm and artificial neural network. *Scientific Reports, 8*, 4895.
Huang, J., Liao, Q., Qoi, M. H., Cowling, B. J., Chang, Z., Wu, P., …, Wei, S. (2018). Epidemiology of recurrent hand, foot and mouth disease, China, 2008–2015. *Emerging Infectious Diseases, 24*. https://doi.org/10.3201/eid2403.171303
Huber, P. J. (1981). *Robust statistics*. New York, NY: Wiley.
Jung, I., Kulldorff, M., & Klassen, A. C. (2007). A spatial scan statistic for ordinal data. *Statistics in Medicine, 26*, 1594–1507.
Kulldorff, M. (1997). A spatial scan statistic. *Communications in Statistics–Theory and Methods, 26*, 1481–1496.
Kulldorff, M., Huang, L., & Konty, K. (2009). A scan statistic for continuous data based on the normal probability model. *International Journal of Health Geographics, 8*, 58.
Last, J. M. (2001). *A dictionary of epidemiology* (4th ed.). Oxford, UK: Oxford University Press.
Marshall, J. B., Spitzner, D. J., & Woodall, W. H. (2007). Use of the local Knox statistic for the prospective monitoring of disease occurrences in space and time. *Statistics in Medicine, 26*, 1579–1593.
Moustakides, G. V. (1986). Optimal stopping times for detecting changes in distributions. *The Annals of Statistics, 14*, 1379–1387.
Noort, S. P., Aguas, R., Ballesteros, S., & Gomes, M. G. (2012). The role of weather on the relation between influenza and influenza-like illness. *Journal of Theoretical Biology, 298*, 131–137.
Opsomer, J., Wang, Y., & Yang, Y. (2001). Nonparametric regressin with correlated errors. *Statistical Science, 16*, 134–153.
Page, E. S. (1954). Continuous inspection schemes. *Biometrika, 4*, 100–114.
Qiu, P. (2014). *Introduction to statistical process control*. Boca Raton, FL: Chapman Hall/CRC.
Roberts, S. W. (1959). Control chart tests based on geometric moving averages. *Technometrics, 1*, 239–250.
Shewhart, W. A. (1931). *The economic control of the quality of manifactured production*. New York, NY: Macmillan.
Sonesson, C. (2007). A CUSUM framework for detection of spacetime disease clusters using scan statistics. *Statistics in Medicine, 26*, 4770–4789.
Unkel, S., Farrington, C. P., & Garthwaite, P. H. (2012). Statistical methods for the prospective detection of infectious disease outbreaks: A review. *Journal of the Royal Statistical Society (Series A), 175*, 49–82.
Wang, Y., Feng, Z., Yang, Y., Self, S., Gao, Y., Longini, I. M., …, Yang, W. (2011). Hand, foot and mouth disease in China: Patterns of spread and transmissibility during 2008–2009. *Epidemiology, 22*, 781–792.
Yang, K., & Qiu, P. (2020). Statistical process control using covariates. *Technometrics*. (revised submission, under review).
Zhao, Y., Zeng, D., Herring, A. H., Ising, A., Waller, A., Richardson, D., & Kosorok, M. R. (2011). Detecting disease outbreaks using local spatiotemporal methods. *Biometrics, 67*, 1508–1517.
Zhou, H., & Lawson, A. B. (2008). EWMA smoothing and Bayesian spatial modeling for health surveillance. *Statistics in Medicine, 27*, 5907–5928.

Chapter 15
Cusp Catastrophe Regression Analysis of Testosterone in Bifurcating the Age-Related Changes in PSA, a Biomarker for Prostate Cancer

Xinguang Chen, Kai Wang, and (Din) Ding-Geng Chen

Abstract Advancing cancer research needs to adapt nonlinear dynamic systems (NDS) approach in addition to the linear dynamic systems (LDS). Dynamic changes in prostate-specific antigen (PSA), a biomarker of prostate cancer showed NDS character but this character has not been examined in literature. In this study, we examine PSA guided by a NDS paradigm. Participants were urology patients diagnosed with either prostate cancer (n = 27) or benign prostate disorder (n = 352) from a tertiary hospital in northcentral Florida. Data were derived from the 2001 to 2015 electronic medical records (EMR). PSA levels (ng/mL) were analyzed with cusp catastrophe mode in which participants' age at the PSA level was used as the asymmetry variable, and testosterone levels (ng/dL) as the bifurcation variable. Modeling analyses were executed in the open source R software. LDS-based linear correlation and regression analyses were also conducted as a comparison purpose. The mean age of the participants was 66.1 (SD = 9.8) years old; the PSA range was 0.05–13.8 with mean = 1.7 (SD = 1.2) ng/mL; and the total-testosterone range was 27.00–1297.00 with mean = 318.0(SD = 191.6) ng/dL. Results from Chen-Chen cusp regression indicate better data-model fit for cusp (R^2 = 0.47) than for linear regression (R^2 = 0.027). Serum PSA was significantly associated with age (a1 = 0.2691, p < .001) and bifurcated by blood testosterone (b1 = 1.0265,

X. Chen (✉)
Department of Epidemiology, College of Public Health and Health Professions, College of Medicine, University of Florida, Gainesville, FL, USA

Global Health Institute, Wuhan University, Wuhan, China
e-mail: jimax.chen@ufl.edu

K. Wang
Harvard University, Cambridge, MA, USA
e-mail: kaiwang@hsph.harvard.edu

(Din) D.-G. Chen
School of Social Work, University of North Carolina, Chapel Hill, NC, USA
e-mail: dinchen@mail.unc.edu

X. Chen, (Din) D.-G. Chen (eds.), *Statistical Methods for Global Health and Epidemiology*, ICSA Book Series in Statistics,
https://doi.org/10.1007/978-3-030-35260-8_15

p < .00) with the estimated cusp point = (age = 63, testosterone = 630 ng/mL). The estimated cusp point was close to the epidemiology data that the risk of prostate cancer started to accelerate at about ages 60–65 years; and testosterone level of 630 ng/mL, closer to the up-limit 800 ng/dL of normal range (280–800) by the American Association of Clinical Endocrinologists (AACE). In conclusion, this is the first study that examined the dynamics of PSA in men and demonstrated that serum PSA level follow the NDS. In addition to confirming the relationship between age, testosterone and PSA, findings of this analysis provide a reasonable explanation of the large PSA-range in healthy men and the small difference in mean PSA between healthy men and men with prostate cancer (1.2 vs. 2.6). There is a need to re-evaluate the role of PSA for prostate cancer screening guided by NDS paradigm.

Keywords Prostate cancer · PSA · Testosterone · Nonlinear dynamics systems · Cusp catastrophe modeling

15.1 Introduction

Worldwide, approximately 1.1 million men diagnosed with prostate cancer every year, one of the leading cancers for men (Bray et al., 2018; Khazaei et al., 2016). In the developed countries, a diagnosis of prostate cancer is based on the prostate biopsies to identify cancer cells located in the prostate tissues (Mottet et al., 2017). To date, more than one million prostate biopsies are performed annually in the United States alone, with the majority revealing no prostate cancer or low-risk prostate cancer that is unlikely to impact survival (Loeb, Carter, Berndt, Ricker, & Schaeffer, 2011). Prostate biopsy, particularly overuse of the procedure is associated with increased risk of medical complications, including pain, bleeding and infections (Borghesi et al., 2017; Loeb et al., 2011, 2012). To reduce unnecessary use of prostate biopsy while not missing men with prostate cancer, a biomarker—prostate specific antigen (PSA) has been identified, reference point established, and widely used as a screening tool in practice (Mottet et al., 2017). Prostate biopsy will be recommended for men whose blood PSA level is ≥4.0 ng/mL. Unfortunately, data from worldwide practice indicate poor sensitivity and specificity of PSA, calling for new evidence supporting the utility of PSA as a screening marker (Andriole et al., 2009; Schröder et al., 2009).

15.1.1 Challenges to Using PSA as Prostate Cancer Screener

Research findings show a large overlap in PSA between men with and without a clinically diagnosed prostate cancer with a large variation coefficient in measured PSA (Habibzadeh, Yadollahie, & Habibzadeh, 2017). To improve the utility of PSA as a screening biomarkers, several PSA derivatives have been proposed for use to aid the screening and early detection of prostate cancer (Gaudreau, Stagg, Soulieres, & Saad, 2016). Typical examples include *PSA velocity* measuring the rate of PSA change over time, *PSA density* assessing the ratio of PSA to prostate volume, age-specific PSA levels and PSA doubling time (Benson, Whang, Olsson, Mcmahon, & Cooner, 1992; Carter et al., 1992; Harris, Dalkin, Martin, Marx, & Ahmann, 1997; Oesterling, Jacobsen, & Cooner, 1995). In addition to PSA, unbounded or free PSA (fPSA), total PSA (tPSA), and % fPSA were proposed and evaluated through randomized trials, with % fPSA showed an improved sensitivity and specificity and being approved by FDA for use (Catalona et al., 1998; Partin et al., 1998). As presented in an updated literature review (Gaudreau et al., 2016), advancements in proteomics and genomics have created lots of opportunities to discover new biomarkers other than SPA with potentials to improve sensitivity and specificity than using PSA alone (Benecchi, 2006; Bjurlin & Loeb, 2013; Carter & Pearson, 1993).

Despite much progress in improving existing PSA-based biomarkers and in discovering new markers, the utility of these markers is often questioned because of unsatisfactory results in practice in assisting screening, diagnosis and treatment (Loughlin, 2014; Partin et al., 1996; Uchio et al., 2016; Vickers, 2013; Vickers & Brewster, 2012). Technically, there is nothing wrong with the selected biomarkers and the evaluation studies to determine the utility of these markers. Randomized controlled design is used for biomarker evaluation, which is termed as gold standard in research and clinical practice. The statistical methods used in analyzing the data, including linear and logistic regression are well-established mathematically and widely used in research. One reason for the controversy about PSA and other biomarkers could be due to the linear dynamic systems we used in our research. Studies to evaluate a biomarker such as PSA naturally assume the kinetics of a biomarker as a linear process (Uchio et al., 2016). When PSA is used as a biomarker, we automatically believe that a men with a higher PSA level is more likely than a man with a lower PSA to have prostate cancer, or if a man experiences an increase in PSA, the likelihood increases for this man to be diagnosed with prostate cancer. However, the relationship between a biomarker (i.e., PSA) and the likelihood to develop prostate cancer could follow a nonlinear and a discrete process with increase and decline in PSA following different paths conditioned on other influential factors as we observed in studying other health and behavioral related issues (Chen & Chen, 2015, 2019; Chen, Lin, Chen, Tang, & Kitzman, 2014).

15.1.2 Age Pattern of PSA Changes

PSA is a small protein named as serine protease, and it is produced by the epithelial cells in the prostate, including normal cells, hyperplastic cells and cancerous cells within the prostatic gland (Nixon, Lilly, Liedtke, & Batjer, 1997). This is one reason why we cannot depend on PSA alone to separate men with and without prostate cancer. PSA level in men's blood increases as age increases (Battikhi & Hussein, 2006; Oesterling et al., 1995; Resim et al., 1999). For example, one study with a large sample (n = 1150) of urologic patients free from prostate cancer and aged 40–79 indicated that the total PSA level (SE) by age groups was 2.4 (0.4) ng/mL for men aged 40–49, 2.7 (0.2) ng/mL for men aged 50–59, 3.6 (0.2) ng/mL for men aged 60–69, and 4.1 (0.23) ng/mL for men aged 70–79 (Battikhi & Hussein, 2006).

Given the age patterns of PSA, researchers proposed age-specific reference ranges for use in practice particularly in the 1990s. For example, a review study by Luboldt, Schindler, and Rubben (2007) suggested using 2.0 ng/mL as cutoff for men age 50 at the first time to recommend for prostate biopsy, 3.0 ng/mL at age 55, and 4.0 ng/mL for any men older than 55. However, as described early in this chapter, adaptations of age-specific references rather than the standard cutoff of 4.0 ng/mL for all have not solved the problem over the utility of PSA in prostate in cancer screening due to unsatisfactory sensitivity-specificity, although with some improvement (Partin et al., 1996). As indicated by Battikhi and Hussein (2006), for urological patients aged 70–79 years old with no prostate cancer, the mean PSA is greater than 4.0 ng/mL, suggesting a large number of non-cancer patients will be misclassified as cancer patients. The large standard error of measured PSA levels across all age ranges suggest that the relationship between PSA and age may follow a nonlinear discrete dynamics rather than a linear continuous dynamics (Chen & Chen, 2015; Guastello & Gregson, 2011).

15.1.3 Relationship Between Testosterone and PSA

Testosterone is a major component of androgens for male reproduction. Total testosterone level declines with age for healthy men. Data from the Massachusetts Male Aging Study indicated that mean (95% CI) ng/ml of total testosterone for heathy men is 538.9 (187.3, 890.4) at age 40–49, 500 (149.9, 847.2) at age 50–59, 501 (178.7, 821.3) at age 60–69, 423.6 (115.3, 734.8) (Mohr, Guay, O'Donnell, & McKinlay, 2005). In addition to declines by age, the testosterone has a very large 95% CI, suggesting large variations in testosterone levels even for men in the same age range. The role of testosterone has long been recognized since the Nobel Prize Award research by Dr. Huggins & Hodges started in 1941 (Huggins & Hodges, 1941), supporting today's androgen deprivation for prostate cancer therapy (Polotti et al., 2017). The effect from androgen reduction in treating prostate cancer makes people to link testosterone levels with PSA, an early biomarker for prostate cancer as previously described in this chapter.

To further understand the role testosterone in prostate cancer for prevention and treatment, several studies report a positive relationship between levels of testosterone and PSA—men with higher testosterone often have higher PSA, although the relationship is not very strong (Elzanaty, Rezanezhad, & Dohle, 2017; Peskoe et al., 2015; Rastrelli et al., 2013). For example, data from the National

Health and Nutrition Examination Survey (NHANCES) indicated that along with increases in total testosterone by quintile from <3.16 ng/mL to ≥6.02 ng/mL, the adjusted PSA level (ng/mL) increased from 0.79 at the first quintile to 1.12 in the third quintile to 1.16 in the last quintile (Peskoe et al., 2015).

In addition to a positive relationship, different results are reported in the literature. For example, in a study by Corona et al. (2010) with a large sample of urologic patients (n = 2291), no significant relationship was found between total testosterone levels and the levels of PSA except a weak positive association for patients younger than 50 years of age. Unfortunately prostate cancer risk is rather low for men younger than 50 years of age. The inconsistent findings from the reported studies and the large variations in testosterone levels among healthy men suggest that the relationship between PSA and testosterone may also follow a nonlinear discrete dynamic process rather than a linear continuous dynamic process. When the relationship between two variables is nonlinear and discrete, findings with weak or inconsistent relationship would be highly likely if such data were analyzed using methods for linear and continuous relationship, such as student t-test, ANVOA and linear regression (Chen & Chen, 2015, 2019).

15.1.4 A Cusp Catastrophe Model of PSA as Function of Age and Testosterone

In the present study, we explored another approach to quantify the relationship of PSA levels with chronological age, and blood testosterone, guided by a nonlinear discrete dynamics. We proposed that changes in circulating PSA level follows a cusp catastrophe process (Thom, 1975). Figure 15.1 depicts the proposed cusp catastrophe model where y-axis indicates PSA level, x1 indicates chronological age, and x2 indicates testosterone level and the curved plane depicts the equilibrium of PSA level in a population. The curved equilibrium plane contains roughly four different regions, including two regions for the stable status of PSA, one region for continuous change in PSA and one region for discrete and sudden change in PSA.

The two stable regions in the figure are marked as *High PSA* and *Low PSA*, within which changes in both age and testosterone results very small changes in PSA. The continuous change region is located backward of the plane, corresponding to the belt area below the label "Equilibrium plane. In this region, testosterone in the blood is low and the relationship between PSA and age following the conventional continuous and linear relationship.

The unstable region is the area located between the two stable regions and marked by the two lines *OQ* (the threshold for sudden jump in PSA level) and *OR* (the threshold line for sudden drop in PSA level). In this region, the relationship between PSA and age becomes more complex with zero- positive and negative associations all likely. Within the cusp region, two men with exact the same age and testosterone level can have very different levels of PSA, one being on the upper part of the curved

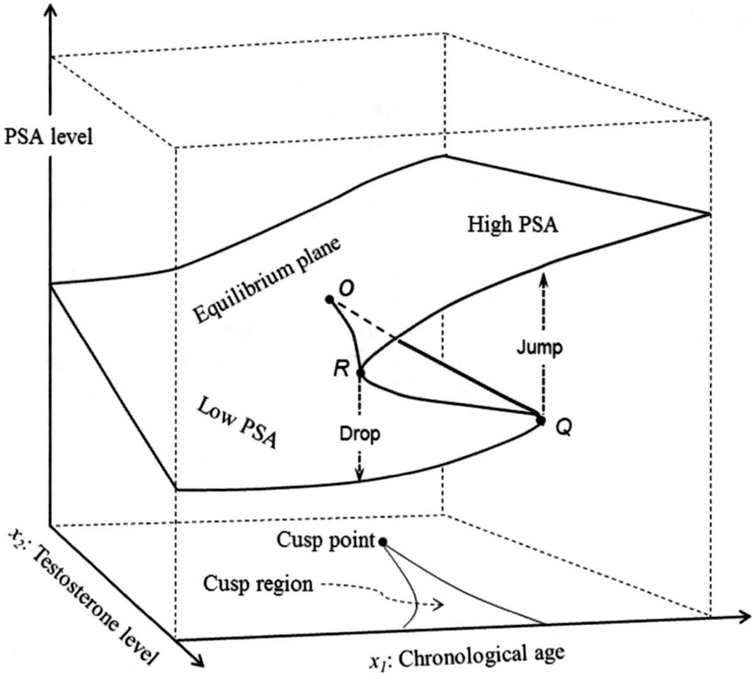

Fig. 15.1 Proposed cusp catastrophe model for PSA dynamics as it relates to chronological age and testosterone levels in men

plane and another being on the lower part of the curved plane. It is this complex relationship of PSA with age and testosterone levels that cannot be captured with the conventional linear modeling methods, such as t-test, ANOVA, and linear and logistic regression.

15.1.5 Purpose of This Study

The purpose of this study is to test the proposed cusp catastrophe model presented in Fig. 15.1 that links PSA with age and testosterone, and to provide new data advancing our understanding of the PSA dynamics and supporting further research for prostate cancer prevention screening and early diagnosis for better treatment outcomes by better using PSA and other data, such as age and testosterone. We will address the research goal using data derived from electronic medical records and new nonlinear discrete paradigms and modeling methodology we established for cusp catastrophe modeling analysis (Chen & Chen, 2015, 2017, 2019).

15.2 Materials

15.2.1 Participants and Data

This study targeted patients with any prostatic disease. We derived data from the Medical Registry Database of a tertiary-level hospital in southeast of the US. The records were linked with medical visits, hospitalizations, drug prescriptions, lab results, and medical diagnoses. Patients from 2001 to 2015 were screened for eligibility. A patient was included as case if he was diagnosed of PCa and had at least one measurement of serum total testosterone prior to the first PCa diagnosis. If a patient was not diagnosed of PCa and had at least one measurement of serum total testosterone prior to the most recent diagnosis of benign prostatic diseases (BPD), he was included as a control. With this criterion, 27 PCa patients and 352 BPD patients were included, yielding a total sample of 379 patients.

15.2.2 Variables and Measurement

Changes in PSA along with age may better be explained with the cusp catastrophe model (Chen & Chen, 2017; Chen et al., 2014). In this model, a man's age is conceptualized as the asymmetry factor, reflecting a fundamental and relatively stable characteristic governing the dynamics of PSA level over time. Changes in circulating testosterone level are conceptualized as the bifurcation factor that has the function to trigger sudden surge or drop in PSA. PSA will increase gradually and continuously, being observed as a linear process, when testosterone level declines normally with age (at the speed below the cusp point). When the age-related decline in blood testosterone accelerates (moving forward) to greater than the cusp point, it will trigger a surge in blood PSA when a man's age passes the threshold line OQ. When the speed of blood testosterone declines from high to low (moving backward), it will trigger sudden drop in blood PSA for all men with their ages below the threshold line OR till the speed of testosterone decline further to below the cusp point.

PSA levels will be stable for men who are outside of the cusp region between the two threshold lines; however, PSA levels may experience sudden increase or decline for men who are within the cusp region. Depending on the direction and age, both sudden increase and sudden declines in blood PSA are likely for men in different age ranges with different speed of testosterone declines. Conventional paradigms and models are effective to characterize only the first part of the PSA dynamics while the cusp catastrophe approach can capture all three characters using one model.

15.3 Statistical Analysis and Cusp Modeling

15.3.1 Statistical Analysis

Descriptive statistics, such as mean and standard deviation (SD), median and inter-quarter range (IQR) were used to describe the study sample. Student t-test and chi-square test were used for simple comparison analysis, and Pearson correlation was used to assess the linear relationship between PSA and other predictors.

15.3.2 Cusp Catastrophe Modeling

A progressive strategy was used to test the proposed cusp catastrophe model of PSA in relation with age and testosterone levels (in Fig. 15.1). We started the analysis with a multiple linear regression modeling analysis in which PSA levels were used as outcome, and age (in years) and testosterone levels (ng/mL) were used as predictors. The linear regression model was used to test the hypothesis that variations in PSA level follow a linear and continuous dynamics.

To prepare for cusp catastrophe modeling, we examined whether PSA levels revealed a bimodality distribution along with the two predictors variables age and testosterone levels. We checked the bimodality using bwplot() function from R. In preparing the violin plot, we categorized both age and testosterone levels into five groups using quintile. The existence of bimodality is a prerequisite for cusp catastrophe modeling (Chen, Wang, & Chen, 2019; Guastello, 1982).

In cusp catastrophe modeling analysis, the blood PSA level (ng/mL) was used as the outcome as in the linear regression model. Age (in year) of the participants was modeled as the asymmetry control variable while testosterone level (ng/mL) was modeled as the bifurcation control variable. We first analyzed the data using the Cobb-Grasman's stochastic density equation cusp catastrophe modeling (SDECusp) (Cobb, 1981, 1998; Grasman, van der Maas, & Wagenmakers, 2009), in which the outcome and the two control variables were modeled as follows:

$$\text{Asymmetry variable}: a = a_0 + a_1\ age \tag{15.1}$$

$$\text{Bifurcation variable}: b = b_0 + b_1\ testosterone \tag{15.2}$$

$$\text{Outcome variable}: y = w_0 + w_1\ PSA \tag{15.3}$$

The analysis was implemented using the published R package "cusp" (Grasman, van der Mass, & Wagenmakers, 2009). The "cusp" package also produces results from alternative linear regression modeling and R^2 based on least square estimates for data-model fitting. This was contrasted with the pseudo-R^2 for cusp catastrophe model estimated using the maximum likelihood method.

Since the Cobb-Grasman's SDECusp implemented using the "cusp" package is degenerative, the estimated parameters can be biased (Grasman et al., 2009; Oliva, Desarbo, Day, & Jedidi, 1987). We thus modeled the same data using the Chen-Chen regression cusp catastrophe model we developed and used in other studies (Chen & Chen, 2017; Chen et al., 2014, 2019). In this modeling approach, the two control variables were modeled as in the Cobb-Grasman's modeling approach (see Eqs. 15.2 and 15.3). However, the outcome variable PSA was modeled as a latent variable:

$$y_i = Y_i + \varepsilon_i, \tag{15.4}$$

where y_i is the PSA measured in the clinic; the true level of PSA Y_i is a latent variable we cannot directly measure or observe; while ε_i represents the errors in measured PSA level. With Eq. 15.4, the procedure to obtain the model parameters is to substitute Y_i to the cusp catastrophe equilibrium equation and let it equal zero:

$$\alpha_i + \beta_i Y_i - Y_i^3 = 0, \tag{15.5}$$

To assess data-model fit, R^2 was also calculated based on the covariance between the observed and model predicted PSA levels. In addition, cusp point was estimated based on the *Cardan discriminant* $\Delta = 27\alpha^2 - 4\beta^3$. With the estimated cusp points, the two threshold lines were estimated and the cusp regions defined by the estimated cusp point and the two threshold lines were presented.

All statistical analyses were conducted using the software R.

15.4 Analytical Findings

15.4.1 Sample Characteristics

Results in Table 15.1 show that among the total sample of 376 patients with complete data, 27 (7.1%) were diagnosed with prostate cancer and the rest with BPD. The subjects were 66.5 (SD = 9.8) years old, 76.0% were white, 2.9% with someone in the family members with prostate cancer. Student t-test indicated extremely significantly higher PSA in subjects with PCa than BPD (4.0 vs. 1.1, $p < .01$).

15.4.2 Results from Linear Correlation Analysis

Results in Table 15.2 show the correlation between PCa and the predictor variables. PCa was positively associated with testosterone ($r = 0.13$, $p < 0.01$) and PSA

Table 15.1 Characteristics of the study sample

Character	PCa	BPD	Total
N (%)	27 (7.1)	351 (92.9)	376 (100)
Age in years			
Median (IQR)	65.0 (60.0, 73.0)	67.0 (60.0, 73.0)	66.5 (60,0, 73.0)
Mean (SD)	66.3 (7.9)	66.1 (10.0)	66.1 (9.8)
Race, n (%)			
White	20 (74.1)	268 (76.1)	228 (76.0)
Black	2 (7.4)	40 (11.4)	42 (11.1)
Other	5 (18.5)	44 (12.5)	49 (12.9)
Family history of PCa			
Yes	1 (3.7)	10 (2.8)	11 (2.9)
No	342 (96.3)	26 (97.2)	368 (97.1)
BMI			
Median (IQR)	25.4 (24.0, 28.7)	27.6 (24.7, 30.9)	27.5 (24.7, 30.8)
Mean (SD)	25.9 (3.3)	28.3 (6.3)	28.2 (6.2)
Testosterone*			
Median (IQR)	362.0 (280.0, 541.0)	316.5 (230.0, 441.0)	318.0 (233.0, 445.0)
Mean (SD)	452.5 (282.6)	351.8 (181..4)	359.0 (191.6)
PSA**			
Median (IQR)	4.0 (2.4, 6.3)	1.1 (0.6, 2.0)	1.2 (0.7, 2.2)
Mean (SD)	4.3 (2.3)	1.6 (1.5)	1.7 (1.2)

Note: *PCa* prostate cancer, *BPD* benign prostate disorder, *BMI* body mass index, *PSA* prostate specific antigen, *IQR* inter-quarter range, *SD* standard deviation. ** P < .01, * P < .05

Table 15.2 Correlations of variables associated with prostate cancer

	Mean (SD)	V1	V2	V3	V4	V5	V6
1. Age in year	66.13 (9.85)						
2. Race	1.37 (0.70)	−0.10					
3. BMI	25.9 (3.3)	−0.22**	−0.06				
4. Family history	0.03 (0.17)	−0.06	−0.00	0.06			
5. Testosterone	358 (192)	0.03	0.04	−0.11	0.08		
6. PSA	1.73 (1.68)	0.14**	−0.02	−0.01	0.08	0.11*	
7. Prostate cancer	0.07 (0.26)	0.01	0.03	−0.08	0.01	0.13**	0.40**

Note: Coding for three categorical variables: Race: 1 = white, 2 = black and 3 = others; family history: 1 = yes, 0 = no; prostate cancer: 1 = yes, 0 = no. ** P < .01, * P < .05

($r = 0.40$, $p < 0.01$). In addition, PSA was positively correlated with age ($r = 0.14$, $p < 0.01$) and testosterone ($r = 0.11$, $p < 0.05$).

15.4.3 Results from Linear Regression Modeling

Results in Table 15.3 indicate that PSA levels were positively associated with age and testosterone whether these two variables were analyzed separately as in Model

Table 15.3 Associations of age and speed of testosterone decline with PSA levels, results from linear regression analysis

Variables	Regression model I Beta (SE)	Regression model II Beta (SE)	Regression model III Beta (SE)
Intercept	0.2554 (0.6290)	−0.0048 (0.8303)	−1.3570 (1.0118)
Age (10 years)	0.2237 (0.0094)*	n/a	0.2156 (0.0093)*
Testosterone level	n/a	0.3053 (0.1441)*	0.2911 (0.1435)*
Data-model fit			
F test (df)	5.70 (1, 357)*	4.48 (1, 357)*	4.94 (2, 356)*
R^2	0.016	0.013	0.027

Note: ** P < .01, * P < .05

I and II, or together as in Model III. According to the results, PSA will increase 0.22 ng/mL with 1 year increase in age; and increase 0.29 ng/mL with addition 1 ng/mL of testosterone.

15.4.4 Bimodality of the PSA Level in Men

Results in Fig. 15.2 suggest the bimodality of blood PSA level along with levels of testosterone (Panel A). At each of the five testosterone levels, participants with different PSA levels tended to clustered in two groups with PSA = 2 as a proximate cutoff. In another word, at the same testosterone level, PSA for a man can be less than 2, not suitable for prostate biopsy or greater than 2, eligible for biopsy.

Likewise, a similar relationship was also revealed between PSA levels and chronological age (Panel B in Fig. 15.2). Across various age ranges, particularly those above median age of 65 (quartile 3), some participants with PSA higher than 2 ng/mL while others with PSA levels lower than 2 ng/mL.

15.4.5 Results from Cobb-Grasman Cusp Modeling

To test the proposed cusp model, we first analyzed our data using the published Cobb-Grasman's stochastic cusp modeling method (Grasman et al., 2009). The main results are summarized in Table 15.4. Results in the table indicate that age was positively associated with PSA (alpha 1 = 0.2068, $p < 0.01$), and this relationship was significantly bifurcated by testosterone level (beta 1 = −0.1293, $p < 0.01$). However, this negative beta 1 coefficient was inconsistent with the results from the correlation and regression analysis reported in Tables 15.2 and 15.3.

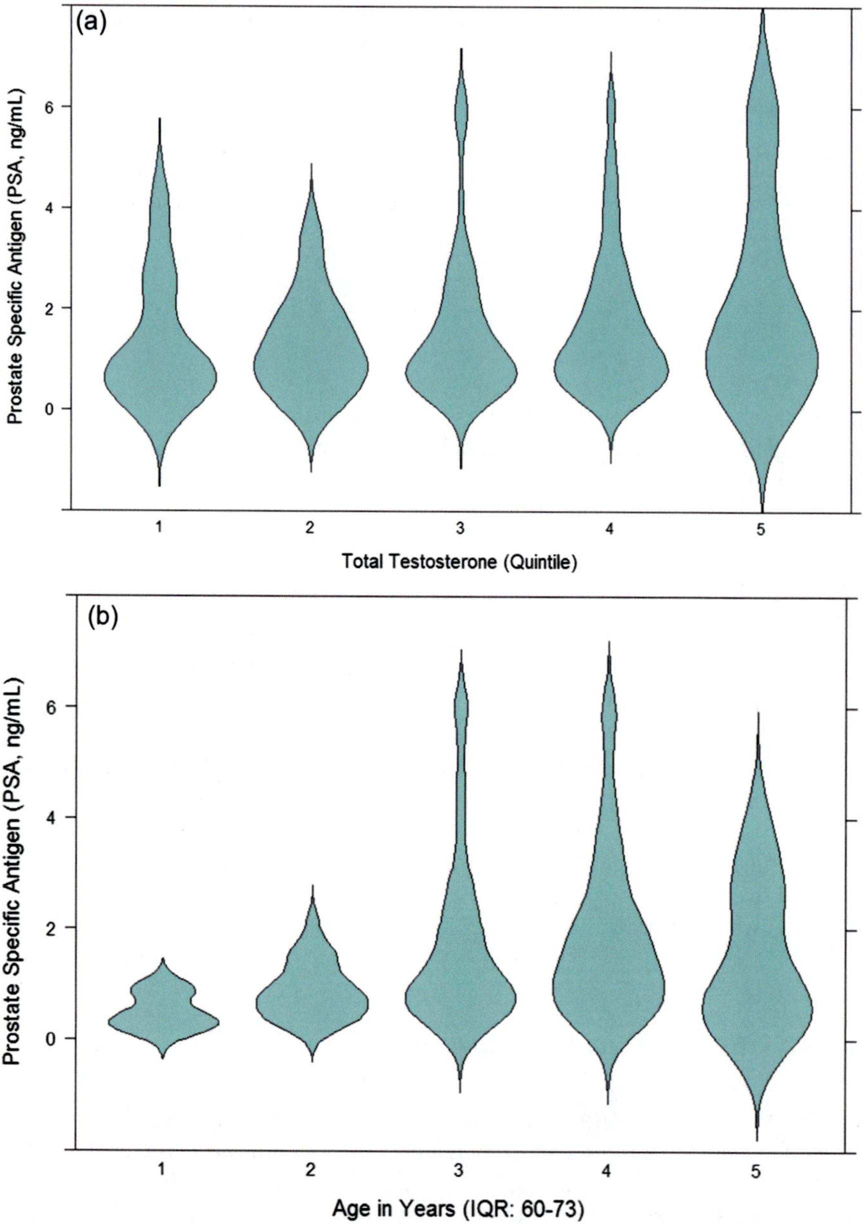

Fig. 15.2 Bimodality of prostate specific antigen (PSA) in relation to testosterone level (Panel **a**) and age (Panel **b**)

Table 15.4 The association of participants' age and testosterone levels with PSA levels: results from Cobb-Grasman SDECusp modeling analysis

Group/variable/parameter	Estimate	SE	Z	p value
Variables centered				
Asymmetry: age in years				
Alpha 0	−1.3287	0.0047	283.86	<0.01
Alpha 1	0.2068	0.0047	44.15	<0.01
Bifurcation: testosterone (ng/dL)				
Beta 0	2.7481	0.0046	597.34	<0.01
Beta 1	−0.1293	0.0046	28.10	<0.01
Outcome: PSA level (ng/mL)				
w0	−1.6595	0.0231	71.74	<0.01
w1	0.6259	0.0222	28.18	<0.01

Note: Non-centered variables produce similar results with the values of the estimated parameters slightly greater than those from the centered variables. $R^2 = 0.027$ from the least square linear regression method and pseudo-$R^2 = 0.32$ from likelihood cusp model, and the difference was statistically highly significant ($p < 0.001$)

Table 15.5 The association of participants' age and testosterone levels with blood PSA levels: results from Chen-Chen RegCusp

Group/variable/parameter	Estimate	SE	Z	p value
Asymmetry: age				
Alpha 0	0.0781	0.0183	4.27	<0.01
Alpha 1	0.1691	0.0179	9.425	<0.01
Bifurcation: T declines				
Beta 0	−1.4390	0.0180	79.88	<0.01
Beta 1	1.0265	0.0181	56.74	<0.01
Cusp point (62 years, testosterone = 630 ng/dL)				

$R^2 = 0.47$, indicating good data-model fit

15.4.6 *Results from Chen-Chen Cusp Regression Modeling*

As the last step, we analyzed the same data using Chen-Chen cusp regression method, the results were presented in Table 15.5. The R^2 was 0.47, suggesting good data-model fit. As shown in in the table, results from Chen-Chen cusp regression modeling first replicated the positively relationship between age and dynamic changes in PSA (alpha 1 = 0.1691, p < .0.1) as well as the effect of testosterone in bifurcating the relationship (beta 1 = 1.0265, p < 0.01) with beta 1 being positive, consistent with the results from correlation and regression analyses.

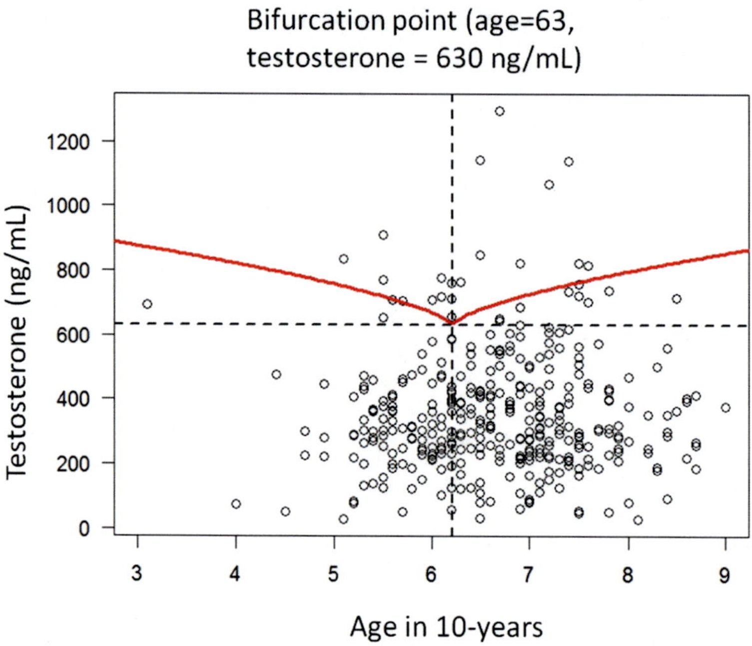

Fig. 15.3 Estimated cusp point, threshold lines and cusp region from Chen-Chen cusp regression modeling analysis

15.4.7 Cusp Point, Threshold Lines and Cusp Region

Based on the parameter estimates in Table 15.5, the estimated cusp point, cusp region and the two threshold lines using the *Cardan discriminant* $\Delta = 27\alpha^2 - 4\beta^3$ are presented in Fig. 15.3. Results in the figure indicate that when testosterone levels by age were below the two threshold lines where $\Delta > 0$, the positive relationship between age and PSA was not bifurcated by testosterone, but continuous. However, when testosterone levels by age were above the two threshold lines where $\Delta < 0$, the relationship between age and PSA was not continuous but bifurcated—at the same age, PSA levels were higher for subjects with higher levels of testosterone and lower for subjects with lower testosterone. This non-continuous region defined by the two threshold lines consists of the cusp region and the cusp point (age = 63 years and testosterone = 630 ng/dL) was the starting point of the cusp region.

15.5 Discussion and Conclusions

To date, few reported studies in the medical and health issues have considered the nonlinear discrete dynamics as guidance to examine the complex relationship among various variables in predicting a health outcome or in developing screening tools using biomarkers, leaving a lot of unsolved questions in medicine and public health. To our knowledge, we are the first to use a nonlinear discrete modeling approach to examine the PSA dynamics as it related to age and testosterone levels. Data for this study were derived from the electronic medical records from academic hospital and managed through the Clinical and Translational Science Institute. Modeling analysis was conducted using the newly established Chen-Chen cusp regression method (Chen & Chen, 2017) with a lot of advantages over the published methods as showing in this and other published studies (Chen & Chen, 2017).

15.5.1 PSA Dynamics Is Nonlinear and Discrete

First and the most important findings of this study is the demonstration of the nonlinear dynamics of PSA in men. Relative to correlation and linear regression that are guided by the linear continuous dynamics approach, the cusp catastrophe modeling guided by the nonlinear discrete dynamics approach performed much better in characterizing the dynamic changes in PSA over age and by testosterone levels. Findings of this study indicate that PSA distribution is not Gaussian but with obvious bimodality, which is consistent with the large variations in measured PSA levels (Adegun, Adebayo, & Atiba, 2015; Arneth, 2009). In addition to the bimodality, the data-model fit is much better for the cusp catastrophe modeling than for the linear regression modeling. With the analysis of the same data, $R^2 = 0.32$ for the Cobb-Grasman cusp modeling, $R^2 = 0.47$ for the Chen-Chen regression cusp modeling, and $R^2 = 0.027$ for the linear regression.

The demonstration of PSA dynamics as a nonlinear discrete process is of great significance to re-consider all published studies in prostate cancer research and practice with a focus on PSA. Findings of this study, including the estimated cusp point indicate that distribution of PSA by age consists of two components, one being continuous for men with testosterone levels lower than 630 ng/dL and other being discrete for men with testosterone greater than 630 ng/dL. We need to consider this evidence in assessing the utility of PSA in preventive screening, screening for prostate biopsy and treatment. Using age-specific reference range of PSA provides an alternative to improve the sensitivity and specificity (Battikhi & Hussein, 2006; Luboldt et al., 2007; Partin et al., 1996); such approach can further be improved by using nonlinear discrete dynamics approach. In addition to PSA, many derived biomarkers such as PSA velocity, PSA density, $\% f$PSA as well as new biomarkers based on genomics and proteomics for prostate cancer. According to our previous research (Chen & Chen, 2015; Chen et al., 2014) and findings of this study, these markers may also follow a nonlinear discrete dynamics (Gaudreau et al., 2016), thus their utility in cancer screening must be reevaluated using nonlinear discrete systems modeling approach.

15.5.2 Co-use of Testosterone and PSA for Screening

Guided by the nonlinear discrete dynamics, findings of this study, particularly the results from Chen-Chen cusp regression modeling approach have demonstrated a consistent and positively relationship of PSA with both age and testosterone levels. This is particularly true for the estimated cusp point, threshold lines and cusp region. First of all, testosterone = 630 ng/dL at the cusp point is reasonable since this level is close to the upper limit of the normal ranges (280, 800 ng/dL) as recommended by the American Association of Clinical Endocrinologists (Petak et al., 2002). Based on the findings on cusp point and threshold lines, sudden increases in PSA is likely for all men aged 63 years or older with testosterone level of 630 ng/dL or higher. The threshold is not fixed but changes with age and testosterone levels. Beyond age 63, either younger or older, testosterone higher than 630 ng/dL will enhance the likelihood for sudden PSA increase. Although the relatively small sample of this study prevented us from further analysis to establish criteria for prostate cancer screening, findings of this study provide useful data for future research with large and representative samples and longitudinal data.

It is worth noting that findings from cusp catastrophe modeling in this study although appearing to be an interaction between age and testosterone in predicting PSA, but it is not. Although findings of this study indicate that the relationship between age and PSA varied by testosterone level, such relationship is assumed to be linear in the conventional statistical and epidemiological analysis. However, as we can see from the estimated threshold lines, the "interaction" is much more complex – it occurred at the cusp point, which is theory-based, therefor can be determined and meaningful; while in the conventional interaction analysis, the cross-point is not theory-based, therefore totally driving by data, and only used to assess the type of interactions (VanderWeele, 2009).

15.5.3 Limitations and Future Research

There are limitations to this study. First, data used for this study were derived from patients attending one hospital in north central Florida, thus the generalizability of the findings from this study needs to be assessed with data from different hospitals located in other areas/places within and outside of the United States. Second, the sample size is relatively small, particularly the number of subjects with prostate cancer (only 27). This prevents us from investigating the relationship between PSA, testosterone level and prostate cancer. In addition, using prostate cancer as outcome requires new methods capable of handling binary variable, which has not been established at the time when this study was conducted. We will further our analysis with focus on prostate cancer using the newly established logisticCusp modeling method introduced in Chap. 16 in this book.

Despite the limitations, this study is the first to model PSA with cusp catastrophe modeling method guided by the nonlinear dynamic systems approach. It is our anticipation that the adaptation of this new approach may generate revolutionary advancement in medical and health research and practice in the era of global health.

References

Adegun, P. T., Adebayo, P. B., & Atiba, S. A. (2015). The likelihood of having serum level of PSA of >= 4.0 ng/mL and >= 10.0 ng/mL in non-obese and obese Nigerian men with LUTS. *Asian Journal of Urology, 2*(3), 158–162. https://doi.org/10.1016/j.ajur.2015.06.004

Andriole, G. L., Crawford, E. D., Grubb, R. L., Buys, S. S., Chia, D., Church, T. R., ... Berg, C. D. (2009). Mortality results from a randomized prostate-Cancer screening trial. *New England Journal of Medicine, 360*(13), 1310–1319. https://doi.org/10.1056/NEJMoa0810696

Arneth, B. M. (2009). Clinical significance of measuring prostate-specific antigen. *Labmedicine, 40*(8), 487–491. https://doi.org/10.1309/Lmeggglz2edwrxuk

Battikhi, M. N. G., & Hussein, I. (2006). Age-specific reference ranges for prostate specific antigen-total and free in patients with prostatitis symptoms and patients at risk. *International Urology and Nephrology, 38*(3–4), 559–564. https://doi.org/10.1007/s11255-006-0073-7

Benecchi, L. (2006). PSA velocity and PSA slope. *Prostate Cancer and Prostatic Diseases, 9*(2), 169–172.

Benson, M. C., Whang, I. S., Olsson, C. A., Mcmahon, D. J., & Cooner, W. H. (1992). The use of prostate specific antigen density to enhance the predictive value of intermediate levels of serum prostate specific antigen. *Journal of Urology, 147*(3), 817–821. https://doi.org/10.1016/S0022-5347(17)37394-9

Bjurlin, M. A., & Loeb, S. (2013). PSA velocity in risk stratification of prostate cancer. *Revista de Urología, 15*(4), 204–206.

Borghesi, M., Ahmed, H., Nam, R., Schaeffer, E., Schiavina, R., Taneja, S., ... Loeb, S. (2017). Complications after systematic, random, and image-guided prostate biopsy. *European Urology, 71*(3), 353–365. https://doi.org/10.1016/j.eururo.2016.08.004

Bray, F., Ferlay, J., Soerjomataram, I., Siegel, R. L., Torre, L. A., & Jemal, A. (2018). Global cancer statistics 2018: GLOBOCAN estimates of incidence and mortality worldwide for 36 cancers in 185 countries. *CA: A Cancer Journal for Clinicians, 68*(6), 394–424. https://doi.org/10.3322/caac.21492

Carter, H. B., & Pearson, J. D. (1993). PSA velocity for the diagnosis of early prostate cancer. A new concept. *The Urologic clinics of North America, 20*(4), 665–670.

Carter, H. B., Pearson, J. D., Metter, E. J., Brant, L. J., Chan, D. W., Andres, R., ... Walsh, P. C. (1992). Longitudinal evaluation of prostate-specific antigen levels in men with and without prostate disease. *JAMA, 267*(16), 2215–2220.

Catalona, W. J., Partin, A. W., Slawin, K. M., Brawer, M. K., Flanigan, R. C., Patel, A., ... Southwick, P. C. (1998). Use of the percentage of free prostate-specific antigen to enhance differentiation of prostate cancer from benign prostatic disease—A prospective multicenter clinical trial. *JAMA-Journal of the American Medical Association, 279*(19), 1542–1547. https://doi.org/10.1001/jama.279.19.1542

Chen, X., & Chen, D. (2015). Cusp catastrophe modeling in medical and health research. In D.-G. Chen & J. Wilson (Eds.), *Innovative statistical methods for public health data*. Cham, Switzerland: Springer.

Chen, D., & Chen, X. (2017). Cusp catastrophe regression and its application in public health and behavioral research. *International Journal of Environmental Research and Public Health, 14*(10), 1220. https://doi.org/10.3390/ijerph14101220

Chen, X., & Chen, D. (2019). Cognitive theories, paradigm of quantum behavior change, and Cusp catastrophe modeling in social behavioral research. *Journal of the Society for Social Work and Research, 10*(1), 127–159. https://doi.org/10.1086/701837

Chen, D., Lin, F., Chen, X., Tang, W., & Kitzman, H. (2014). Cusp catastrophe model: A nonlinear model for health outcomes in nursing research. *Nursing Research, 63*(3), 211–220. https://doi.org/10.1097/NNR.0000000000000034

Chen, X., Wang, Y., & Chen, D. (2019). Nonlinear dynamics of binge drinking among U.S. high school students in grade 12: Cusp catastrophe modeling of national survey data. *Nonlinear Dynamics, Psychology, and Life Sciences, 23*(4), 465–490. (Revised submission).

Cobb, L. (1981). Parameter-estimation for the cusp catastrophe model. *Behavioral Science, 26*(1), 75–78. https://doi.org/10.1002/bs.3830260107

Cobb, L. (1998). *An introduction to cusp surface analysis.* Technical report. Louisville: Kentucky Aetheling Consultants.

Corona, G., Boddi, V., Lotti, F., Gacci, M., Carini, M., De Vita, G., & Maggi, M. (2010). The relationship of testosterone to prostate-specific antigen in men with sexual dysfunction. *Journal of Sexual Medicine* 7(1): 284–292. https://doi.org/10.1111/j.1743-6109.2009.01549.x.

Elzanaty, S., Rezanezhad, B., & Dohle, G. (2017). Association between serum testosterone and PSA levels in middle-aged healthy men from the general population. *Current Urology, 10*(1), 40–44. https://doi.org/10.1159/000447149

Gaudreau, P. O., Stagg, J., Soulieres, D., & Saad, F. (2016). The present and future of biomarkers in prostate cancer: Proteomics, genomics, and immunology advancements. *Biomarkers in Cancer, 8*(Suppl 2), 15–33. https://doi.org/10.4137/BIC.S31802

Grasman, R. P., van der Maas, H. L., & Wagenmakers, E. J. (2009). Fitting the cusp catastrophe in R: A cusp package primer. *Journal of Statistical Software, 32*(8), 1–27.

Guastello, S. J. (1982). Moderator regression and the cusp catastrophe: Application of two-stage personnel selection, training, therapy, and policy evaluation. *Behavioral Science, 27*(3), 259–272.

Guastello, S. J., & Gregson, A. M. (2011). *Nonlinear dynamical systems analysis for the behavioral sciences using real data.* Boca Raton: CRC Press/Taylor & Francis Group.

Habibzadeh, P., Yadollahie, M., & Habibzadeh, F. (2017). What is a "diagnostic test reference range" good for? *European Urology, 72*(5), 859–860. https://doi.org/10.1016/j.eururo.2017.05.024

Harris, C. H., Dalkin, B. L., Martin, E., Marx, P. C., & Ahmann, F. R. (1997). Prospective longitudinal evaluation of men with initial prostate specific antigen levels of 4.0 ng./ml. or less. *The Journal of Urology, 157*(5), 1740–1743.

Huggins, C., & Hodges, C. V. (1941). Studies on prostatic cancer. I. The effect of castration, of estrogen and androgen injection on serum phosphatases in metastatic carcinoma of the prostate. *Cancer Research, 1*(4), 293–297.

Khazaei, S., Rezaeian, S., Ayubi, E., Gholamaliee, B., Pishkuhi, M. A., Khazaei, S., … Hanis, S. M. (2016). Global prostate cancer incidence and mortality rates according to the human development index. *Asian Pacific Journal of Cancer Prevention, 17*(8), 3793–3796.

Loeb, S., Carter, H. B., Berndt, S. I., Ricker, W., & Schaeffer, E. M. (2011). Complications after prostate biopsy: Data from SEER-Medicare. *The Journal of Urology, 186*(5), 1830–1834. https://doi.org/10.1016/j.juro.2011.06.057

Loeb, S., van den Heuvel, S., Zhu, X., Bangma, C. H., Schroder, F. H., & Roobol, M. J. (2012). Infectious complications and hospital admissions after prostate biopsy in a European randomized trial. *European Urology, 61*(6), 1110–1114. https://doi.org/10.1016/j.eururo.2011.12.058

Loughlin, K. R. (2014). PSA velocity: A systematic review of clinical applications. *Urologic Oncology, 32*(8), 1116–1125.

Luboldt, H., Schindler, J. F., & Rubben, H. (2007). Age-specific reference ranges for prostate-specific antigen as a marker for prostate cancer. *EAU-EBU Update Series, 5*, 38–48.

Mohr, B. A., Guay, A. T., O'Donnell, A. B., & McKinlay, J. B. (2005). Normal, bound and nonbound testosterone levels in normally ageing men: Results from the Massachusetts

Male Ageing Study. *Clinical Endocrinology, 62*(1), 64–73. https://doi.org/10.1111/j.1365-2265.2004.02174.x

Mottet, N., Bellmunt, J., Bolla, M., Briers, E., Cumberbatch, M. G., De Santis, M., ... Cornford, P. (2017). EAU-ESTRO-SIOG guidelines on prostate cancer. Part 1: Screening, diagnosis, and local treatment with curative intent. *European Urology, 71*(4), 618–629. https://doi.org/10.1016/j.eururo.2016.08.003

Nixon, R. G., Lilly, J. D., Liedtke, R. J., & Batjer, J. D. (1997). Variation of free and total prostate-specific antigen levels: The effect on the percent free/total prostate-specific antigen. *Archives of Pathology & Laboratory Medicine, 121*(4), 385–391.

Oesterling, J. E., Jacobsen, S. J., & Cooner, W. H. (1995). The use of age-specific reference ranges for serum prostate-specific antigen in men 60 years old or older. *Journal of Urology, 153*(4), 1160–1163. https://doi.org/10.1016/S0022-5347(01)67538-4

Oliva, T. A., Desarbo, W. S., Day, D. L., & Jedidi, K. (1987). GEMCAT: A general multivariate methodology for estimate catastrophe models. *Behaivoral Sciences, 32*, 121–137.

Partin, A. W., Brawer, M. K., Subong, E. N. P., Kelley, C. A., Cox, J. L., Bruzek, D. J., ... Chan, D. W. (1998). Prospective evaluation of percent free-PSA and complexed-PSA for early detection of prostate cancer. *Prostate Cancer and Prostatic Diseases, 1*(4), 197–203. https://doi.org/10.1038/sj.pcan.4500232

Partin, A. W., Criley, S. R., Subong, E. N. P., Zincke, H., Walsh, P. C., & Oesterling, J. E. (1996). Standard versus age-specific prostate specific antigen reference ranges among men with clinically localized prostate cancer: A pathological analysis. *Journal of Urology, 155*(4), 1336–1339. https://doi.org/10.1016/S0022-5347(01)66260-8

Peskoe, S. B., Joshu, C. E., Rohrmann, S., McGlynn, K. A., Nyante, S. J., Bradwin, G., ... Platz, E. A. (2015). Circulating total testosterone and PSA concentrations in a nationally representative sample of men without a diagnosis of prostate cancer. *Prostate, 75*(11), 1167–1176. https://doi.org/10.1002/pros.22998

Petak, S. M., Nankin, H. R., Spark, R. F., Swerdloff, R. S., Rodriguez-Rigau, L. J., & American Association of Clinical, Endocrinologists. (2002). American Association of Clinical Endocrinologists Medical Guidelines for clinical practice for the evaluation and treatment of hypogonadism in adult male patients—2002 update. *Endocrine Practice, 8*(6), 440–456.

Polotti, C. F., Kim, C. J., Chuchvara, N., Polotti, A. B., Singer, E. A., & Elsamra, S. (2017). Androgen deprivation therapy for the treatment of prostate cancer: A focus on pharmacokinetics. *Expert Opinion on Drug Metabolism & Toxicology, 13*(12), 1265–1273. https://doi.org/10.1080/17425255.2017.1405934

Rastrelli, G., Corona, G., Vignozzi, L., Maseroli, E., Silverii, A., Monami, M., ... Maggi, M. (2013). Serum PSA as a predictor of testosterone deficiency. *Journal of Sexual Medicine, 10*(10), 2518–2528. https://doi.org/10.1111/jsm.12266

Resim, S., Cek, M., Gurbuz, Z. G., Fazlioglu, A., Caskurlu, T., Uras, A. R., & Sevin, G. (1999). Serum PSA and age-specific reference ranges in patients with prostatism symptoms. *International Urology and Nephrology, 31*(2), 221–228.

Schröder, F. H., Hugosson, J., Roobol, M. J., Tammela, T. L. J., Ciatto, S., Nelen, V., ... Auvinen, A. (2009). Screening and prostate-cancer mortality in a randomized European study. *New England Journal of Medicine, 360*(13), 1320–1328. https://doi.org/10.1056/NEJMoa0810084

Thom, R. (1975). *Structural stability and morphogenesis*. New York, NY: Benjamin-Addison-Wesley.

Uchio, E., Aslan, M., Ko, J., Wells, C. K., Radhakrishnan, K., & Concato, J. (2016). Velocity and doubling time of prostate-specific antigen: Mathematics can matter. *Journal of Investigative Medicine, 64*(2), 400–404.

VanderWeele, T. J. (2009). Sufficient cause interactions and statistical interactions. *Epidemiology, 20*(1), 6–13. https://doi.org/10.1097/EDE.0b013e31818f69e7

Vickers, A. J. (2013). Counterpoint: Prostate-specific antigen velocity is not of value for early detection of cancer. *Journal of the National Comprehensive Cancer Network, 11*(3), 286–290.

Vickers, A. J., & Brewster, S. F. (2012). PSA velocity and doubling time in diagnosis and prognosis of prostate cancer. *British Journal of Medical and Surgical Urology, 5*(4), 162–168.

Chapter 16
Logistic Cusp Catastrophe Regression for Binary Outcome: Method Development and Empirical Testing

(Din) Ding-Geng Chen and Xinguang Chen

Abstract Cusp catastrophe models are unique to advance life sciences, psychology and behavioral studies. Extensive progresses have been made to utilize this modeling technique for continuous outcome and there is no development for binary data. To fill this gap, this chapter is then aimed to develop a cusp catastrophe modelling method for binary outcome. Building upon our previous research on the nonlinear regression cusp (RegCusp) catastrophe model for continuous outcome, we propose a logistic cusp catastrophe regression (LogisticCusp). LogisticCusp is based on the principles of logistic regression for binary outcome variable y (yes/no) being expressed as a latent binary variable Y through a logit link. This latent regression provides a mathematical connection between an observed outcome variable as a binomially distributed random variable and the deterministic cusp catastrophe at its equilibrium. By connecting the two, Y in the LogisticCusp is considered as one of the true roots of the deterministic cusp catastrophe model determined using the Maxwell or Delay conventions. We validate the method using a 5-step Monte-Carlo simulation with two predictors and three parameters for both bifurcation and asymmetry control variables. We further tested the method with binge drinking behavior in youth with data from the Monitoring the Future Study. Results from 5000 Monte-Carlo simulations indicate that the parameter estimates obtained through LogisticCusp are unbiased and efficient using maximum likelihood estimation with quasi-Newton numerical search algorithm. Results from empirical testing with real data are consistent with those estimated using other methods. LogisticCusp adds a new tool for researchers to examine many issues in

(Din) D.-G. Chen (✉)
School of Social Work, University of North Carolina, Chapel Hill, NC, USA
e-mail: dinchen@email.unc.edu

X. Chen
Department of Epidemiology, College of Public Health and Health Professions, College of Medicine, University of Florida, Gainesville, FL, USA

Global Health Institute, Wuhan University, Wuhan, China
e-mail: jimax.chen@ufl.edu

X. Chen, (Din) D.-G. Chen (eds.), *Statistical Methods for Global Health and Epidemiology*, ICSA Book Series in Statistics,
https://doi.org/10.1007/978-3-030-35260-8_16

psychology, life sciences, and behavioral studies, particularly, issues in medicine and public health with the powerful cusp catastrophe modeling for binary outcome.

Keywords Cusp catastrophe model · Logistic cusp catastrophe regression · Bifurcation · Asymmetry · Binary outcome

16.1 Background

Up to date, the statistical models commonly used to examine medical, health, psychological, and socio-behavioral outcomes depends on the linear regression and continuous change approach (Chen & Chen, 2015, 2019; Chen, Stanton, Chen, & Li, 2013). However, in the real world, these outcomes are rarely linear and continuous because of the nature of the medical, health, and behavioral outcomes and the multiple, complex influences of environmental, behavioral, psychological, and biological factors (Chen, Lin, Chen, Tang, & Kitzman, 2014; Chen et al., 2010; Witkiewitz, van der Maas, Hufford, & Marlatt, 2007; Xu & Chen, 2016). What might appear to be small and inconsequential changes in one of these factors can lead to abrupt and sudden changes in an outcome (Thom, 1975). Under these conditions, a linear and continuous approach seriously limits the predictability of the influence of hypothesized factors on a particular outcome variable (Chen & Chen, 2015, 2019; Chen, Wang, & Chen, 2019) and therefore a new paradigm to incorporate nonlinear and discrete behaviors is needed to fill this knowledge gap.

16.1.1 Cusp Catastrophe for Nonlinear Discrete Systems

To account for nonlinearity and discrete characteristics in low-dimensional scenarios, researchers often turn to natural extensions of a linear regression model, including the kernel regression or regression/smoothing splines (Berk, 2008; Faraway, 2009; Guastello & Gregson, 2011). In addition to these nonparametric methods, other techniques for use with high-dimensional data include additive models, multivariate adaptive regression splines, random forests, neural networks, and support vector machine. These techniques have been discussed extensively elsewhere (Chen & Chen, 2017; Faraway, 2009). Despite much strength, these nonparametric methods do not have a mechanism to identify and incorporate a medical, health and behavior outcomes with sudden and discrete changes and multi-modes. Cusp catastrophe model is one that is capable to quantify such a mechanism.

As a complement to many traditional analytical approaches, the cusp catastrophe model offers distinct advantages given its capacity to not only simultaneously handle complex linear and nonlinear relationships in a high-order probability density function but also to incorporate sudden jumps in outcome measures, as outlined in Zeeman (Zeeman, 1977) and Gilmore (Gilmore, 1981). Catastrophe theory was proposed in the 1970s (Thom, 1975) to understand a complicated set of behaviors that included gradual, continuous changes as well as sudden and discrete or catastrophic changes in general. The cusp catastrophe model has been used extensively in a wide range of research fields, including the modeling of tobacco use (Xu & Chen, 2016), adolescent alcohol use (Clair, 1998), changes in adolescent substance use (Mazanov & Byrne, 2006), binge drinking among high school and college students (Chen et al., 2019; Guastello, Aruka, Doyle, & Smerz, 2008) adult population (White, Tapert, & Shukla, 2017) and problem drinking among persons living with HIV (Witkiewitz et al., 2007), sexual initiation and condom use among young adolescents (Chen et al., 2010, 2013), nursing turnover (Wagner, 2010), HIV prevention (Xu, Chen, Yu, Joseph, & Stanton, 2017), therapy and program evaluation (Guastello, 1982), health outcomes (Chen et al., 2014), and accident process (Guastello, 1989; Guastello & Lynn, 2014).

16.1.2 Established Methods for Cusp Catastrophe Modeling

Historically, three main implementation approaches have been established for data analysis to conduct cusp catastrophe modeling.

The first method test the outcome variable if it follows cusp catastrophe by inserting regression coefficients into the deterministic cusp model and the method was operationalized by Guastello using a *polynomial regression approach* (Guastello, 1982; Guastello et al., 2008). This method is straight forward to understand and the analysis can be completed using any software packages with regression analysis functionality (Guastello & Gregson, 2011).

The second method uses a *stochastic differential equation* from Cobb and his colleagues (Cobb, 1981; Cobb & Zacks, 1985; Grasman, van der Maas, & Wagenmakers, 2009) with likelihood estimation implemented in an R package "cusp". Since the method was established by Cobb and implemented through Grasman's work, this approach has been named as Cobb-Grasman cusp modeling (Chen et al., 2019).

The third method takes a different approach to solve the deterministic cusp catastrophe model with a statistical approach. Different from the Cobb-Grasman's approach described above, in this method, the deterministic cusp catastrophe is directly casted into the classical multiple regression with the outcome variable being measured with a latent variable and the two control variables each being measured as linear combination. In this modeling approach, method for estimation of the cusp region is also provided (Chen & Chen, 2017). This Chen-Chen method has been used in modeling harm perception and social influence on binge drinking among high school students in the United States (Chen et al., 2019). In Chap. 15 of this book, this method was used to model prostate-specific antigen (PSA), a biomarker of prostate cancer in men.

16.1.3 Need for Methods to Model Binary Data

All the methods described above for cusp catastrophe modeling are for continuous outcome variables, and no one method is available for other types of outcomes, to the best of our knowledge. To fill this methodology gap, in this chapter we attempted a method to analyze binary outcome with cusp catastrophe model. In our previous research, we developed a regression-based approach to solve for cusp catastrophe model for continuous outcomes (Chen & Chen, 2017) and used it in analyzing binge drinking among youth (Chen et al., 2019). We used the same regression-based approach in this new method with the continuous outcome being replaced by binary outcome for cusp catastrophe modeling of binary data in the framework of statistical logistic regression.

16.2 An Overview of the Cusp Catastrophe Model

Catastrophe theory was proposed in the 1970s by Thom (1975) and popularized over the next two decades by several leading researchers (Cobb, 1981; Cobb & Ragade, 1978; Cobb & Watson, 1980; Cobb & Zacks, 1985; Gilmore, 1981; Thom & Fowler, 1975; Zeeman, 1977). Thom (1975) originally proposed the catastrophe theory to understand complicated phenomena that included both gradual, continuous change and sudden, discontinuous or catastrophic change.

16.2.1 Deterministic Cusp Model

To apply this model in research, the deterministic cusp catastrophe model can be specified with three components: two control factors (i.e., α and β) and one outcome variable (i.e., y). This model is defined by a dynamic system:

$$\frac{dy}{dt} = -\frac{dV\,(y; \alpha, \beta)}{dy} \tag{16.1}$$

where V, commonly called the potential function, is defined as

$$V\,(y; \alpha, \beta) = -\alpha y - \frac{1}{2}\beta y^2 + \frac{1}{4}y^4 \tag{16.2}$$

In this potential function V, α is the asymmetry or normal control factor, and β is the bifurcation or splitting control factor. Both α and β are linked to determine the outcome variable y in a three-dimensional response surface. When the right side of Eq. (16.1) moves toward zero, change in the outcome y also tends toward zero with change in time; this status is called equilibrium. In general, the behavior of the outcome y (i.e., how y changes with time t) is complicated, but all subjects tend to move toward equilibrium the surface.

16.2.2 *Characteristics of the Cusp Catastrophe Model*

Figure 16.1 graphically depicts the equilibrium surface that reflects the response plan of the outcome measure (y) at various combinations of the asymmetry control factor (the measure of α in Fig. 16.1) and the bifurcation control factor (the measure of β in Fig. 16.1).

As shown in Fig. 16.1, dynamic changes in y have two stable regions (attractors), which are the lower area in the front left (lower stable region) and the upper area in the front right (upper stable region). Beyond these stable regions, y becomes sensitive to changes in α and β. The unstable region can be projected to the control plane (α, β) as the *cusp region*. The cusp region is characterized by line OQ (the ascending threshold) and line OR (the descending threshold) of the equilibrium

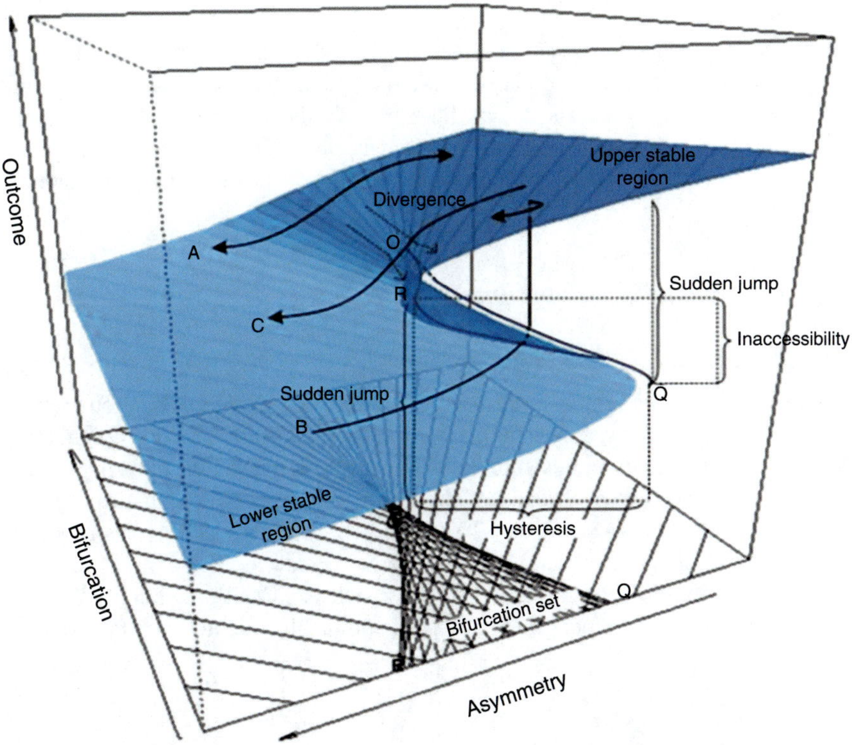

Fig. 16.1 Cusp catastrophe model for outcome (y) in the equilibrium plane with an asymmetry control variable (the measure of α) and a bifurcation control variable (the measure of β)

surface. In this region, y becomes highly unstable with regard to changes in α and β, jumping between the two stable regions when (α, β) approaches the two threshold lines OQ and OR. In Fig. 16.1, paths A, B, and C depict three typical but distinct pathways of change in the health outcome measure (y). Path A shows that in situations where $y < O$, a smooth relation exists between y and α. Path B shows that in situations when $y > O$, if α increases to reach and pass the ascending threshold link OQ, y will suddenly jump from the low stable region to the upper stable region of the equilibrium plane. Path C shows that a sudden drop occurs in y as α declines to reach and pass the descending threshold line OR.

The cusp catastrophe model can be used as both a qualitative and a quantitative analytical method in research to investigate the relationship between predictors and outcome variables (e.g., behaviors or health outcomes). The qualitative approach focuses on identifying the five catastrophe elements (i.e., catastrophe flags) outlined by Gilmore (1981), whereas the quantitative approach uses numerical data to statistically fit the model.

16.3 Implementation of a Cusp Catastrophe Model

As described in the Introduction, since the introduction of the cusp catastrophe model, three quantitative approaches have been developed and used to implement the model for data analysis: Guastello's polynomial regression, Cobb-Grasman stochastic differential equation implemented in an R package "cusp", and Chen-Chen approach to cast the cusp catastrophe model into the nonlinear regression.

16.3.1 Guastello's Polynomial Approach

Specifically, as the first implementation, Guastello's approach is derived by reformulating the cusp dynamic system in Eq. (16.1) in the differential equation form into a difference equation system as outlined in Guastello (1982), Guastello et al., 2008). Since its first publication, this approach has been widely used in analyzing research data because this approach can be implemented in common statistical software packages, including SAS, SPSS, STATA, and R. This approach makes it possible the first time for many researchers to modeling social and behavioral issues with cusp catastrophe modeling. Guastello's approach is suitable for longitudinal data with outcome variables measured at two time points that are not vary far from each other.

16.3.2 Cobb-Grasman's Approach

As the second approach in implementing the cusp catastrophe model is Cobb-Grasman's stochastic differential equation method (named thereafter as "SDE-Cusp"). In this SDECusp approach, the deterministic cusp model in Eq. (16.1) is first extended with a probabilistic/stochastic Wiener process. With this extension, the modeling process incorporates measurement errors in the outcome variable. Using this approach, the response surface of cusp catastrophe is modeled as a probability density function where the bimodal nature of the outcome corresponds to the two states of outcome variable. Mathematically, Cobb and his colleagues (Cobb & Ragade, 1978; Cobb & Watson, 1980; Cobb & Zacks, 1985; Hartelman, van der Maas, & Molenaar, 1998; Honerkamp, 1994) cast the deterministic cusp model in Eq. (16.1) into a stochastic differential equation (SDE) as follows:

$$dz = \frac{\partial V(z, \alpha, \beta)}{\partial z} dt + dW(t) \tag{16.3}$$

where $dW(t)$ is a white noise Wiener process with variance σ^2.

This extension is in fact a special case of general stochastic dynamical systems modeling with a constant diffusion function defined by $dW(t)$. Since the model Eq. (16.2) cannot be solved analytically, computational implementation of this stochastic model is limited. However, at the equilibrium state when time (t) approaches the infinity, it is easier to estimate the probability density function of the corresponding limiting stationary stochastic processes. In other words, the probability density function of the outcome measure (y) can be expressed as follows:

$$f(y) = \frac{\Psi}{\sigma^2} \exp\left[\frac{\alpha(y-\lambda) + \frac{1}{2}\beta(y-\lambda)^2 - \frac{1}{4}(y-\lambda)^4}{\sigma^2}\right] \tag{16.4}$$

where the parameter ψ is a normalizing constant and λ is used to determine the origin of y.

With this probability density function, the regression predictors α and β can be incorporated as linear combinations to replace the canonical asymmetry factor (i.e., α) and bifurcation factor (i.e., β). Note that as a distribution for a limiting stationary stochastic process, this probability density function in Eq. (16.3) is independent from time t, thus it can be used to model cross-sectional relationship with the advantage to detect and quantify its potential cusp nature comprising both sudden and continuous states. Moreover, the probability density function allows the well-known statistical theory of maximum likelihood to be used for model parameter estimation and statistical inference. *R* Package "cusp" has been developed to implement this SDECusp (Grasman et al., 2009). This SDECusp model with R package "cusp" is extremely well-suited for use with cross-sectional data. We have used this SDECusp model extensively for research and publications (Chen, Lin, et al., 2014; Chen et al., 2013; Diks & Wang, 2016; Katerndahl, Burge, Ferrer, Wood, & Becho, 2015; Xu & Chen, 2016; Xu et al., 2017; Yu et al., 2018).

16.3.3 Chen-Chen's Cusp Regression Approach

As the third approach, Chen and Chen (2017) developed a cusp catastrophe nonlinear regression model ("RegCusp") for continuous data as a conceptual model that is guided by the statistical theory of nonlinear regression models (Seber & Lee, 2003). Following Eq. (16.1), the RegCusp model can be formulated as following:

$$y_i = Y_i + \varepsilon_i, \tag{16.5}$$

where y_i ($i = 1, \ldots$,n) are the observed outcome values and ε_i are the residuals from n observations, and are assumed to be normally distributed as $\epsilon_i \sim N(0, \sigma^2)$.

Mathematically, it can be seen that the latent variable Y_i in Eq. (16.5) is one of the real roots of the deterministic cusp catastrophe equation:

$$\alpha_i + \beta_i Y_i - Y_i^3 = 0, \tag{16.6}$$

where α_i and β_i are two control variables which is discussed later in the section of cusp catastrophe conventions. For any observed data with p independent variables $(x_1, \ldots, x_p)$ and the outcome variable y_i, the variables α_i and β_i are the control variables for ith subject.

In modeling analysis, these two control variables α_i and β_i are modeled in a way similarly to the Cobb-Grasman (Cobb & Zacks, 1985; Grasman et al., 2009):

$$\alpha_i = a_0 + a_1 x_{1i} + \cdots + a_p x_{pi} = \sum_{j=0}^{p} a_j x_{ji} \tag{16.7}$$

$$\beta_i = b_0 + b_1 x_{1i} + \cdots + b_p x_{pi} = \sum_{j=0}^{p} b_j x_{ji} \tag{16.8}$$

With the formulations of Eqs. (16.5)–(16.8), a nonlinear regression method can be used to estimate the model parameters of $\boldsymbol{a} = (a_0, a_1, \ldots, a_p)$, $\boldsymbol{b} = (b_0, b_1, \ldots, b_p)$ from Eqs. (16.7) and (16.8). The model parameters can be estimated using maximum likelihood estimation with the likelihood function formulated as follows:

$$L\left(\boldsymbol{a}, \boldsymbol{b}, \sigma^2 | data\right) = \left(\frac{1}{\sqrt{2\pi\sigma}}\right)^n \exp\left(-\frac{\sum_{i=1}^{n} (z_i - Z_i)^2}{2\sigma^2}\right) \tag{16.9}$$

With the likelihood function defined in Eq. (16.10), the theory of likelihood estimation can be readily applied to estimate RegCusp parameters as well as the associated statistical inferences on parameter significance and model selection.

16.4 Cusp Catastrophe Modeling of Binary Data

To establish the logistic cusp catastrophe regression model, we start with the binary data structure, then introduce logistic cusp catastrophe regression, conventions and algorithm for parameter estimation, and the method for cusp region estimation.

16.4.1 The Binary Data Structure

Suppose data from n participants are available as $data = (y_i, x_{1i}, \ldots, x_{pi})$ $(i = 1, \ldots, n)$ where y_i is observed binary outcome with 0/1 from the ith participants, $x_{1i}, \ldots, x_{pi}$ are the corresponding p-independent variables. Then y_i will be binary distributed as:

$$y_i \sim Binary\,(p_i) \tag{16.10}$$

where $p_i = \Pr(y_i = 1)$ is the probability to observe category 1.

16.4.2 The Binary Cusp Catastrophe Model

We make use of the logistic type of regression to model the logit of p_i to the latent variable Y_i, such that

$$p_i = \frac{\exp(Y_i)}{1 + \exp(Y_i)} \tag{16.11}$$

is one of the real roots of the deterministic cusp catastrophe equation:

$$\alpha_i + \beta_i Y_i - Y_i^3 = 0, \tag{16.12}$$

where α_i and β_i are two control variables which is discussed later in the section of cusp catastrophe conventions.

The two control variables of α_i and β_i are modeled in a way similarly to SDECusp with the linear combination of multiple independent variables in Eqs. (16.7) and (16.8)

16.4.3 Maximun Likelihood Estimation

With the formulations of Eqs. (16.10) to (16.12), a maximum likelihood procedure can be developed to estimate the model parameters of $\boldsymbol{a} = (a_0, a_1, \ldots, a_m)$, $\boldsymbol{b} = (b_0, b_1, \ldots, b_m)$ from Eq. (16.7) and (16.8) as well as the associated statistical inferences on parameter significance and model selection. Based on the theory of maximum likelihood estimation, the parameters of $\boldsymbol{a} = (a_0, a_1, \ldots, a_m)$, $\boldsymbol{b} = (b_0, b_1, \ldots, b_m)$ are estimated by solving the system of gradient equations and their associated variances can be obtained by the Fisher information matrix or Hessian matrix.

Specifically, we construct the likelihood function from Eq. (16.10) as follows:

$$L(\boldsymbol{a}, \boldsymbol{b}|data) = \prod_{i=1}^{n} p_i^{y_i}(1 - p_i)^{1-y_i} \tag{16.13}$$

To maximize the likelihood function defined in Eq. (16.13) is equivalent to maximize the log-likelihood function as follows:

$$\begin{aligned} logL(\boldsymbol{a}, \boldsymbol{b}|data) &= \sum_{i=1}^{n} \left[y_i \log(p_i) + (1 - y_i)\log(1 - p_i)\right] \\ &= \sum_{i=1}^{n} \left[y_i Y_i + \log(1 - p_i)\right] \end{aligned} \tag{16.14}$$

16.4.4 Cusp Catastrophe Conventions

The cusp catastrophe model is not the traditional statistical model in which each combination of independent variables is associated with one and only one outcome value. In fact, the RegCusp model formulated from Eq. (16.6) and the LogisticCusp model formulated from Eq. (16.12) could have one, two, or three roots for each α_i and β_i combinations depending on the locations on the control plan, defined by Eqs. (16.7) and (16.8). There three roots can be solved analytically as follows:

$$\begin{aligned} &Y_1 = \frac{1}{6}\frac{\nabla^{2/3} + 12\beta}{\nabla^{1/3}} Y_2 = \frac{1}{12}\frac{\sqrt{3}I\nabla^{2/3} - 12\sqrt{3}I\beta - \nabla^{\frac{2}{3}} - 12\beta}{\nabla^{1/3}}, \quad \text{and} \\ &Y_3 = -\frac{1}{12}\frac{\sqrt{3}I\nabla^{\frac{2}{3}} - 12\sqrt{3}I\beta + \nabla^{\frac{2}{3}} + 12\beta}{\nabla^{1/3}} \end{aligned} \tag{16.15}$$

where $I = \sqrt{-1}$ as the imaginary unit, $\nabla = 108\alpha + 12\sqrt{3\Delta}$ and $\Delta = 27\alpha^2 - 4\beta^3$ is the well-known *Cardan discriminant*. Which one to choose to fit the likelihood function in Eq. (16.13) for the latent variable Y in Eq. (16.12) would have to be determined using the Cardan discriminant.

From Eq. (16.15), it can be derived that when $\Delta > 0$, Eq. (16.12) has one real root; but when $\Delta \leq 0$, Eq. (16.12) has three real roots. Among these three roots, there are three cases: (a) if $\alpha = \beta = \Delta = 0$, the three roots are the same, which is referred as the *cusp point* (labeled O in Fig. 16.1); (b) if $\Delta = 0$, but $\alpha \neq 0$ *or* $\beta \neq 0$, two roots are the same, which are the two lines OQ and OR forming the boundary for the cusp region (Fig. 16.1); and (c) if $\Delta < 0$, and $\alpha \neq 0$ *or* $\beta \neq 0$, the three roots are distinct, which characterizes the cusp region between OQ and OR also indicated in Fig. 16.1. Therefore, this LogisticCusp model is no longer within the traditional domain of mathematical and statistical modeling. Further investigation is needed to identify the statistical properties of this LogisticCusp model.

To select the correct root for the cusp catastrophe model described by Eq. (16.12), we used two modeling conventions: *delay convention* and *Maxwell convention*. The delay convention is used to select the root from the cusp surface of $\frac{dV(y;\alpha,\beta)}{dy} = 0$ in Eq. (16.1) that are close to the observed y. The Maxwell convention is used to select the roots on the cusp surface of $\frac{dV(y;\alpha,\beta)}{dy} = 0$ in Eq. (16.1) corresponding to the minimum of the associated potential function $V(y; \alpha, \beta) = \alpha y + \frac{1}{2}\beta y^2 - \frac{1}{4}y^4$.

16.4.5 Cusp Region Estimation

Based on the discussion above, the boundary of the cusp region depicted in Fig. 16.1 can be constructed from $\Delta = 0$. Since $\Delta = 27\alpha^2 - 4\beta^3$, this can be solved at $\beta = \sqrt[3]{27\alpha^2/4}$. Therefore for the asymmetric parameter α from a range of lower limit (say, $\alpha_{Lower\ Limit}$) to upper limit (say, $\alpha_{Upper\ Limit}$), β can be calculated by at $\beta = \sqrt[3]{27\alpha^2/4}$ which would correspond to the two lines OQ and OR forming the boundary for the cusp region (Fig. 16.1).

When $\alpha = \beta = 0$, then $\Delta = 0$ which would be the cusp point as commonly referred as the *cusp point* (labeled O in Fig. 16.1). When $\Delta < 0$, the values of (α, β) are within the cusp region and when $\Delta > 0$, the values of (α, β) are outside the cusp region.

This cusp region under (α, β) coordinate system can be easily transformed into the original data coordinate system of the interest based on the estimated Eqs. (16.7) and (16.8). For example, if the interest is for (x_1, x_2), we can plug the estimated Eqs. (16.7) and (16.8) with x_1 and x_2 varying and the other xs fixed into $\beta = \sqrt[3]{27\alpha^2/4}$ and solve for x_2 as a function of x_1. This is illustrated in the real data analysis in Sect. 4.

16.4.6 Numeric Search Algorithms for Parameter Estimates

There are several methods to be used to maximize the log-likelihood function in Eq. (16.13). We make use of R function "optim". The default method is an implementation of that of Nelder and Mead (1965) which uses only function values and is robust but relatively slow. It will work reasonably well for non-differentiable functions. Another commonly-used method is a quasi-Newton method (also known as a variable metric algorithm), specifically that published simultaneously in 1970 by Broyden, Fletcher, Goldfarb and Shanno which is named as BFGS. The BFGS uses function values and gradients for the optimization. Specifically, with the log-likelihood function in Eq. (16.14), the parameters of $\boldsymbol{a} = (a_0, a_1, \ldots, a_p)$, $\boldsymbol{b} = (b_0, b_1, \ldots, b_p)$ are estimated by solving the system of 2p + 2 gradients as:

$$\begin{pmatrix} \frac{\partial logL}{\partial a} \\ \frac{\partial logL}{\partial b} \end{pmatrix}_{(2p+2)\times 1} = \left(\frac{\partial logL}{\partial a_0}, \frac{\partial logL}{\partial a_1}, \ldots, \frac{\partial logL}{\partial a_j}, \ldots, \frac{\partial logL}{\partial a_p}, \frac{\partial logL}{\partial b_0}, \frac{\partial logL}{\partial b_1}, \ldots, \frac{\partial logL}{\partial b_j}, \ldots, \frac{\partial logL}{\partial b_p}\right)' = 0 \tag{16.16}$$

where $(.)'$ in Eq. (16.16) denotes the vector transpose and the partial derivatives in Eq. (16.16) can be derived as $\begin{cases} \frac{\partial logL}{\partial a_j} = \sum_{i=1}^{n} \left[y_i \frac{\partial Y_i}{\partial a_j} - \frac{1}{1-p_i} \frac{\partial p_i}{\partial a_j} \right] \\ \frac{\partial logL}{\partial b_j} = \sum_{i=1}^{n} \left[y_i \frac{\partial Y_i}{\partial b_j} - \frac{1}{1-p_i} \frac{\partial p_i}{\partial b_j} \right] \end{cases}$ for all $j = 0, 1, \ldots, p$. In addition, the partial derivatives of $\frac{\partial Y_i}{\partial a_j}$ and $\frac{\partial Y_i}{\partial b_j}$ in the gradients can be derived from Eq. (16.12) as $\frac{\partial Y_i}{\partial a_j} = -\frac{x_{ji}}{\beta_i - 3Y_i^2}$ and $\frac{\partial Y_i}{\partial b_j} = -\frac{x_{ji} Y_i}{\beta_i - 3Y_i^2}$. Also the partial derivatives of $\frac{\partial p_i}{\partial a_j}$ and $\frac{\partial p_i}{\partial b_j}$ in the gradients can be derived from Eq. (16.11) as $\frac{\partial p_i}{\partial a_j} = p_i (1 - p_i) \frac{\partial Y_i}{\partial a_j}$ and $\frac{\partial p_i}{\partial b_j} = p_i (1 - p_i) \frac{\partial Y_i}{\partial b_j}$.

Equation (16.16) is highly complicated and it's obvious that there are no analytical solutions to solve the $2p + 2$ gradients from Eq. (16.16) to estimate the $2p + 2$ parameters of $\boldsymbol{a} = (a_0, a_1, \ldots, a_p)$ and $\boldsymbol{b} = (b_0, b_1, \ldots, b_p)$. Therefore, a numerical iterative search algorithm has to be used to obtain the parameter estimators from Eq. (16.16). We make use of Newton's method (Nocedal & Wright, 1999) to solve Eq. (16.8) iteratively using following iterative scheme with a large number of iterations of $s = 1, \ldots, S$ (i.e. S > 1000):

$$\begin{pmatrix} a^{(s+1)} \\ b^{(s+1)} \end{pmatrix} = \begin{pmatrix} a^{(s)} \\ b^{(s)} \end{pmatrix} - \begin{pmatrix} \frac{\partial^2 logL}{\partial a^2}, & \frac{\partial^2 logL}{\partial a \partial b} \\ \frac{\partial^2 logL}{\partial a \partial b}, & \frac{\partial^2 logL}{\partial b^2} \end{pmatrix}^{-1}_{\begin{pmatrix} a^{(s)} \\ b^{(s)} \end{pmatrix}} \begin{pmatrix} \frac{\partial logL}{\partial a} \\ \frac{\partial logL}{\partial b} \end{pmatrix}_{\begin{pmatrix} a^{(s)} \\ b^{(s)} \end{pmatrix}} \tag{16.17}$$

Note that in the right side of Eq. (16.17), $\begin{pmatrix} \frac{\partial logL}{\partial a} \\ \frac{\partial logL}{\partial b} \end{pmatrix}$ and $\begin{pmatrix} \frac{\partial^2 logL}{\partial a^2}, & \frac{\partial^2 logL}{\partial a \partial b} \\ \frac{\partial^2 logL}{\partial a \partial b}, & \frac{\partial^2 logL}{\partial b^2} \end{pmatrix}$ are the gradient vector in Eq. (16.16) and the Hessian matrix evaluated at the sth iteration of the parameters $\begin{pmatrix} a^{(s)} \\ b^{(s)} \end{pmatrix}$. The Hessian matrix is a $(2p + 2) \times (2p + 2)$ matrix with its elements of the associated second derivatives. Specifically, in the Hessian matrix,

- The upper-left matrix $\frac{\partial^2 logL}{\partial a^2}$ is a $(p + 1) \times (p + 1)$ matrix with diagonal elements as $\frac{\partial^2 logL}{\partial a_j^2} = \sum_{i=1}^{n} \left[y_i \frac{\partial^2 Y_i}{\partial a_j^2} - \frac{1}{1-p_i} \frac{\partial^2 p_i}{\partial a_j^2} + \frac{1}{(1-p_i)^2} \left(\frac{\partial p_i}{\partial a_j} \right)^2 \right]$ for all $j = 1, \ldots, p$, and the off-diagonal elements as $\frac{\partial^2 logL}{\partial a_j \partial a_k} = \sum_{i=1}^{n} \left[y_i \frac{\partial^2 Y_i}{\partial a_j \partial a_k} - \frac{1}{1-p_i} \frac{\partial^2 p_i}{\partial a_j \partial a_k} + \frac{1}{(1-p_i)^2} \frac{\partial p_i}{\partial a_j} \frac{\partial p_i}{\partial a_k} \right]$ for all $j, k = 1, \ldots, p$ and $j \neq k$.
- The upper-right matrix $\frac{\partial^2 logL}{\partial a \partial b}$ is the same as the lower-left matrix which is a $(p + 1) \times (p + 1)$ matrix with elements as $\frac{\partial^2 logL}{\partial a_j \partial b_k} = \sum_{i=1}^{n} \left[y_i \frac{\partial^2 Y_i}{\partial a_j \partial b_k} - \frac{1}{1-p_i} \frac{\partial^2 p_i}{\partial a_j \partial b_k} + \frac{1}{(1-p_i)^2} \frac{\partial p_i}{\partial a_j} \frac{\partial p_i}{\partial b_k} \right]$ for all $j, k = 1, \ldots, p$.
- The lower-right matrix $\frac{\partial^2 logL}{\partial b^2}$ is a $(p + 1) \times (p + 1)$ matrix with diagonal elements as $\frac{\partial^2 logL}{\partial b_j^2} = \sum_{i=1}^{n} \left[y_i \frac{\partial^2 Y_i}{\partial b_j^2} - \frac{1}{1-p_i} \frac{\partial^2 p_i}{\partial b_j^2} + \frac{1}{(1-p_i)^2} \left(\frac{\partial p_i}{\partial b_j} \right)^2 \right]$ for all $j = 1, \ldots, p$, and the off-diagonal elements as $\frac{\partial^2 logL}{\partial b_j \partial b_k} = \sum_{i=1}^{n} \left[y_i \frac{\partial^2 Y_i}{\partial b_j \partial b_k} - \frac{1}{1-p_i} \frac{\partial^2 p_i}{\partial b_j \partial b_k} + \frac{1}{(1-p_i)^2} \frac{\partial p_i}{\partial b_j} \frac{\partial p_i}{\partial b_k} \right]$ for all $j, k = 1, \ldots, p$ and $j \neq k$.
- In addition, all the second-order derivatives $\frac{\partial^2 Y_i}{\partial a_j^2}$, $\frac{\partial^2 Y_i}{\partial a_j \partial a_k}$, $\frac{\partial^2 Y_i}{\partial b_j^2}$, $\frac{\partial^2 Y_i}{\partial b_j \partial b_k}$, $\frac{\partial^2 p_i}{\partial a_j^2}$, $\frac{\partial^2 p_i}{\partial a_j \partial a_k}$, $\frac{\partial^2 p_i}{\partial b_j^2}$ and $\frac{\partial^2 p_i}{\partial b_j \partial b_k}$ in the above calculations of Hessian matrix can be similarly obtained using the first-order derivatives from the calculations in Eq. (16.16).

We name the above estimation process as "LogisticCusp" with respect to the "RegCusp" in Chen and Chen (2017).

16.5 Test the Logistic Cusp Catastrophe Model Through Monte-Carlo Simualtion

As the first step to examine the logistic cusp regression method described above, we conducted Monte Carlo simulation studies with known parameters.

16.5.1 Model Settings for Simulation

To conduct Monte Carlo simulation, surrogate data are generated using Eqs. (16.10) to (16.12) with the number of observations $n = 300$. Two (i.e., $p = 3$) independent variables x_1 and x_2 are simulated independently from the standard normal distribution.

To test whether the novel model can correctly distinguish and determine the model variables, we make use of the true parameters of $\boldsymbol{a} = (2, 2, 0)$, $\boldsymbol{b} = (2, 0, 2)$ from Eqs. (16.3) and (16.4) where $a_2 = 0$ in Eq. (16.3) to represent the correct model selection of x_1 from Eq. (16.3) and $b_1 = 0$ to represent the correct model selection of x_2 from Eq. (16.4).

16.5.2 Steps of Simulation Study

The simulation is an iterative process, and it was completed in the following seven consecutive steps:

Step 1: With $n = 300$, simulate x_1 and x_2 from the standard normal distribution;
Step 2: With the true parameters $\boldsymbol{a} = (2, 2, 0)$ and $\boldsymbol{b} = (2, 0, 2)$ and the x_1 and x_2 from Step 1, calculate α_i and β_i from Eqs. (16.7) and (16.8);
Step 3: With the α_i and β_i from Step 2, solve Eq. (16.12) to obtain Y_i and select the one root corresponding to the Maxwell convention, or the minimum of the associated potential function $\mathrm{V}(Y_\mathrm{i}, \alpha_i, \beta_i)$;
Step 4: With the selected $\mathrm{Y_i}$ from Step 3, generate the outcome variable $\mathrm{y_i}$ using Eq. (16.10);
Step 5: Using the data generated from Steps 1 through 4, the objective function can be formed to estimate the parameters $\boldsymbol{a}$ and $\boldsymbol{b}$ based on Eq. (16.13) using maximum likelihood estimation.
Step 6: Repeated Steps 1 to 5 for a large number of simulations (we used 5000 times) and record the estimated parameters

Following the steps described above, we first investigated the default Nelder and Mead optimization and we found that the estimation from the maximum likelihood is unbiased, but lack of efficiency of the Fisher information matrix for variance estimation. We further investigated the gradients and Hessian matrix from Eqs. (16.16) and (16.17) with the quasi-Newton (BFGS) and we found that BFGS produced very satisfactory variance estimation. As a routine, we run the simulation for 100,000 times to obtain the modeling results.

Table 16.1 Summary of the result for BFGS from 100,000 simulations

Parameter	True	Mean	Median	ECP
a_0	2.0000	2.0412	2.0191	0.8491
a_1	2.0000	2.0486	2.0231	0.7649
a_2	0.0000	0.0129	0.0170	0.7176
b_0	2.0000	2.0199	2.0114	0.8341
b_1	0.0000	0.0032	0.0121	0.7721
b_2	2.0000	2.0370	2.0180	0.6823

16.5.3 Results and Interpretation

Table 16.1 summarizes the main results from the simulation analysis. It can be seen from Table 16.1 that the parameters are estimated unbiased (i.e., the "Mean" and "Median" of the 100,000 estimated parameters are close to the "True" values) and the empirical coverage probabilities (ECP) are very reasonable with more than 70%. We also investigated this BFGS estimation with 200,000 simulations, similar conclusions are found.

Results from the simulation studies indicate that the LogisticCusp performed quit well to estimate the known parameters of *a*s and *b*s for the asymmetry and the bifurcation control variables, including the intercept and the slope with small differences between the known values and estimates. For example, the true value for b_1 is 2.0000, and the mean estimate is 2.0370.

16.6 Modeling Analysis with Real Data: Binge Drinking

We have known from the above simulation studies that the logistic cusp catastrophe regression works well. To further demonstrate the utility of the newly established method, we analyze real data using the logistic cusp regression method that validated from the Monte-Carlo simulations.

16.6.1 Data Sources and Variables

Data used for empirical testing were 1122 youth lifetime drinkers derived from the 2015 Monitoring the Future Study: A Continuing Study of American Youth (12th-Grade Survey) (ICPSR 36408, URL: https://www.icpsr.umich.edu/icpsrweb/ICPSR/studies/36408). Of the total sample, 48.6% were male, and 50.1% were White and 24.4% were Black, 39.8% less than 18 years of age and 60.2% were older than 18. The response variable in this study is the number of drinks (denoted by "*y*") in binge drinking. Based on self-reported data, 848 (75.6%) did not engage in binge drinking in the past month, 130 (11.6%) engaged once, 72 (6.4%) engaged twice and 72 (6.4%) engaged in three or more times. A binary variable if binge drinking (y/n) (denoted by "y_2") was created for modeling with participants who engaged in binge drinking at least once in the past month as yes; otherwise no.

Perception of alcohol harm was modeled as the asymmetry variable (denoted by "x_1"). The variable was measured using responses to the question: "How much do you think people risk harming themselves (physically or in other ways), if they: (1) Take one or two drinks nearly every day? (2) Take four or five drinks nearly every day? (3) Have five or more drinks once or twice each weekend? Answer options to these questions were: 0 (*no risk*), 1 (*slight risk*), 2 (*moderate risk*), 3 (*great risk*). Items were reverse coded and mean scores (range: 0–3) were computed for analysis such that 0 (*most risk or highest level of harm*) and 3 (*least risk or lowest level of harm)*. This measure was used in MTF's research (Johnston, O'Malley, Miech, Bachman, & Schulenberg, 2017) and reported studies indicate perceived harm is a significant predictor of alcohol use in adolescents (Pedersen, Fjaer, & Gray, 2016).

Frequency of drinking in social settings was modeled as the bifurcation variable (denoted by "x_2") based on the responses to the question: "When you used alcohol during the last year, how often did you use it in each of the following situations?" (1) With 1 or 2 other people; and (2) at a party. Answer options to the questions were 0 (*not at all*), 1 (*few times*), 2 (*sometimes*), 3 (*most times*), and 4 (*every time*). The highest frequency (range: 0–4) at either of the two settings was used for modeling analysis. Social setting has been reported as an influential factor for alcohol use in high school and college students (Weitzman, Nelson, & Wechsler, 2003).

16.6.2 Modeling Analysis

Modeling analysis was conducted using the R program we developed and used in the simulation studies presented in Sect. 4. For comparison purposes, we analyzed the same data with Cobb-Grasman's SDECusp and Chen-Chen's RegCusp. In the modeling analysis the asymmetry variable is the perceive alcohol as less risk, and the bifurcation variable is the social setting for drinking. We consider two types of outcome variable of binge drinking, y, as continuous variable and y_2, as the binary variable. Using continuous outcome, y, we can fit the typical multiple linear regression ("Linear Regression"), the stochastic cusp catastrophe model ("SDECusp") and the regression cusp ("RegCusp") catastrophe model. With the binary outcome, y_2, we can fit the LogisticCusp model in this chapter.

16.6.3 Parameter Estimates and Comparison

Results in Table 16.2 summarizes the parameter estimates and their associated standard errors with standardized data on y, x_1 and x_2. Parameter estimates from the linear regarrison and the three cusp catastrophe modeling methods are all

Table 16.2 Results from linear and 3 cusp regression modeling methods

Model	Binge drinking (outcome, y)	Perceived alcohol as less risk (x_1)	Social setting for drinking (x_2)	Cusp point estimated
Linear regression	Continuous (y)	$a_1 = 0.187$ (0.028)***	$b_1 = 0.299$ (0.028)***	NA
SDECusp	Continuous (y)	$a_0 = -0.595$ (0.031)*** $a_1 = 0.169$ (0.023)***	$b_0 = 3.739$ (0.087)*** $b_1 = -0.221$ (0.043)***	(−1.545, 15.950)
RegCusp	Continuous (y)	$a_0 = -0.002$ (0.035) $a_1 = 0.132$ (0.034)***	$b_0 = -0.821$ (0.033)*** $b_1 = 0.916$ (0.035)***	(1.082, 2.483)
LogisticCusp	Dichotomous (y_2)	$a_0 = 0.129$ (0.002)*** $a_1 = 1.252$ (0.037)***	$b_0 = -0.886$ (0.008)*** $b_1 = 2.948$ (0.017)***	(0.996, 1.982)

Note: values in the parenthesis are standard error

statistically highly statistically significant at p-value <0.001, except the a_0 from the RegCusp that is not ($p > 0.05$).

16.6.4 Comparison of the Estimated Cusp Regions

With SDECusp, RegCusp and LogisticCusp models, we can estimate the cusp point in the cusp region as denoted by point O in Fig. 16.1. This can be done by setting the estimated α and β in Eqs. (16.7) and (16.8) to be zero and solving for the corresponding values of x_1 and x_2 which would be the estimated cusp point as described in Section "Cusp Region Estimation". As seen in Table 16.2, the cusp point is estimated at (−1.545, 15.950) for SDECusp catastrophe model which is out of data region. The estimated cusp point using RegCusp and BinaryCusp are (1.082, 2.483) and (0.996, 1.982), respectively. The cusp point estimated using these two method are reasonable compared to the cusp point estimated with the SDECusp method. The estimated cusp point from the SDECusp was far off the data range of the two predictor variables with x_1 ranging from 0 to 3 and x_2 from 0 to 4. According to the cusp point estimated with the RegCusp, sudden changes in binge drink behavior would occur only when x_1, the perceived alcohol harm was slightly greater than 1 (somewhat harmful); and x_2, the frequency of drinking in social settings was about in the middle between 2 (sometimes) and 3 (most times). If results from LogisticCusp is used, the values in the two control variables reduced a bit. Sudden changes in binge drinking would occur when x_1 is approaching 1.0 (perceive alcohol use as "somewhat harmful) and x_2 is approaching 2 (sometimes

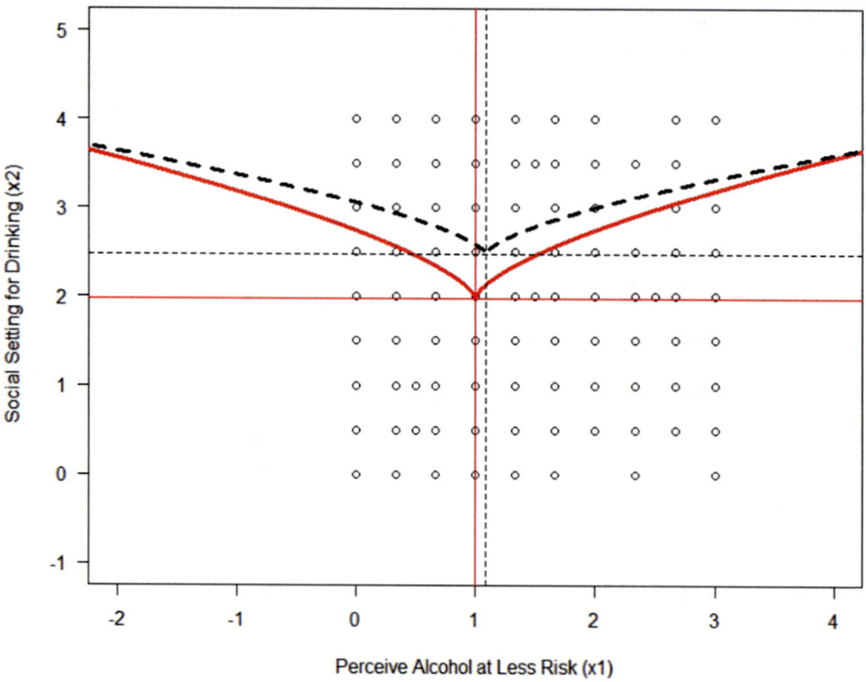

Fig. 16.2 Estimated cusp point along with cusp region for both RegCusp (black line) and LogisticCusp (red line) models

drinking in social settings). In another word, with a binary outcome, the estimated sudden change becomes more sensitive than with a continuous outcome.

Figure 16.2 graphically illustrates the estimated cusp points and the associated cusp regions for both RegCusp and LogisticCusp models. As seen in Fig. 16.2, the dashed lines are for RegCusp model where the estimated cusp point is at ((1.082, 2.483) and the solid lines are for LogisticCusp model where the estimated cusp point is at (0.996, 1.982).

16.7 Discussion and Conclusions

In this chapter, we report our research in successfully establishing the LogisticCusp method for modeling binary outcome variables. The method is grounded on the well-established logistic regression to solve for high-order cusp catastrophe models. The innovative use of a latent binary variable creates a mathematical bridge linking the deterministic cusp catastrophe with a statistical logistic regression. By application of the log likelihood method and numerical search approach with either Maxell or delayed convention, unbiased parameter estimates can be obtained; and by application of the bootstrapping, correct model variances can also be estimated. In addition to validation through simulation, we empirically test the method using data from national probability sample of youth with a binary variable for binge drinking. Binary variables are more common than continuous variables in research. The LogisticCusp provide a new and only tool, the first time for researchers to examine challenge questions with binary outcome variables. Binary variables are widely used by researchers in almost all scientific fields in addition to life sciences, psychology and behavioral studies.

There are several advantages with the LogisticCusp method we developed. First, all binary variables suitable for logistic regression can be used for cusp catastrophe modeling to nonlinearity and discreteness of a phenomenon. Second, both the asymmetry and bifurcation variables in a logistic cusp regression can be modeled as either a single or multi-variate variable, greatly enhancing the flexibility for modeling analysis. Research from this and previous analysis (Chen et al., 2019) also indicate adequate validity of the estimated the cusp point, and the corresponding cusp region and the two threshold lines with the LogisticCusp method. In addition to assessing the validity of the estimated parameters, determination of the threshold lines provide important data guiding practice to avoid sudden changes moving toward unfavorable outcomes and to promote sudden changes leading to favorable outcomes. Third, as in other method, R^2 or the variances explained by a cusp model can also be estimated as in the traditional regression analysis, facilitating model comparisons to help determine whether a study variable is nonlinear discrete or linear and continuous. Last, the method can be executed in R, free of charge.

There are a couple of limitations to the LogisticCusp method. Like many statistical methods with numerical search for parameter solutions, the LogisticCusp method is sensitive to initial values. Several measures can be used to help determine initial values: a) Generate initial values using parameter estimates for the same data but using other methods such as linear regression, logistic regression, RegCusp, and SDECusp. (b) Check if the estimated cusp point, cusp region and the two threshold lines are within the data range with a meaningful interpretation. Another limitation is the variance estimation. Like in RegCusp, the estimated variances tended to be too small for LogisticCusp. Despite that the bootstrapping provides as a remedy to this issue, we will conduct further research to understand this issue.

Despite these limitations, the establishment of the regression-based approach, including the LogisticCusp in this study and the RegCusp in our previous studies (Chen & Chen, 2017; Chen, Chen, & Zhang, 2016) provide an innovative and highly needed approach for researchers to solve for a deterministic cusp catastrophe model with a statistical method capable of handling sampling and measurement errors. In addition, the accurate estimation of the cusp point, cusp research and the threshold lines advanced cusp catastrophe modeling from qualitatively detecting the cusp to quantitatively describing cusp catastrophe. It is our anticipation that the application of the regression-based cusp catastrophe modeling methods we established will provide a set of great analytics to advance medical, health, social and behavioral studies.

Acknowledgments This research was support in part by National Institute of Health (NIH) Eunice Kennedy Shriver National Institute of Child Health and Human Development (NICHD, R01HD075635, PIs: Chen X and Chen D).

References

Berk, R. A. (2008). *Statistical learning from a regression perspective*. Berlin: Springer. (ISBN 978-0-387-77500-5).

Chen, D., & Chen, X. (2017). Cusp catastrophe regression and its application in public health and behavioral research. *International Journal of Environmental Research and Public Health, 14*(10), 1220. https://doi.org/10.3390/Ijerph14101220

Chen, D., Chen, X., Lin, F., Tang, W., Lio, Y. L., & Guo, T. Y. (2014). Cusp catastrophe polynomial model: Power and sample size estimation. *Open Journal of Statistics, 4*(10), 803–813. https://doi.org/10.4236/ojs.2014.410076

Chen, D., Chen, X., & Zhang, K. (2016). *An exploratory statistical cusp catastrophe model*. Paper presented at the 2016 IEEE International Conference on Data Science and Advanced Analytics Montreal, QC, Canada.

Chen, D., Lin, F., Chen, X., Tang, W., & Kitzman, H. (2014). Cusp catastrophe model: A nonlinear model for health outcomes in nursing research. *Nursing Research, 63*(3), 211–220. https://doi.org/10.1097/NNR.0000000000000034

Chen, X., & Chen, D. (2015). Cusp catastrophe modeling in medical and health research. In D. G. Chen & J. Wilson (Eds.), *Innovative statistical methods for public health data*. Cham: Springer International.

Chen, X., & Chen, D. (2019). Cognitive theories, paradigm of quantum behavior change, and cusp catastrophe modeling in social behavioral research. *Journal of the Society for Social Work and Research, 10*(1), 127–159. https://doi.org/10.1086/701837

Chen, X., Lunn, S., Harris, C., Li, X. M., Deveaux, L., Marshall, S., … Stanton, B. (2010). Modeling early sexual initiation among young adolescents using quantum and continuous behavior change methods: Implications for HIV prevention. *Nonlinear Dynamics, Psychology, and Life Sciences, 14*(4), 491–509.

Chen, X., Wang, Y., & Chen, D. (2019). Nonlinear dynamics of binge drinking among U.S. high school students in grade 12: Cusp catastrophe modeling of national survey data. *Nonlinear Dynamics, Psychology, and Life Sciences, 23*(4), 465–490. *Revised submission.*

Chen, X. G., Stanton, B., Chen, D., & Li, X. M. (2013). Intention to use condom, cusp modeling, and evaluation of an HIV prevention intervention trial. *Nonlinear Dynamics, Psychology, and Life Sciences, 17*(3), 385–403.

Clair, S. (1998). A cusp catastrophe model for adolescent alcohol use: An empirical test. *Nonlinear Dynamics, Psychology, and Life Sciences, 2*, 217–241.

Cobb, L. (1981). Parameter-estimation for the cusp catastrophe model. *Behavioral Science, 26*(1), 75–78. https://doi.org/10.1002/bs.3830260107

Cobb, L., & Ragade, R. K. (1978). Applications of catastrophe theory in the behavioral and life sciences. *Behavioral Science, 23*, 291–419.

Cobb, L., & Watson, B. (1980). Statistical catastrophe theory: An overview. *Mathematical Modelling, 1*(4), 311–317. https://doi.org/10.1016/0270-0255(1080)90041-X

Cobb, L., & Zacks, S. (1985). Applications of catastrophe-theory for statistical modeling in the biosciences. *Journal of the American Statistical Association, 80*(392), 793–802. https://doi.org/10.2307/2288534

Diks, C., & Wang, J. X. (2016). Can a stochastic cusp catastrophe model explain housing market crashes? *Journal of Economic Dynamics & Control, 69*, 68–88. https://doi.org/10.1016/j.jedc.2016.05.008

Faraway, J. J. (2009). *Linear model with R*. Abingdon: Taylor & Francis.

Gilmore, R. (1981). *Catastrophe theory for scientists and engineers*. New York: Wiley.

Grasman, R. P., van der Maas, H. L., & Wagenmakers, E. J. (2009). Fitting the cusp catastrophe in R: A cusp package primer. *Journal of Statistical Software, 32*(8), 1–27.

Guastello, S. J. (1982). Moderator rgression and the cusp catastrophe: Application of two-stage personnel selection, training, therapy, and policy evaluation. *Behavioral Science, 27*(3), 259–272.

Guastello, S. J. (1989). Catastrophe modeling of the accident process—Evaluation of an accident reduction program using the occupational hazards survey. *Accident Analysis and Prevention, 21*(1), 61–77. https://doi.org/10.1016/0001-4575(89)90049-3

Guastello, S. J., Aruka, Y., Doyle, M., & Smerz, K. E. (2008). Cross-cultural generalizability of a cusp catastrophe model for binge drinking among college students. *Nonlinear Dynamics, Psychology, and Life Sciences, 12*(4), 397–407.

Guastello, S. J., & Gregson, A. M. (2011). *Nonlinear dynamical systems analysis for the behavioral sciences using real data*. Boca Raton, FL: CRC/Taylor & Francis Group.

Guastello, S. J., & Lynn, M. (2014). Catastrophe model of the accident process, safety climate, and anxiety. *Nonlinear Dynamics, Psychology, and Life Sciences, 18*(2), 177–198.

Hartelman, P. A. I., van der Maas, H. L. J., & Molenaar, P. C. M. (1998). Detecting and modelling developmental transitions. *British Journal of Developmental Psychology, 16*, 97–122. https://doi.org/10.1111/j.2044-835X.1998.tb00751.x

Honerkamp, J. (1994). *Stochastic dynamical system: Concepts, numerical methods*. New York, NY: VCH.

Johnston, L. D., O'Malley, P. M., Miech, R. A., Bachman, J. G., & Schulenberg, J. E. (2017). *Monitoring the Future national survey results on drug use, 1975–2016: Overview, key findings on adolescent drug use*. Ann Arbor: Institute for Social Research, The University of Michigan.

Katerndahl, D. A., Burge, S. K., Ferrer, R. L., Wood, R., & Becho, J. (2015). Modeling outcomes of partner violence using cusp catastrophe modeling. *Nonlinear Dynamics, Psychology, and Life Sciences, 19*(3), 249–268.

Mazanov, J., & Byrne, D. G. (2006). A cusp catastrophe model analysis of changes in adolescent substance use: Assessment of behavioural intention as a bifurcation variable. *Nonlinear Dynamics, Psychology, and Life Sciences, 10*(4), 445–470.

Nelder, J. A., & Mead, R. (1965). A simplex algorithm for function minimization. *Computer Journal, 7*, 308–313.

Nocedal, J., & Wright, S. J. (1999). *Numerical optimization*. Berlin: Springer. ISBN 0-387-98793-2.

Pedersen, W., Fjaer, E. G., & Gray, P. (2016). Perceptions of harms associated wih tobacco, alcohol, and cannabis among students from the UK and Norway. *Contemporary Drug Problems, 43*, 47–61.

Seber, G. A., & Lee, A. J. (2003). *Linear regresson analysis* (2nd ed.). New York, NY: Wiley-Science.

Thom, R. (1975). *Structural stability and morphogenesis*. New York, NY: Benjamin-Addison-Wesley.

Thom, R., & Fowler, D. H. (1975). *Structural stability and morphogenesis: An outline of a general theory of models*. New York, NY: W. A. Benjamin.

Wagner, C. M. (2010). Predicting nursing turnover with catastrophe theory. *Journal of Advanced Nursing, 66*(9), 2071–2084. https://doi.org/10.1111/j.1365-2648.2010.05388.x

Weitzman, Nelson, T. F., & Wechsler, H. (2003). Taking up binge drinking in college: The influences of person, social group, and environment. *The Journal of Adolescent Health, 32*(1), 26–35.

White, A. M., Tapert, S., & Shukla, S. D. (2017). Binge drinking, predictors, patterns and consequences. *The Journal of the National Institute on Alcohol Abuse and Alcoholism, 39*(1), e1–e3.

Witkiewitz, K., van der Maas, H. L. J., Hufford, M. R., & Marlatt, G. A. (2007). Nonnormality and divergence in posttreatment alcohol use: Reexamining the Project MATCH data "another way". *Journal of Abnormal Psychology, 116*(2), 378–394. https://doi.org/10.1037/0021-843X.116.2.378

Xu, Y., & Chen, X. (2016). Protection motivation theory and cigarette smoking among vocational high school students in China: A cusp catastrophe modeling analysis. *Global Health Research and Policy, 1*, 3. https://doi.org/10.1186/s41256-016-0004-9

Xu, Y., Chen, X., Yu, B., Joseph, V., & Stanton, B. (2017). The effects of self-efficacy in bifurcating the relationship of perceived benefit and cost with condom use among adolescents: A cusp catastrophe modeling analysis. *Journal of Adolescence, 61*, 31–39. https://doi.org/10.1016/j.adolescence.2017.09.004

Yu, B., Chen, X., Stanton, B., Chen, D. D., Xu, Y., & Wang, Y. (2018). Quantum changes in self-efficacy and condom-use intention among youth: A chained cusp catastrophe model. *Journal of Adolescence, 68*, 187–197. https://doi.org/10.1016/j.adolescence.2018.07.020

Zeeman, E. C. (1977). *Catastrophe theory: Selected papers 1972–1077*. Boston, MA: Addison-Wesley.

Correction to: Statistical Methods for Global Health and Epidemiology

Xinguang Chen and (Din) Ding-Geng Chen

Correction to:
X. Chen, (Din) D.-G. Chen (eds.),
Statistical Methods for Global Health and Epidemiology,
ICSA Book Series in Statistics,
https://doi.org/10.1007/978-3-030-35260-8

This book was inadvertently published without appendix in chapters 8 and 13. The original chapters have been corrected.

The changes in Chapters 8 and 13 caused a change in the page numbers of the subsequent chapters (i.e., Chapters 9–16), but the contents of those chapters remain unchanged.

The updated version of these chapters can be found at
https://doi.org/10.1007/978-3-030-35260-8_8
https://doi.org/10.1007/978-3-030-35260-8_13

X. Chen, (Din) D.-G. Chen (eds.), *Statistical Methods for Global Health and Epidemiology*, ICSA Book Series in Statistics,
https://doi.org/10.1007/978-3-030-35260-8_17

Index

X. Chen, (Din) D.-G. Chen (eds.), *Statistical Methods for Global Health and Epidemiology*, ICSA Book Series in Statistics,
https://doi.org/10.1007/978-3-030-35260-8

Printed in the United States
By Bookmasters